Special Care in Dentistry

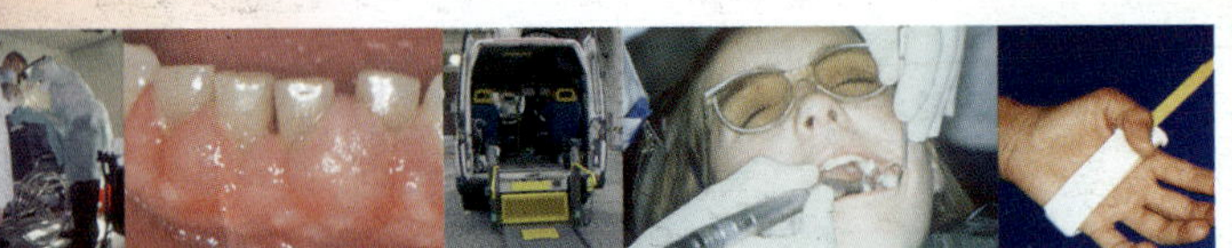

Commissioning Editor: Michael Parkinson
Development Editor: Hannah Kenner
Project Manager: Frances Affleck
Design Direction: George Ajayi
Illustration Manager: Gillian Murray
Illustrator: Oxford Illustrators

Special Care in Dentistry

HANDBOOK OF ORAL HEALTH CARE

Crispian Scully CBE PhD MD MDS MRCS FDSRCPS FFDRCSI FDSRCS FDSRCSE FRCPath FMedSci DSc

Dean and Director of Studies and Research, Eastman Dental Institute
University College London, UK
Adjunct Professor, University of Helsinki, Finland

Pedro Diz Dios PhD MD MDS

Senior Lecturer, Head of Department, Special Needs Unit, School of Medicine and Dentistry, University of Santiago de Compostela, Spain

Navdeep Kumar PhD FDSRCS

Honorary Lecturer, Special Needs Dentistry, Oral Medicine Unit, Division of Maxillofacial Diagnostic, Medical and Surgical Sciences, Eastman Dental Institute
University College London, UK

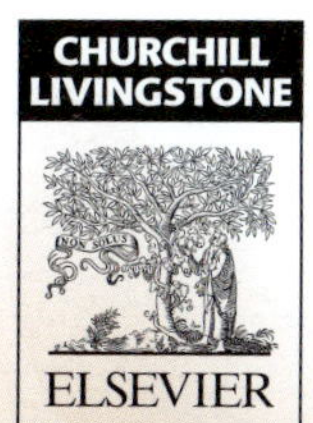

Edinburgh London New York Oxford Philadelphia St Louis Sydney Toronto 2007

CHURCHILL
LIVINGSTONE
ELSEVIER

First published 2007

ISBN 10: 0 443 071519
ISBN 13: 978 0 443 07151 5

British Library Cataloguing in Publication Data
A catalogue record for this book is available from the British Library

Library of Congress Cataloging in Publication Data
A catalog record for this book is available from the Library of Congress

Notice

Knowledge and best practice in this field are constantly changing. As new research and experience broaden our knowledge, changes in practice, treatment and drug therapy may become necessary or appropriate. Readers are advised to check the most current information provided (i) on procedures featured or (ii) by the manufacturer of each product to be administered, to verify the recommended dose or formula, the method and duration of administration, and contraindications. It is the responsibility of the practitioner, relying on their own experience and knowledge of the patient, to make diagnoses, to determine dosages and the best treatment for each individual patient, and to take all appropriate safety precautions. To the fullest extent of the law, neither the Publisher nor the Authors assume any liability for any injury and/or damage to persons or property arising out of or related to any use of the material contained in this book.

The Publisher

Printed in China

Preface

Improvements in medical and social care during the last 20 years have increased the life expectancy of many people, including those with previously life-threatening disorders. However, many of these individuals remain vulnerable and require particular attention to ensure that both general and oral health care provision meet their special needs.

It is estimated that there are currently nearly 10 million people living with disability in the UK. These special needs populations include individuals with developmental or acquired physical or learning disabilities, those with medical problems such as bleeding disorders, individuals with mental health problems or dental phobias, socially excluded individuals, such as the homeless, and frail and functionally dependent elders. The impact of oral, dental and craniofacial diseases in these groups may be considerable, resulting in compromised general health, social well-being, and quality of life. However, evidence suggests that these individuals have an increased risk of experiencing oral disease, and have greater oral preventive and treatment needs, as compared to the general population. Furthermore, there is gathering evidence that the psychosocial problems that these individuals may experience as a result of their oral disease may lead to an accelerated deterioration in both general and oral health. Furthermore, these people may develop anxieties or phobias from exposure to health care encounters, creating further barriers.

Hence special care dentistry poses unique challenges, not only in terms of the spectrum of people encountered, but also in relation to the need for an inventive and carefully planned approach suited to each individual's needs. To ensure that these individuals receive the same high standards of dental and oral health care as their unaffected cohorts, it is important that adequate attention is paid both to improving access and adapting the design of clinical facilities. Furthermore, detailed medical and social histories are essential, consent issues may need to be considered, and the care plan should be continually updated to adapt to the individual's changing special needs.

Although there is an increasing awareness of the importance of oral health for those with special needs and the potential hazards in operative intervention, there are currently limited resources available within state health services and specialised units. Many dental personnel outside of these units are reluctant to undertake treatment for patients with special needs, and yet in some cases, this care is often not beyond the skills of many practitioners. Nevertheless, most remain anxious about providing care – not least because of their perceived lack of knowledge regarding the implications of the disability in question.

Fortunately, the importance of special care dentistry is achieving greater recognition in many countries. For example, in the USA, the Social Security Act was amended in 2004 to require States to provide oral health services to children, aged, blind and disabled individuals under the Medicaid program. The specialty is now recognised in the UK. Furthermore, there are now special care training programmes in several countries for dentists and professionals complementary to dentistry, there are journals devoted to the area, academic departments, and national and international societies. Organisations supporting people with disabilities are also working closely to improve oral health care provision, (http://www.disabilitynow.org.uk) and specialised centres are becoming available (e.g. Mun-H-Center, in Goteborg, Sweden).

This book covers the management of the oral health needs of many groups of individuals with disabilities. The care of individuals with special needs due to social exclusion (e.g. the homeless), and aspects of oral health care related to religion or ethnicity are beyond the remit of this text. The aim of the book is to outline a practical approach for the safe dental management of individual patients with special needs (termed service users by some), and highlight which patients should be referred for treatment in community clinics, hospital units or by specialists.

We do not attempt to be comprehensive, nor to present details of practical dental or other procedures, but rather to present the main problems to be considered in providing oral health care for patients with special needs. We start by outlining the general aspects of access, the Disability Discrimination Act, and issues of consent, behaviour management and treatment modification, whilst acknowledging that normalisation is desirable, and in every way possible such patients should be treated in the same way as people without disability. We then discuss the various conditions alphabetically and, for each condition, cover the most important aspects of behavioural management and operative dentistry. Finally, we highlight the main orofacial problems encountered in these groups. We intend this book not to replace but to complement care paths already established, such as the several guidelines of the British Society for Disability and Oral Health (http://www.bsdh.org.uk/guidelines.html) and the National Oral Health Information Clearinghouse (NOHIC), a service of the National Institute of Dental and Craniofacial Research (http://www.nohic.nidcr.nih.gov/index.asp). More detail about medical aspects can be found elsewhere (Scully C, Cawson RA 2004 Medical problems in dentistry, 5th edition. Elsevier Churchill Livingstone, Edinburgh). More detail about oral lesions (Scully C 2004 Oral and maxillofacial medicine. Wright, Edinburgh. Scully C, Flint S, Porter SR, Moos K 2004 Oral and maxillofacial diseases, 3rd edition. Taylor and Francis, London) and the range of diseases much less commonly encountered can be found elsewhere (www.rarediseases.org).

We do not presume to have all the answers and, in this field in particular, there is a dearth of an evidence base at the level of randomised controlled trials. Therefore, most of what is included is written on the basis of lower levels of evidence, but not least from our personal experiences over many years, working in primary care, and in secondary or tertiary referral centres, and in units caring for individuals with conditions ranging from mainly learning disabilities, to those dealing with physical disabilities such as cerebral palsy, and those focusing on medical problems such as cardiac disease, HIV and haemophilia.

We trust the book will prove of value to the whole of the dental team working with people who have special needs; to students, GDPs and GPs; to trainees studying for Diploma or Membership examinations in Special Care Dentistry; and for those studying for Memberships in Dental Surgery.

CS
PD
NK

ADVISORS

Advice has generously been given by colleagues, including:
Jeremy Bagg (Glasgow),
Inmaculada Tomás Carmona (Santiago de Compostela),
Marie-France Davison (London),
Andrew Eder (London),
John Huw Evans (London),
Javier Fernández Feijoo (Santiago de Compostela),
John Hobkirk (London),
Kishor Gulabivala (London),
Jacobo Limeres Posse (Santiago de Compostela)
Andrew Smith (Glasgow),
Christopher Tredwin (London),
Richard Tucker (London),
David Wiesenfeld (Melbourne).

Drug doses must always be checked in a formulary before administration. Doses must be reduced for children. Doses may need to be reduced in the elderly or in some medical conditions. Contraindications must always be checked and the patient warned of any possible adverse effects.

Contents

1. INTRODUCTION

2. APPROPRIATE ORAL HEALTH CARE

3. SPECIFIC PROBLEM AREAS; ALPHABETICALLY ARRANGED

4. MAIN OROFACIAL PROBLEMS

Chapter 1

INTRODUCTION

DEFINITIONS

The most commonly cited definitions relevant to the field of special care in dentistry are those of the World Health Organization in 1976 and 1980, which drew a distinction between ■ impairment, ■ disability and ■ handicap. These were defined in 1976:

An *impairment* is any loss or abnormality of psychological, physiological or anatomical structure or function.

A *disability* is any restriction or lack (resulting from an impairment) of ability to perform an activity in the manner or within the range considered normal for a human being.

A *handicap* is a disadvantage for a given individual, resulting from an impairment or a disability, that prevents the fulfilment of a role that is considered normal (depending on age, sex and social and cultural factors) for that individual.

According to activists in the disability movement, the WHO definitions did not distinguish between the physical and social implications of the terms 'disability' and 'impairment'. They maintained that impairment refers to physical or cognitive limitations that an individual may have, such as the inability to walk or speak. In contrast, disability refers to socially imposed restrictions, that is, the system of social constraints that are imposed on those with impairments by the discriminatory practices of society.

Thus, the Union of the Physically Impaired Against Segregation defined impairment and disability in the following manner:

An *impairment* is lacking part of or all of a limb, or having a defective limb, organism or mechanism of the body.

A *disability* is the disadvantage or restriction of activity caused by contemporary organisation, which takes no or little account of people who have physical impairments and thus excludes them from the mainstream of social activities.

Furthermore, according to the United Nations Standard Rules on the equalisation of opportunities for persons with disabilities, the term '*disability*' summarises a great number of different functional limitations occurring in any population, in any country, of the world. People may be disabled by physical, intellectual or sensory impairment, medical conditions or mental illness. Such impairments, conditions or illnesses may be permanent or transitory in nature. The term '*handicap*' means the loss or limitation of opportunities to take part in the life of the community on an equal level with others. It describes the encounter between the person with a disability and the environment.

The purpose of this term is to emphasise the focus on the shortcomings in the environment and in many organised activities in society – for example, information, communication and education – which prevent persons with disabilities from participating on equal terms.

In view of the above, in 1980, the WHO adopted an International Classification of Impairments, Disabilities, and Handicaps, which provided a more precise and at the same time relativistic approach. WHO (1980) definitions then are:

- An *impairment* is a loss or abnormality of structure or function including psychological functioning. Examples are • reduced visual acuity • diminished hearing capacity • lack of muscular control • decreased learning ability • an inability to concentrate.
- A *disability* is a restriction or lack of ability to perform an activity within the range considered normal for a human being. Some prefer the term difficulty, as in 'learning difficulty'. A person is considered to have a disability if there is a physical or mental impairment which 'substantially' limits one or more major life activities which include, but are not limited to: • breathing • caring for oneself • concentrating • hearing • interacting with other people • learning • lifting • performing manual tasks • reaching • reading • seeing • speaking • standing • thinking • walking • working.
- A *handicap* is a disadvantage resulting from an impairment or disability that limits or prevents the fulfilment of a normal role.

This terminology recognises the necessity of addressing both the individual needs (such as rehabilitation and technical aids) and the shortcomings of the society (various obstacles for participation). In other words, an impairment is a loss or abnormality; a disability is a functional limitation of ability; a handicap is something which is imposed on a disability which makes it more limiting than it must necessarily be. The example of haemophilia A illustrates this well. It is an X-linked genetic disorder, in which blood coagulation factor VIII is lacking. The defect (the disease) causes a bleeding tendency (the impairment), resulting in haemarthroses along with movement problems (the disability). As a consequence of this, dental staff and other people may be reluctant to treat affected patients (thus creating a handicap).

Although the WHO Classification (1980) makes a clear distinction between 'impairment', 'disability' and 'handicap', and has been extensively used, some users have expressed concern that in its definition of the term 'handicap' the classification may still be considered too medical and too centred on the individual, and may not adequately clarify the interaction between societal conditions or expectations and the abilities of the individual. Furthermore, many individuals do not like the term 'learning disability' and prefer the term 'people with learning difficulties'. This is the term used by People First, an international advocacy organisation. In the UK, the Warnock Committee suggested the term 'learning difficulties' to cover specific problems with learning in children that might arise as a result of factors such as medical and emotional problems.

CAUSES OF DISABILITY

Disabilities may be classified in a variety of ways, such as in Box 1.1. Developmental disabilities are caused by impairments that occur during

Box 1.1 Disability and impairment

Disabilities	Impairments
Physical	Mobility, Respiratory
Mental	Emotional, Social
Sensory	Hearing, Visual
Cognitive	Learning, Attention

development (birth to age 18) and include intra-uterine infections, metabolic defects, fetal alcohol syndrome, chromosomal abnormalities, birth hypoxia, autism, cerebral palsy, and postnatal infections such as meningitis or encephalitis. Acquired disabilities are caused by impairments sustained after these developmental years, such as traumatic brain injury, spinal cord damage, multiple sclerosis, arthritis and Alzheimer's disease.

Further reading • Gelbier S 2004 History of the British Society for Disability and Oral Health and British Society of Dentistry for the Handicapped. J Disability Oral Health 5(2):Suppl, 43 • Stanfield M, Scully C, Davison M F, Porter S R 2003 The oral health of clients with learning disability: changes following relocation from hospital to community. Br Dent J 194:271–277 • http://www.mdx.ac.uk/www/study/mhhtim.htm
• http://www.reddisability.org.uk/DisFamous.htm
• http://www.friendlyreports.org.uk

ACCESS AND LEGAL BACKGROUND

The main obstacle or barrier to health care (including oral health care) has been access, but changes stemming from the Americans with Disabilities Act 1990 (ADA) and the Disability Discrimination Act 1995 (DDA) have, and are, changing this significantly. The ADA is a federal law that prohibits discrimination against a person with a disability who is seeking employment or access to services, including dental services. Similarly, in the UK, under the DDA it is unlawful to treat a person with disability less favourably for a reason related to that person's disability (unless it can be justified). The DDA defines a person with disability as 'a person who has or has had a physical or mental impairment which has a substantial and long-term adverse effect upon his or her ability to carry out normal day-to-day activities'.

Service providers (an expression which includes all dental staff), are placed under a duty not to discriminate by refusing to provide good facilities or services or providing them at a lower standard or in a worse manner, or offering a service on worse terms than would be offered to other members of the public. In the UK, the Disability Rights Commission (DRC) is an independent body established in April 2000 by Act of Parliament to stop discrimination and promote equality of opportunity for disabled people.

Further reading • www.disabilityaware.org
• http://www.legislation.hmso.gov.uk/acts/acts 1995/1995050.htm.
• http://www.drc-gb.org/thelaw/drcact.asp

IMPLICATIONS OF THE DISABILITY LEGISLATION

From October 1, 2004, all providers of dentistry in the UK have been expected to take reasonable steps to make their dental practices accessible to people with disability. They are expected to remove, alter or provide means of avoiding physical features that make it impossible or unreasonably difficult for people with disability to use their services. This includes possible alterations to the building design or construction, the approach and access to and exit from the building, e.g. ramp access for wheelchairs, parking bays for those with disabilities and modifications to fixtures and fittings, furniture and furnishings, and equipment and materials.

Another example is that any 'no dogs' policy or rule would have to be amended to allow entry to service animals such as guide dogs or hearing dogs – the disabled person must be permitted to bring service animals into the premises, but not necessarily into the surgery. Dental staff are thus required to make reasonable modifications to facilitate access to the premises by persons with disabilities, unless it can be shown that taking those steps would result in an 'undue burden' or fundamentally alter the nature of the services provided. The law prohibits imposing a surcharge on a person with a disability for the cost of such auxiliary aids and services.

Dental staff must treat the person with a disability on the same basis as they treat non-disabled patients. For example, if the person with a disability requires a procedure for which a non-disabled patient would ordinarily be referred, the person with a disability may legally be referred. However, if the person with a disability poses a 'direct threat' (significant risk that cannot be eliminated using special procedures) to the health or safety of others, you may refuse to admit that person to your premises, e.g. an aggressive patient who may need to be treated in hospital under general anaesthesia.

Dental staff must communicate in such a way that the person can understand what is being said to them. Communication includes facial expression and body language as well as verbal expression. The essential rule in communicating with anyone who has a disability is to address them directly. A caregiver, family member, partner or companion should also be present to provide information that the patient cannot perhaps provide – but an effort always should be made to include the patient in the discussion.

Further reading • Scully C, Cawson R A 2004 Medical problems in dentistry, 5th edn. Churchill Livingstone, Edinburgh • Scully C, Kalantzis A 2005 Oxford handbook of dental patient care. Oxford University Press, Oxford • World Health Organization 1976 Document A29/INFDOCI/1, Geneva, Switzerland. Union of the Physically Impaired Against Segregation. Fundamental Principles of Disability, London, 1976. • World Health Organization 1980 International Classification of Impairments, Disabilities, and Handicaps: A manual of classification relating to the consequences of disease. WHO, Geneva • http://www.radar.org.uk/RANE/Templates/ frontpage.asp?lHeaderID=227 • http://www.disabilityalliance.org/ • http://www.scdonline.org/ • http://www.scope.org.uk • http://www.hmso.gov.uk/acts/acts2001/20010010.htm • http://www.drc-gb.org

Chapter 2

APPROPRIATE ORAL HEALTH CARE

Provision of oral health care for individuals with special needs involves not only the delivery of safe and appropriate dental care but also focuses on the need to improve the oral health status of these populations by employing effective preventive measures. These objectives can be facilitated by the development of clinical guidelines and integrated care pathways to help overcome barriers to oral health care.

BARRIERS TO ORAL HEALTH CARE

The barriers to oral health care for people with special needs can be classified by illustrating the role of the dental profession and its interaction with individuals and society and government, as follows:

Barriers with reference to the individual ■ Lack of perceived need ■ Anxiety or fear, which may be heightened by previous dental or medical encounters ■ Financial considerations ■ Lack of access (e.g. Fig. 2.1).

Barriers with reference to the dental profession ■ Inappropriate manpower resources ■ Uneven geographical distribution ■ Training inappropriate to changing needs and demands ■ Insufficient sensitivity to patient attitudes and needs.

Barriers with reference to society ■ Insufficient public support of attitudes conducive to health ■ Inadequate oral health care facilities ■ Inadequate oral health manpower planning ■ Insufficient support for research.

Barriers with reference to government ■ Lack of political will ■ Inadequate resources (e.g. Fig. 2.2) ■ Low priority.

The key to removing these barriers and improving oral health care provision for people with special needs is education of the individual, the dental profession, society and government as to the importance of oral health and its positive effects on general health.

GOALS

Whilst perfect oral health is the ideal goal, five important objectives when providing oral health care are: ■ enabling patients to care for their own oral

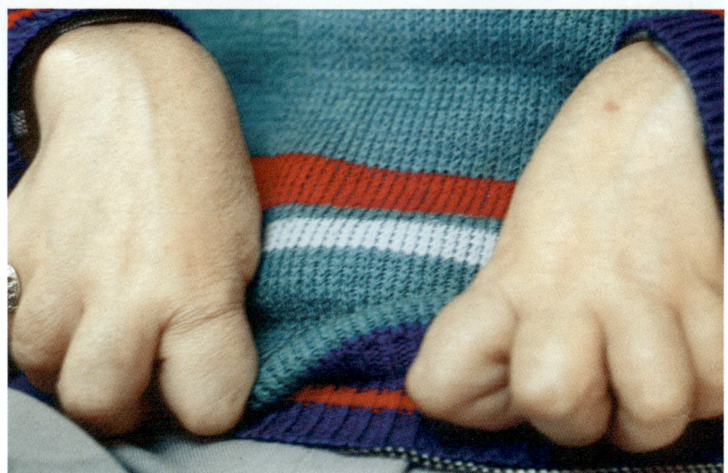

Figure 2.1 **Impaired physical access**

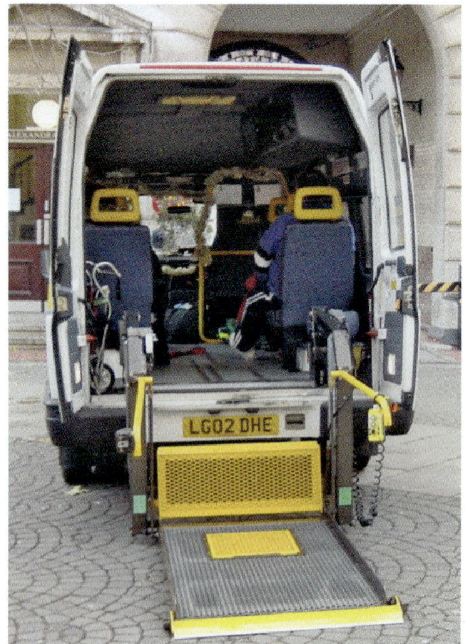

Figure 2.2 **Transport vehicles adapted to accommodate wheelchairs**

health, with or without assistance ■ keeping patients free from pain and acute disease ■ maintaining effective oral function ■ retaining aesthetics ■ causing no harm.

THE PEOPLE INVOLVED IN PROVIDING CARE

Although the dentist may be the team leader, dental care professionals are essential to successful provision of care. Care may also involve the following groups: ■ parents/carers ■ social services/social work departments ■ health visitors ■ general medical practitioner ■ paediatric consultant/ other hospital specialists ■ school teachers and assistants ■ colleagues in paediatric dentistry, oral surgery, oral medicine, periodontics, endodontics, prosthodontics, orthodontics.

A multidisciplinary team approach to patient care leads to a more effective sharing of resources, generates more creative responses to problems involving patient care, heightens communication skills, produces new approaches to learning and clinical practice, and results in the formulation of a practical and appropriate treatment plan. Furthermore, involvement of other professionals ensures that they appreciate the importance of oral health care and its relationship to general health, and dispels the misconception that oral disease and tooth loss are unavoidable consequences of certain disabilities.

TREATMENT PLANNING

While patients from a specific special needs group may have several treatment needs in common with other members of that group, each patient should be considered and treated as an individual with a distinctive set of treatment needs. The development of individualised treatment plans may involve several members of the multidisciplinary team, as outlined above.

In order to facilitate appropriate oral health care, it is important to: ■ obtain a careful medical, dental, family and social history ■ determine the oral/dental needs of the patient ■ obtain informed consent to any investigations that may be needed ■ obtain informed consent to the resulting treatment plan.

The main objectives when formulating a treatment plan include: ■ early assessment of oral health ■ realistic methods of oral hygiene intervention – a dental hygienist can be particularly helpful in delivering advice and support ■ dietary advice – liaise with a dietician where appropriate ■ formulation of an oral health care plan – this should include preventative measures to minimise further oral disease ■ management of current oral disease – this may include the management of dental emergencies, in addition to stabilisation of oral health status ■ regular oral examination – the frequency of these examinations must be individually assessed in terms of the risk of further oral disease.

Medical history An apparently fit patient attending for dental treatment may have a serious systemic disease and may be taking medication which may further compromise the provision of care. Many patients with life-threatening diseases now survive as a result of advances in surgical and medical care. Either or both can significantly affect the dental management or even the fate of the patient. These problems may be compounded by the fact that patients are seen briefly and medical support is lacking in most primary care dental surgeries. A detailed medical history is essential in order to: ■ determine any effect on oral health ■ assess the fitness of the patient for the procedure ■ decide on the type of behaviour and pain control required ■ decide how treatment may need to be modified ■ warn of any possible emergencies that could arise ■ determine any possible risk to staff or other patients/visitors.

The history must be reviewed before any surgical procedure, general anaesthetic, conscious sedation or local anaesthetic is given, and at each new course of dental treatment.

Preoperative assessment An arbitrary guideline to assist in the selection of appropriate treatment modalities for a patient may be based on the Classification of Physical Status of the American Society of Anesthesiology (ASA) (Table 2.1).

According to the current guidelines, dental treatment must be significantly modified if the patient has an ASA score of III or IV. Of note, a relatively high percentage of the population aged between 65 and 74 years (23.9%) and 75 or over (34.9%) has an ASA score of III or IV.

Preoperative planning Good preoperative assessment and organisation will assist in anticipating potential hazards when providing oral care, and also help to ensure measures are in place to manage emergencies quickly and efficiently. In most situations dentistry is safe, provided that the patient is healthy and the procedure is not dramatically invasive. Risks arise when these conditions do not apply and the dental team attempts anything over-ambitious in terms of their skill, knowledge or available facilities. It is helpful to formulate a checklist to ensure that factors such as transport, disabled parking and the need for accompanying carers are considered prior to the first treatment appointment. It may also be of benefit to devise a treatment plan consisting of a preoperative, operative and postoperative phase, to ensure that other factors (such as the provision of preoperative antibiotics for the prophylaxis of infective endocarditis) are also considered (Table 2.2).

Analgesia and behaviour management Morbidity is minimal when local anaesthesia (LA) is used. Sedation is more hazardous than local anaesthesia; it must be carried out by adequately trained personnel and with due consideration of the possible risks. General anaesthesia (GA), whether intravenous or inhalational, leads to impaired control of vital functions and is thus only carried out by a qualified anaesthetist, and permitted only in a hospital with appropriate facilities.

CONSENT

Consent in relation to dentistry is the expressed or implied agreement of the patient to undergo a dental examination, investigation or treatment. The law in relation to consent is evolving and there are significant variations between countries. However, the principles remain essentially the same:

Table 2.1 **Classification of Physical Status of the American Society of Anesthesiology (ASA)**

ASA	Definition	Dental treatment modifications
I	Normal, healthy patient	None
II	A patient with mild systemic disease, e.g. well controlled diabetes, anticoagulation, mild asthma, hypertension, epilepsy, pregnancy, anxiety	Medical advice may be helpful. Often few treatment modifications needed, unless GA or major surgery is needed.
III	A patient with severe systemic disease limiting activity but not incapacitating, e.g. chronic renal failure, epilepsy with frequent seizures, uncontrolled hypertension, uncontrolled diabetes, severe asthma, stroke	Medical advice is helpful. Dental care should focus on elimination of acute infection and chronic disease, prior to medical/surgical procedure (e.g. haemodialysis patients). Patients are often best treated in a hospital-based clinic where expert medical support is available.
IV	A patient with incapacitating disease that is a constant threat to life, e.g. cancer, unstable angina or recent myocardial infarct, arrhythmia, recent cerebrovascular accident, end-stage renal disease, liver failure	Medical advice is indicated. All potential dental problems should be corrected prior to medical/surgical procedure to deal with basic problem (e.g. radiotherapy to head and neck, or organ transplant). Patients are often best treated in a hospital-based clinic where expert medical support is available. Emergency dental care is usually indicated.
V	Moribund patient not expected to live more than 24 hours with or without treatment	Medical advice is essential. Patients are often best treated in a hospital-based clinic where expert medical support is available. Emergency dental care is usually indicated.

- Before you examine, treat or care for competent adult patients you must obtain their consent.
- Adults are always assumed to be competent unless demonstrated otherwise. If you have doubts about their competence, the question to ask is: 'can this patient understand and weigh up the information needed to make this decision?' Unexpected decisions do not prove the patient is incompetent, but may indicate a need for further information or explanation.
- Patients may be competent to make some health care decisions, even if they are not competent to make others.
- Giving and obtaining consent is usually a process, not a one-off event. Patients can change their minds and withdraw consent at any time.

Table 2.2 **Example of clinic appointment schedule**

Special care service				
Patient	Last name			
	First name			
	Date of birth			
	Unit number			
	Telephone			
	Mobile			
	Fax			
	E-mail			
Systemic disease	Main problems			
Communication difficulties	Main problems			
Appointment		Date Hour	Date Hour	Date Hour
Treatment planned	Restorative			
	Surgical			
	Mixed			
Support required	Transport			
	Disabled parking			
	Special seating			
	Caregiver present			
	Additional staff			
	Other			
Appropriate dental care	Antibiotic prophylaxis*			
	Blood tests (e.g. INR)			
	BP monitoring			
	Cardiac monitoring			
	Medical assessment			
	Others			
Drugs to avoid	No restraints			
	Drugs*			
	LA			
Behaviour control	Relative analgesia			
	IV sedation			
	GA			
	Others			

*Specify drugs, doses and time of administration.

To give valid consent, patients must receive sufficient information about their condition and proposed treatment. It is the dentist's responsibility to explain all the relevant facts to the patient, and to ascertain that they understand them. The information given to patients must, as a minimum, include:

- The nature, purpose, benefits and risks of the treatment.
- Alternative treatments and their relative benefits and risks.
- All aspects of the procedure expected to be carried out.
- The prognosis if no treatment is given.

If the patient is not offered as much information as they reasonably need to make their decision, and in a form they can understand, their consent may not be valid. For example, information for those with visual impairment may be provided in the form of audio tapes, braille, or large print.

Consent can be written, oral or non-verbal. A signature on a consent form does not itself prove the consent is valid; the point of the form is to record the patient's decision, and also increasingly the discussions that have taken place. Your Trust or organisation may have a policy setting out when you need to obtain written consent.

There are several legal tests that have been described in relation to consent. The *Bolam* test states that a doctor who: 'acted in accordance with a practice accepted as proper by a responsible body of medical men skilled in that particular art is not negligent if he is acting in accordance with such a practice, merely because there is a body of opinion which takes a contrary view.' However a judge may on certain rare occasions choose between two bodies of medical opinion, if one is to be regarded as 'logically indefensible' (*Bolitho* principle). The main alternative to the *Bolam* test is the '*prudent-patient test*' widely used in North America. According to this test, doctors should provide the amount of information that a 'prudent patient' would want.

In the UK, competent adults, namely a person aged 18 and over who has the capacity to make their own decisions about treatment, can consent to dental treatment. They are also entitled to refuse treatment, even where it would clearly benefit their health. The defence of 'emergency' is to allow restraint where you must act quickly to prevent the patient from harming themselves or others (or committing a crime). Emergency treatment to save life or to prevent serious harm to the patient must always be given, if the patient is unable to give consent, e.g. owing to unconsciousness. Another example is that of a patient running amok, who you could restrain, before you have the chance to fully assess the situation. Furthermore, the UK Mental Health Act 1983 (sections 63, 57) enables dental treatment of someone suffering from a mental disorder, to prevent further deterioration of their mental health (e.g. treatment of a dental abscess).

Minors aged 16 and 17, and children below 16 who are *Gillick* competent (understand fully what is involved in the proposed procedure), may also consent to treatment without their parents' authorisation, although their parents will ideally be involved. Legally, a parent can consent if a competent child refuses, but it is likely that taking such a serious step will be rare.

Adults without capacity cannot give consent to treatment. Mental capacity legislation has been the subject of debate and legislative change around the world. Currently, in England and Wales, no-one can authorise treatment on behalf of an adult. However, patients without capacity to consent may receive dental treatment if it is in the patient's *best interests*, with the views of relatives and carers taken into account. In contrast, *The Adults with Incapacity (Scotland) Act 2000*, which came into effect in 2002, allows a competent adult to nominate a person, known as a welfare attorney or proxy, to make medical decisions on their behalf if and when they lose the capacity to make those decisions for themselves. The Act also provides for a general power to treat a patient who is unable to consent to the treatment in question. In order to bring that power into effect, the medical practitioner primarily responsible for treatment must have completed a certificate of incapacity before any treatment is undertaken, other than in an emergency. *The Mental Health (Care and Treatment) (Scotland) Act 2003* was passed by the Scottish parliament in March 2003, with most of it coming into effect in April 2005. It allows for medical/dental intervention to prevent serious deterioration in the patient's mental health condition or to prevent the patient from harming themselves.

The new *Mental Capacity Act (England and Wales)* received Royal Assent in April 2005 and will probably come into force in April 2007. It is central to the legal issues around treating patients over the age of 16 who lack capacity to consent to treatment. The Act is particularly significant in two ways relevant to consent to medical management:

- It will, for the first time, allow consent to be given or withheld for the medical treatment of patients who lack capacity, by another person (typically a close relative). [Under current law there is no proxy consent (and therefore no relevant lack of consent) for adult patients who lack capacity.]
- It provides, again for the first time, for statutory recognition of 'advance directives'. These are statements made by a person whilst competent (i.e. whilst having legal capacity) about the treatment that they would want, or not want, in specified situations, in the future were they to lack capacity at the time the treatment would be relevant.

The information provided is an example of UK law. It is important to remember that the legal situation with regard to consent varies around the world and is subject to continued debate and development.

Further reading • Bridgman A M, Wilson M A 2000 The treatment of adult patients with mental disability. Part 1: Consent and duty. Br Dent J 189(2):66–68 • Bridgman A M, Wilson M A 2000 The treatment of adult patients with a mental disability. Part 2: Assessment of competence. Br Dent J 189(3):143–146 • http://www.markwalton.net/ • http://www.markwalton.net/guidemha/index.asp?

ORAL HEALTH IN PEOPLE WITH DISABILITIES

- A healthy mouth is important in maintaining quality of life for patients with disabilities.
- The evidence is that there is significant unmet need in many people with disabilities and that the care offered does not always match that for other people.

- Most oral disease is caused by:
  - frequent dietary consumption of refined carbohydrates, causing dental caries
  - infrequent or inadequate removal of dental bacterial plaque, causing gingivitis, periodontitis and halitosis.
- A preventive approach is essential.
- Key workers assigned to a patient should be aware of the importance of preventive dental advice as part of the overall care plan.
- Regular oral examination by a dental professional is important.
- The frequency of these examinations must be individually assessed.
- Early intervention can minimise future oral disease, pain, and the need for operative intervention and the associated use of anaesthesia and other drugs.
- The key points for an oral health plan for patients with disabilities are:
  - early assessment of oral health
  - individual care plans drawn up following liaison with family and other health care providers for each case
  - establish a good diet in liaison with a dietician – minimise refined carbohydrates, confectionery and between-meal snacking
  - establish realistic methods of oral hygiene:
    - teeth should be cleaned at least twice daily, using a fluoridated toothpaste and a small-headed toothbrush
    - if the patient is unable to rinse and spit, chlorhexidine gel (gluconate) may be used in place of toothpaste
    - there are various aids available to help patients or their carers maintain a clean, comfortable oral environment; a dental hygienist can be particularly helpful in delivering advice and support
    - dentures should be assessed for fit and comfort as ill-fitting dentures can rub and cause discomfort and ulceration. Dentures (complete and partial) should be removed after every meal, rinsed in cold running water to remove food debris and checked for sharp edges and cracks. They should be replaced in the mouth after the mouth has been checked for food debris and wiped or rinsed clean. At night, dentures should be cleaned with a toothbrush and left to soak in fresh tap water overnight.

KEY CONSIDERATIONS FOR DENTAL MANAGEMENT

Many people with disability are amenable to routine treatment in the dental surgery, but more time may be required. Some people with disabilities require special facilities or an escort to facilitate dental treatment. In patients who are medically compromised, preventive oral health care and the avoidance of non-essential surgery and other invasive procedures are particularly important.

Special issues that may need to be considered include: ■ modifications required to routine treatment procedures ■ accommodating a person who has hearing or visual impairment ■ treating a person who uses a wheelchair ■ managing/accommodating the behaviour of a patient who has difficulty cooperating ■ ensuring airway patency ■ referral for treatment and consultation by specialists.

The treatment modifications indicated to take into account these issues depend not only upon the skill and experience of the team(s) involved, but also on the: ■ type and severity of concurrent disease, its treatment and complications (clearly the more invasive and prolonged the operative interference, and the more severe the medical condition, the more are the risks to the patient) ■ type of pain control or behaviour management needed ■ extent and duration of operative interference ■ extent of interference with normal feeding and life postoperatively.

Communication with the medical team and other care providers can be crucial and ensures optimal care. This is particularly important in relation to: ■ assessment of competency/consent ■ timing and sequencing of dental, medical, surgical and other treatment; nurses, social workers or support coordinator, psychologists, physicians and surgeons may need to be involved ■ use of sedation or general anaesthesia ■ antibiotic prophylaxis ■ control of bleeding tendency ■ potential drug interactions.

Unfortunately, there are few, if any, randomised controlled trials in this field, so the level of evidence available on which to base clinical decisions is not always of the highest (Box 2.1). Most evidence is from levels 3–5.

Behaviour management

Although many patients can be managed using conventional techniques, some may require the implementation of behavioural management strategies, ranging from adapting the clinical environment to create an empathic relaxed environment, to full general anaesthesia. This is particularly true when undertaking complicated procedures, which the patient's medical, psychological or behavioural conditions prevent from being performed in the normal manner.

People with autism, Down syndrome or other learning disabilities, or systemic medical conditions, commonly need behavioural support. Furthermore, demanding, manipulative and resistant behaviours may be seen, particularly in some psychiatric patients and those with dementia or learning disability. The family, partner or caregivers should be consulted to help determine the patient's needs, and help prepare such patients for treatment.

Some behaviour management strategies are: ■ creating a quiet, caring, empathetic relaxed environment ■ scheduling appointments at the appropriate time of day ■ behaviour modification techniques:

Box 2.1 The five levels of evidence

1a.	Systematic review of multiple randomised controlled trials (RCTs)
1b.	Individual well-designed RCT
2a.	Systematic review of cohort studies
2b.	Individual cohort study, or low quality RCT
3a.	Systematic review of case-control studies
3b.	Individual case-control studies
4.	Non-analytical studies (case series)
5.	Opinions of expert committees or respected authorities

• desensitisation (progressive desensitisation may be effective with some anxious individuals – this modality should at least be attempted • positive reinforcement • voice control • distraction via music or television • physical or chemical restraint – rarely.

Many patients with disabilities can readily be treated under local anaesthesia (LA), but this is not the case in some patients who move uncontrollably or who cannot cooperate. A step-wise approach should be employed, whereby the least invasive form of pain and behaviour control is attempted prior to the more potentially dangerous methods of sedation or general anaesthesia (GA).

Intervention (restraint) The question of the use of intervention (restraint) for those unable to comply with routine care, particularly in people with disabilities – and especially in those with learning disability or dementia – is highly controversial. Indeed, this is the area in special care dentistry that often excites the most controversy and passion. No consensus exists regarding either the definition of restraint or what constitutes the use of restraints. Nevertheless, restraint is often divided into 'physical restraint' or 'chemical restraint'. Physical restraint refers to one person holding another person's arms, legs or head to control movements and prevent self-injury by the patient, but also encompasses the use of devices such as mouth props, blankets, straps, Papoose boards, pedi-wraps, and tape ('mechanical restraint'). Chemical restraint refers to the use of sedation or general anaesthesia.

Considerations as to the use of chemical restraints include: ■ can and will the patient cooperate? ■ can and will the patient take the medications orally? ■ what are the potential drug interactions or adverse effects? ■ what is the opinion of the patient's physician and other care providers? ■ is informed consent from the patient possible, and has it been obtained?

Conscious sedation (CS) requires an appropriately trained team and monitoring equipment, with the ability to respond to complications. CS can be a very effective and safe modality, and it is disappointing that it may be less attractive to some parents than is GA.

GA should normally be the last resort in the behavioural management armamentarium but, for those patients who have greatest difficulty in cooperating, it can be the most ideal method, permitting a higher standard of technical dentistry to be achieved, since the anaesthetic team manages the patient's medical status and vital signs while the dental team can concentrate on the dentistry. GA may also be used to carry out more complex procedures and, by saving time, may enable more comprehensive treatment to be provided.

Most people with disabilities can be safely managed under general anaesthesia for dental treatment in a hospital setting with minimal morbidity. Nevertheless, there is little doubt that GA is more dangerous than CS. Intraoperative complications are uncommon, but may include non-fatal ventricular arrhythmias, slight falls in blood pressure, hypertension (greater than 20% of preoperative value), laryngospasm and minor airway problems resulting in a desaturation of oxygen to a level below 85%. However, to use GA presupposes the assistance of an anaesthetist, the presence of other essential facilities and emergency support, and absence of any medical contraindications.

When physical restraints are used, it is generally accepted that they should not: ■ cause any physical injury to the patient ■ be used for the convenience of the staff ■ be used except when absolutely necessary ■ be more restrictive than necessary ■ be used as punishment.

The British Institute of Learning Disabilities summarises key policy principles on physical interventions as follows:

1. Any physical intervention should be consistent with the legal obligations and responsibilities of care agencies and their staff and the rights and protection afforded to people with learning disabilities under law.
2. Working within the 'legal framework', services are responsible for the provision of care, including physical interventions, which are in a person's best interest.

Values

3. Physical interventions should only be used in the best interests of the patient.
4. Patients should be treated fairly and with courtesy and respect.
5. Patients should be helped to make choices and be involved in making decisions that affect their lives.
6. There should be experiences and opportunities for learning that are appropriate to the person's interests and abilities.

Prevention of challenging behaviour

7. Challenging behaviours can often be prevented by the careful management of setting conditions.
8. The interaction between environmental setting conditions and personal setting conditions should be explored for each patient who presents a challenge. Setting conditions should be modified to reduce the likelihood of challenging behaviour occurring (primary prevention).
9. Secondary prevention procedures should be developed to ensure that problematic episodes are properly managed with non-physical interventions before patients become violent.
10. For each patient who presents a challenge there should be individualised strategies for responding to incidents of violence and reckless behaviour. Where appropriate, the strategy should include directions for using physical interventions.
11. Individualised procedures should be established for responding to patients who are likely to present violent or reckless behaviour. The procedures should enable care staff to respond effectively to violent or reckless behaviours while ensuring the safety of all concerned.

Promoting the best interests of patients

12. Physical interventions should only be used in conjunction with other strategies designed to help patients learn alternative non-challenging behaviours.
13. Planned physical interventions should be justified in respect of: what is known of the client from a formal multidisciplinary assessment; alternative

approaches which have been tried; an evaluation of the potential risks involved; reference to a body of expert knowledge and established good practice.

14. The use of physical interventions should be subject to regular review.

Physical intervention and risk assessment

15. The potential hazards associated with the use of physical interventions should be systematically explored using a risk assessment procedure. Physical interventions should not involve unreasonable risk.

Minimising risk and promoting the wellbeing of patients

16. Physical interventions should be employed using the minimum reasonable force.
17. Any single physical intervention should be employed for the minimum duration of time.
18. For individual patients, physical interventions should be sanctioned for the shortest period of time consistent with the patient's best interests.
19. Physical interventions should not cause pain.
20. Patients should have individual assessments to identify contraindications of physical interventions before they are approved.
21. Patients who receive a physical intervention should be routinely assessed for signs of injury or psychological distress.

Management responsibilities

22. Service managers are responsible for developing and implementing policies on the use of physical interventions.
23. The use of any procedure should be clearly set out in the form of written guidance for staff.
24. Service managers are responsible for ensuring that all incidents involving the use of physical interventions are clearly, comprehensively and promptly recorded.
25. All patients and their families and representatives should have ready access to an effective complaints procedure.
26. Careful consideration should be given to the impact of resource management on the use of physical interventions.

Employers' responsibility towards staff

27. Employers and managers are responsible for the safety and wellbeing of staff.
28. Staff should be encouraged to monitor all physical interventions and to report any incidents that give cause for concern.

Staff training

29. Staff who may be required to use physical interventions should receive regular training on knowledge, skills and values.
30. Training should be provided by an instructor with appropriate experience and qualifications.
31. Staff should only employ physical interventions they have been trained to use.

32. Staff deployment should be organised to ensure that appropriately trained staff are available to respond to any incident requiring physical intervention.

Further reading ● Bridgman A M 2000 Mental incapacity and restraint for treatment: present law and proposals for reform. J Med Ethics 26(5):387–392 ● Bridgman A M, Wilson M A 2000 The treatment of adult patients with a mental disability. Part 3: The use of restraint. Br Dent J 189(4):195–198 ● Carr K R, Wilson S, Nimer S, Thornton J B Jr 1999 Behavior management techniques among pediatric dentists practicing in the southeastern United States. Pediatr Dent 21(6):347–353 ● Connick C, Palat M, Pugliese S 2000 The appropriate use of physical restraint: considerations. ASDC J Dent Child 67(4):231, 256–262 ● Connick C, Pugliese S, Willette J, Palat M 2000 Desensitization: strengths and limitations of its use in dentistry for the patient with severe and profound mental retardation. ASDC J Dent Child 67(4):250–255 ● Connick C M, Bates M L, Barsley R E 1999 Dental treatment guidelines for use of restraints within the nine Louisiana developmental centers. Louisiana State University Dental Health Resources Program. LDA J 58(2):23–26 ● Geary J L, Kinirons M J, Boyd D, Gregg T A 2000 Individualized mouth prop for dental professionals and carers. Int J Paediatr Dent 10(1):71–74 ● Kupietzky A 2004 Strap him down or knock him out: Is conscious sedation with restraint an alternative to general anaesthesia? Br Dent J 196(3):133–138 ● Limeres J, Vázquez E, Medina J, Tomás I, Feijoo JF, Diz P 2003 Evaluación preanestésica de discapacitados severos susceptibles de tratamiento odontológico bajo anestesia general. Medicina Oral 8:353–360 ● Scully C, Kumar N 2002 Dentistry for those requiring special care. Primary Dental Care 10:17–22 ● Scully C 2004 The medically compromised patient: an overview. In: Prabhu S R (ed) Textbook of oral medicine. Oxford University Press, New Delhi, p236–244 ● Tyrer G L 1999 Referrals for dental general anaesthesia: how many really need GA? Br Dent J 187:440–443
● http://www.bild.org.uk./physical_interventions/summary_of_principles.htm
● http://www.friendlyreports.org.uk

Prevention

Prevention of oral disease is of paramount importance for individuals with disabilities, not least to prevent disease and complications such as pain but also to obviate the need for operative intervention.

Prevention programmes must be started at as early an age as feasible and reinforced on a long-term basis, incorporating them into other daily programmes such as rehabilitation, education and occupational therapy. Dental recalls should be planned in accordance with the individual patient's needs: people with severe dental disease or a predisposition to it (e.g. xerostomia predisposing to caries) may need to be seen every 2–3 months.

Patients should be involved in maintaining their own oral hygiene as much as possible, but carers may need to assist. Education of the family members, partner or other care providers may be critical for ensuring regular and appropriate supervision of diet and oral hygiene. Caregivers may well need dental health education, and should be shown how to properly position the person for oral hygiene care. Chairs, pillows, head rests, bean bags, and other devices may be helpful.

Dietary counselling is crucial, to avoid caries and erosion. Ideally, patients should brush their teeth after each meal and before bedtime, but at least twice daily is acceptable. Brushes can be modified to assist people with physical disabilities to brush their own teeth. Electric toothbrushes may improve patient compliance in patients with physical or mental disabilities. Other aids helpful to many people include:

- Fluoride toothpastes, mouth rinses or gels, which may be beneficial in controlling caries. Patients who might swallow a rinse can benefit from application with a toothbrush, cotton bud or sponge-sticks. Additional topical fluorides such as professional applications of varnish are indicated when the caries rate is high.
- Chlorhexidine mouth rinses or gels, which may be beneficial in controlling gingivitis and periodontitis. Patients who might swallow a rinse can benefit from application with a toothbrush, cotton bud or sponge-sticks. Intermittent use (e.g. weekends or every other day) may help to minimise problems with staining.

Where cooperation is good:

- Tooth flossing is recommended daily, although a second person may need to assist.
- Disclosing solutions may be beneficial in promoting behavioural changes.
- Fissure sealants may be beneficial.

Further reading ● Diz Dios P, Fernández Feijoo J 2000 Pacientes especiales en atención primaria. In: Suárez Quintanilla J (ed) Odontología en atención primaria. Instituto Lácer de Salud Buco-Dental, Barcelona ● Eirea M, Diz P, Vázquez E, Castro M et al 1996 Effectiveness of a new toothbrush design for physically impaired patients. Stoma 40:37–42 ● Rutkauskas J S (ed) 1994 Practical considerations in special patient care. Dent Clin North Amer 38(3):361–584 ● Helpin M L, Rosenberg H M 1997 Dental care: beyond brushing and flossing. In: Children with disabilities, 4th edn. Brookes Publishing Co., Baltimore, p643–656 ● http://www.nohic.nidcr.nih.gov/poc/publication/careguide.aspx

Access and positioning

Access to oral health for individuals with special needs has been limited in the past, but legislation such as the Disability Discrimination Act (DDA) 1995 has improved the situation. Special attention should be paid to non-ambulatory, home-bound, and institutionalised patients who may need access to portable dentistry programmes (domiciliary care) and treatment facilities based inside institutions. Patients with severe disabilities generally benefit from short dental appointments but there is a balance between this, achieving an adequate amount of treatment, and the difficulties and costs encountered with transporting patients to the dental surgery on repeated occasions.

Patients using a wheelchair may have to be transferred from their wheelchair to the dental chair. In these situations, it is an essential requirement that all staff have training in manual handling, and that such training should also include the safe use of equipment to assist transfer (e.g. sliding board, turntable, and hoist). Where patients need to be treated in their wheelchairs, the surgery layout should provide enough space for this. Furthermore, surgeries may be designed with tilting floor ramps/platforms, and dental units which can directly lift wheelchairs are now available.

Operative procedures and the airway Individuals with disabling conditions may not possess the ability or reflexes to adequately protect their own airway during operative procedures in the mouth. This may be due to their specific disabling condition or their inability to cooperate. Such a patient might inadvertently swallow or aspirate dental restorations, materials or instruments. It is vital therefore that, if a rubber dam cannot be used, these patients are properly positioned at 45 degrees to prevent aspiration, and not placed in a supine position. The use of the rubber dam may in any event be contraindicated because of the patient's inability to control or swallow oral secretions (e.g. severe Parkinson's disease).

Surgery Surgery can be undertaken on the conscious patient only where the patient can remain both still and cooperative. However, simple procedures may sometimes be performed if the patient who moves involuntarily is appropriately restrained, either with consent having been obtained or in their best interests. In others, sedation or GA is required.

Special care should be taken in patients requiring antibiotic prophylaxis and in those with bleeding tendencies. In all patients having surgery, consideration should be given to ensuring an adequate escort postoperatively, and to minimising complications and the need for further procedures such as suture removal.

Further reading ● Chalmers J M, Kingsford Smith D, Carter K D 1998 A multidisciplinary dental program for community-living adults with chronic mental illness. Spec Care Dentist 18(5):194–201 ● Harrison M G, Roberts G J 1998 Comprehensive dental treatment of healthy and chronically sick children under intubation general anaesthesia during a 5-year period. Br Dent J 184(10):503–506 ● Frassica J J, Miller E C 1989 Anesthesia management in pediatric and special needs patients undergoing dental and oral surgery. Int Anesthesiol Clin 27(2):109–115.

Treatment modification

Restorative dentistry Patients with disabilities may be more likely to have dental anomalies, such as hypodontia, and to suffer from tooth wear, erosion, and caries. While prevention plays a key role, expedient restoration of the dentition (if dental disease has already occurred) can be crucial, as it will help to minimise the need for advanced restorative procedures in the longer term. Furthermore, it is often critical to prevent tooth loss, particularly when dentures would be poorly tolerated.

However, clinical work can be very difficult as access to the oral environment is often limited and patient tolerance and concentration may be reduced. The use of rotatory instruments may be especially hazardous in patients with uncontrollable movements or those unable to be cooperative. Individuals with disabling conditions may not tolerate the rubber dam or cooperate during restorative procedures without the aid of chemical restraints such as sedation or general anaesthesia. The choice of restorative material and technique may require modification. Restoration by indirect techniques may not be possible, so the choice is often limited to amalgam, resin composite and glass ionomer. Glass ionomer restorations may be particularly appropriate for patients with a high caries rate, since they adhere to tooth substance and release fluoride. Stainless steel crowns may be appropriate for restoring severely damaged teeth when the patient's lack of cooperation precludes more complicated restorative procedures. In addition, alternative techniques, such as the atraumatic restorative treatment technique (ART), or a chemo-mechanical caries removal technique (Carisolv®) may be employed. These may reduce the need for local anaesthesia.

Further reading • Gryst M E, Mount G J 1999 The use of glass ionomer in special needs patients. Aust Dent J 44(4):268–274 • Jones J A, Mash L K, Niessen L C 1993 Restorative considerations for special needs patients. Dent Clin North Am 37(3):483–495.

Periodontics Individuals with disabling conditions may not possess the ability to adequately maintain good oral hygiene, which can lead to periodontal diseases and/or halitosis. It is frequently not possible to improve the level of plaque control with standard toothbrushes, because of the patient's impaired cognition, mobility and manual dexterity. Electric toothbrushes may, therefore, be easier and more effective under these circumstances. Chlorhexidine spray or mouthwashes, used twice daily, can provide significant assistance with plaque control. Chlorhexidine at a concentration of 0.06% appears to be as effective in reducing plaque accumulation as a 0.12% concentration. Regular, routine scaling usually improves gingival health considerably, however there is little indication for sophisticated periodontal surgery. If there are certain cardiac defects, antibiotic cover may be indicated.

Other factors contributing to periodontal diseases include gingival enlargement caused by some drugs, e.g. phenytoin or ciclosporin, or by one of the genetic syndromes. Gingivectomy may sometimes be justifiable for aesthetic and social reasons, or if the enlarged gingival tissues interfere with occlusion or effective oral hygiene. Electrosurgery or laser surgery may be considered instead of the external bevel gingivectomy where periodontal packs may not be well retained or tolerated. Gingival enlargement is likely to recur, particularly if there is inadequate improvement in oral hygiene. Therefore, frequent recall examinations and prophylaxis, as often as every 2 or 3 months, can be justified.

Further reading • Craig D C, Boyle C A, Fleming G J, Palmer R 2000 A sedation technique for implant and periodontal surgery. J Clin Periodontol 27(12):955–959.

Endodontics Maintaining severely damaged or worn teeth is critical in individuals with disabling conditions who cannot tolerate removable prostheses. Endodontic treatment should be considered when a tooth is restorable and the patient can cooperate. Sedation or general anaesthesia may facilitate endodontic treatment, particularly of anterior teeth, in those patients who are less cooperative. There is no convincing evidence that poor systemic health compromises the chances of a successful endodontic outcome – only one study has implicated diabetes as potentially reducing the success of root canal treatment.

The use of rubber dam and one-appointment procedures are advisable when possible. When radiographs cannot be obtained, an apex locator can be helpful in determining working length. Rotary instrumentation may facilitate effective and speedier canal preparation, but root canal irrigation should not be compromised. Irrigant delivery may be enhanced using endosonics.

Provided that canal preparation is well controlled, obturation may be simplified by using commercially available, thermoplasticised gutta-percha on a carrier.

Further reading • Battrum D E, Gutmann J L 1994 Comprehensive endodontics for special needs patients: a case report. Univ Tor Dent J 8(1):7–9 • Scully C, Gulabivala K, Ng P 2003 Systemic complications of endodontic manipulations. In: Glick M (ed) Endodontic topics, vol 4. Blackwell, Copenhagen, p60–68.

Fixed prosthodontics The provision of fixed prosthodontics involving teeth or implants may be appropriate if the patient can cooperate and adequate oral hygiene can be maintained by the patient and/or caregiver. If the patient is unable to cooperate, so precluding more complicated procedures for restoring severely damaged teeth, long-term provisional restorations or stainless steel crowns may be more appropriate. Although technique sensitive, resin-bonded bridges can also be useful as treatment is generally quicker and less invasive.

Replacement of anterior teeth with fixed prosthodontics is generally contraindicated for the patient who has severe epilepsy or is likely to suffer trauma – as in some patients with severe learning disability or dementia, or those who suffer self-harm – as restorations or abutment teeth may fracture.

Further reading • Gilmour A G, Morgan C L 2003 Restorative management of the elderly patient. Prim Dent Care 10(2):45–48 • Jones J A, Mash L K, Niessen L C 1993 Restorative considerations for special needs patients. Dent Clin North Am 37(3):483–495.

Removable prosthodontics Removable prostheses can be a helpful solution to the restoration of occlusal function and appearance in many people with disability. Implant-stabilised prostheses can be advantageous if peri-implant health can be adequately maintained. However, conventional removable prostheses are contraindicated for patients with severe epilepsy, who may inhale foreign bodies during a convulsion. Such prostheses are also not indicated for the patient with insufficient muscle control or physical or mental capacity to adapt to them. These patients include some with learning disability, dementia, stroke, or movement disorders (Parkinson's disease, Huntington's chorea or tardive dyskinesia). Patients must also be capable of recognising, inserting, removing, and cleaning their denture. Any prosthesis for a person with epilepsy should be constructed of radio-opaque material, whilst those for patients with a learning disability or dementia should be marked with their identity as they can be mislaid or lost.

Impression taking can also be difficult, but may be facilitated by using a viscous material, such as composition or a putty-type silicone material. If the patient objects violently, these materials can be readily removed without leaving unset material in the oropharynx. If patients will not keep their mouths open, a mouth prop on alternate sides and sectional impressions may overcome the difficulty. However, in patients with severe cerebral palsy, stridor can be caused by a bite block.

Registration of occlusal records can be very difficult if cooperation is lacking, and some people with more severe disabilities tend to have a deterioration of breathing function when using a bite registration block. Those patients who are incapable of managing complete dentures can become 'dentally impaired' in addition to their other disabilities.

Further reading ● Jones J A, Mash L K, Niessen L C 1993 Restorative considerations for special needs patients. Dent Clin North Am 37(3):483–495 ● Paunovich E D, Aubertin M A, Saunders M J, Prange M 2000 The role of dentistry in palliative care of the head and neck cancer patient. Tex Dent J 117(6):36–45 ● Thomson W M, Brown R H, Williams S M 1992 Dentures, prosthetic treatment needs, and mucosal health in an institutionalised elderly population. NZ Dent J 88(392):51–55.

Implants Early clinical studies on osseointegrated implants (OI), which provided much of the evidence base for their success, employed strict patient selection criteria. These studies excluded many systemic disorders, which it was believed might contraindicate implant treatment. However, in recent years the justification for some of these assumptions has been challenged, as – perhaps unsurprisingly – the evidence for any increased failure rates of implant treatment in medically compromised patients is quite sparse. There appear to be apparently few absolute contraindications to implant treatment, but a number that may increase the risk of treatment failure or complications.

In all patients with disabilities in whom OI are considered, it would clearly be prudent to weigh carefully the cost–benefit analysis. Furthermore, it is crucial to undertake the procedures with strict asepsis, to minimise trauma and take especial care in avoiding stress and undue haemorrhage. Crucially, the patient must be able to maintain an excellent standard of oral hygiene. Treatment modifications may be indicated (Table 2.3).

Orthodontics Comprehensive treatment of patients with orofacial clefts is best carried out within a multidisciplinary team which includes, in addition to orthodontists, oral and maxillofacial, ENT and plastic surgeons; paediatric dentists; people to assist oral rehabilitation; and speech therapists. Active orthodontic treatment is provided at the appropriate stages in the patient's growth and development, and may extend from shortly after birth until early adulthood.

Orthognathic surgery involves cooperation between orthodontists and maxillofacial surgeons. The aim of such treatment is to correct serious malformations of skeletal jaw structures, from patients for whom conventional orthodontic treatment is insufficient to correct the abnormal jaw relationship, to patients suffering from syndromes which affect the jaw and skull growth (e.g. Crouzon's or Apert's syndrome, hemifacial microsomia and other asymmetry malformations), to patients with tumours or growth disorders which impair normal jaw development.

Further reading ● AlSarheed M, Bedi R, Hunt N P 2003 Orthodontic treatment need and self-perception of 11–16-year-old Saudi Arabian children with a sensory impairment attending Special Schools. J Orthod 30:29–34 ● AlSarheed M, Bedi R, Hunt N P 2004 The views and attitudes of parents of children with a sensory impairment towards orthodontic care. Eur J Orthod 26:87–91 ● Onyeaso C O 2003 Orthodontic treatment need of mentally handicapped children in Ibadan, Nigeria, according to the dental aesthetic index. J Dent Child (Chic) 70(2):159–163 ● Waldman H B, Perlman S P, Swerdloff M 2000 Orthodontics and the population with special needs. Am J Orthod Dentofacial Orthop 118(1):14–17.

Table 2.3 **Implants in various conditions**

Condition	Evidence that condition is a contraindication to implants	Implant success rate compared with that in healthy population (level of evidence)	Other considerations	Management modifications that may be indicated
Alcoholism	–	Similar (5)	Tobacco use, bleeding problem, osteoporosis, impaired immunity, malnutrition, behavioural problems	May not be a good risk group
Bleeding disorder	Medical advice should be taken first	Similar (5)	Possibility of blood-borne infections	May not be a good risk group, medical advice should be taken first
Bone disease (osteoporosis, osteopenia)	–	Similar (4)	–	Sinus lifts may be contraindicated
Cardiac disease	Medical advice should be taken first	Similar (5)	May be anticoagulated. Poor risk for general anaesthesia (GA)	Avoid GA Give endocarditis prophylaxis
Corticosteroid therapy	–	Similar (5)	May be impaired immunity	Consider parenteral corticosteroid cover. Consider antimicrobial prophylaxis

Table 2.3 **Implants in various conditions—cont'd**

Condition	Evidence that condition is a contraindication to implants	Implant success rate compared with that in healthy population (level of evidence)	Other considerations	Management modifications that may be indicated
Diabetes mellitus	–	Slightly reduced (2a)	Microvascular disease. Osteoporosis	Avoid hypoglycaemia Use chlorhexidine Consider antibiotic prophylaxis
Immunocompromised patients	Medical advice should be taken first	Similar (4)	May be blood-borne infections	Use chlorhexidine Consider antibiotic prophylaxis
Mucosal disease	–	Similar (4)	–	–
Neuropsychiatric disorders	Medical advice should be taken first	Similar (4)	Behavioural	–
Radiotherapy or chemotherapy	–	Reduced (1b) Similar (3b)	Prognosis	Surgery 21 days before DXR. DXR <66 Gy (ORN) or <50. Hyperbaric oxygen. Defer implants 8 months. Consider antimicrobial cover
Xerostomia	–	Similar (4)	–	–

Chapter 3

SPECIFIC PROBLEM AREAS

ACROMEGALY

Definition Acromegaly is a chronic, progressive disorder caused by growth hormone (GH) hypersecretion after normal growth cessation. Excess GH production before epiphyseal closure results in gigantism.

General aspects

Aetiopathogenesis GH hypersecretion is usually caused by an eosinophilic adenoma of the anterior pituitary. Other uncommon causes include pancreatic islet cell tumours and some lung endocrine tumours that produce GH stimulating factors.

Clinical presentation ■ Excess tissue growth (Fig. 3.1): ● supra-orbital ridge (prominent) ● nose (broadened) ● skin (thickening) ● macroglossia ● mandible (spaced teeth, prognathism) ● hands and feet (large) ■ Systemic complications due to organ enlargement: ● diabetes ● hypertension ● cardiomyopathy ■ Local effects of pituitary tumour (headache, visual defects).

Diagnosis Diagnosis is confirmed by clinical, laboratory and radiographic findings: ■ plasma GH – raised ■ oral glucose tolerance test – fails to suppress GH ■ serum insulin-like growth factor 1 – raised ■ CT and MRI.

Treatment ■ Neurosurgery and/or radiation ■ Dopamine agonists (bromocriptine) and somatostatin analogues (sandostatin).

Prognosis Acromegalic patients have a decreased life expectancy, because of cardiovascular diseases, tumours and endocrine problems. Cardiac failure is the major cause of death.

Oral findings

■ The skull is thickened and the paranasal air sinuses are enlarged ■ Mandibular enlargement leads to class III malocclusion with spacing of the teeth and thickening of all soft tissues, but most conspicuously of the face ■ Enlargement of the dental bases leads to relatively sudden ill-fitting dentures ■ Macroglossia and thick lips are due to soft tissue growth

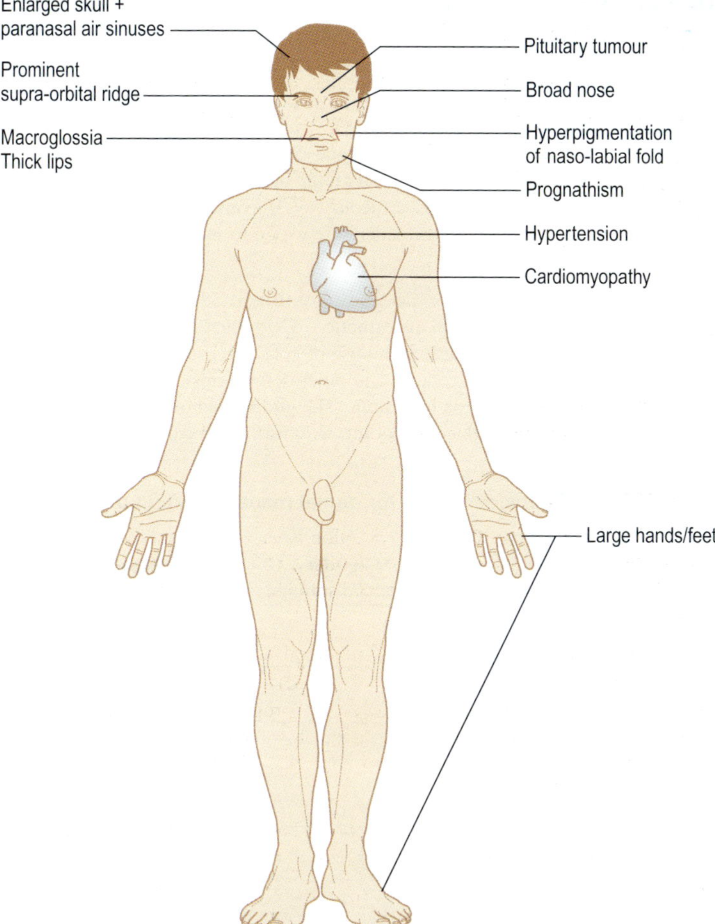

Figure 3.1 **Clinical presentation of acromegaly**

■ Apical hypercementosis ■ Sialosis ■ Hyperpigmentation of the naso-labial fold ■ Progressive periodontal disease has been described – probably related to dental malposition and tissue enlargement.

Dental management

Risk assessment Dental management may be complicated by:
■ visual impairment ■ cardiomyopathy ■ cardiac arrhythmias
■ hypertension ■ diabetes mellitus ■ hypopituitarism.

Rarely, acromegalics have Cushing's syndrome or hyperparathyroidism due to associated multiple endocrine adenoma syndrome.

Preventive dentistry and patient education The abnormal skeletal growth may result in carpal tunnel syndrome, and an enlarged tongue, leading to difficulty with toothbrushing. An electric toothbrush may be beneficial in these circumstances.

Patient access and positioning Obstruction of the upper airway may be associated with sleep apnoea and fatigue. Such patients should be seen later in the day when they are rested, with the dental chair positioned more upright to avoid further collapse of the airway. If available, longer dental chairs, or chairs which can be extended, are useful to increase patient comfort during treatment.

Pain and anxiety control **Local anaesthesia** Hyperpituitarism does not affect the selection of local anaesthetic. **Conscious sedation** There are no contraindications regarding the use of conscious sedation.
General anaesthesia Kyphosis and other deformities affecting respiration may make general anaesthesia hazardous. The glottic opening may be narrowed and the cords' mobility reduced. A goitre may further embarrass the airway.

Table 3.1 **Key considerations for dental management in acromegaly (see text)**

	Management modifications*	Comments/possible complications
Risk assessment	2	Blindness, diabetes, hypertension, arrhythmias
Preventive dentistry and education	1	Carpal tunnel syndrome, enlarged tongue
Pain and anxiety control		
– Local anaesthesia	0	
– Conscious sedation	0	
– General anaesthesia	1/4	Kyphosis, narrow glottis
Patient access and positioning		
– Access to dental office	0	
– Timing of treatment	1	Sleep apnoea, fatigue
– Patient positioning	1	Longer dental chair
Treatment modification		
– Oral surgery	0	
– Implantology	0	
– Conservative/Endodontics	0	
– Fixed prosthetics	0	
– Removable prosthetics	0	
– Non-surgical periodontology	0	
– Surgical periodontology	0	
Hazardous and contraindicated drugs	0	

*0 = No special considerations. 1 = Caution advised. 2 = Specialised medical advice recommended in some cases. 3 = Specialised medical advice mandatory. 4 = Only to be performed in hospital environment. 5 = Should be avoided.

Treatment modification **Surgery** Orthognathic surgery may be considered, although fatalities have followed such surgery in the past, because of airway obstruction. **Periodontology** Early treatment and regular review are important to control periodontal disease progression.

Drug use No antibiotics or analgesics are contraindicated.

Further reading ● Brennan M D, Jackson I T, Keller E E, Laws E R Jr, Sather A H 1985 Multidisciplinary management of acromegaly and its deformities. JAMA 253:682–683 ● Whelan J, Redpath T, Buckle R 1982 The medical and anaesthetic management of acromegalic patients undergoing maxillo-facial surgery. Br J Oral Surg 20:77–83.

ADDISON'S DISEASE

Definition Addison's disease is adrenocortical hypofunction due to the destruction or dysfunction of the adrenal cortex. It may be:
■ primary – occurs when at least 90% of the adrenal cortex has been destroyed, and leads to low levels of both cortisol and aldosterone
■ secondary – due to low levels of adrenocorticotrophic hormone (ACTH), which causes a drop in the adrenal glands' production of cortisol but not aldosterone.

General aspects

Aetiopathogenesis ■ Main cause is autoimmune (sometimes also associated with diabetes, Graves' disease, pernicious anaemia, vitiligo or hypoparathyroidism), particularly in women ■ Rare causes include adrenal tuberculosis, histoplasmosis or tumours ■ Secondary adrenocortical hypofunction may also follow an abrupt withdrawal from systemic corticosteroid therapy.

Clinical presentation ■ Low cortisol leads to: ● skin and mucosal hyperpigmentation (due to raised ACTH in primary disease; part of ACTH molecule is similar to melanocyte stimulating hormone) (Fig. 3.2) ● hypotension (weakness, lethargy, tiredness, collapse) ● weight loss ■ Adrenocortical hypofunction may lead to shock and death if the individual is stressed as, for example, by an operation, infection or trauma.

Diagnosis ■ Postural hypotension ■ Plasma cortisol level – low ■ Plasma sodium – low ■ Plasma potassium – high ■ ACTH stimulation test – impaired ■ Adrenal antibodies.

Treatment ■ Glucocorticoids (cortisone or cortisol) and mineralocorticoids (fludrocortisone).

Prognosis Untreated patients may survive several months or years, followed by a progressive wasting of the body and death. Patients on steroid replacement therapy enjoy a normal life.

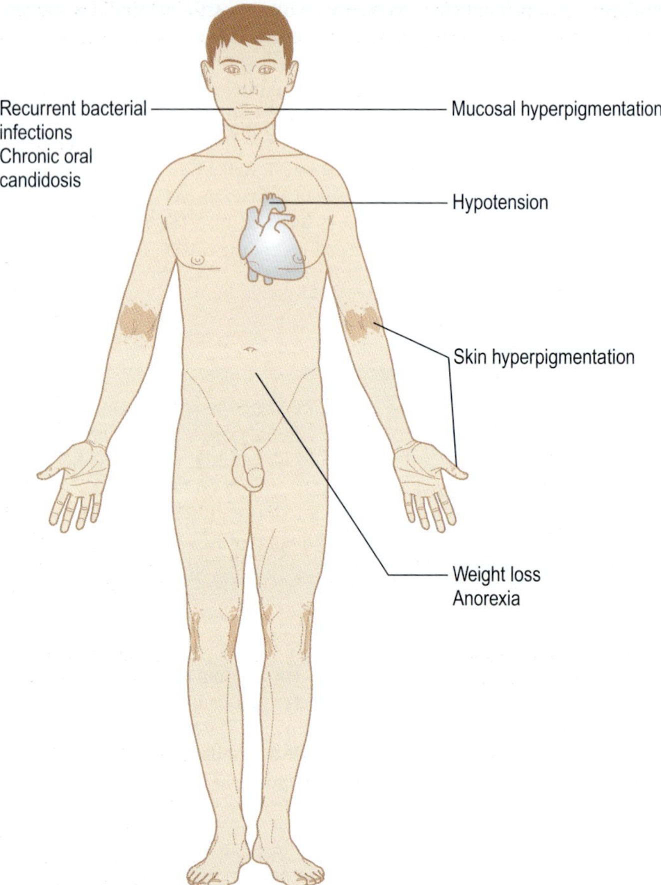

Figure 3.2 **Clinical presentation of Addison's disease**

Oral findings

■ Pigmentation of the mucosae of a brown or black colour is seen in over 75% of patients with Addison's disease. Hyperpigmentation predominantly affects areas that are normally pigmented or exposed to trauma (for example in the buccal mucosa at the occlusal line, or the tongue, and occasionally, the gingivae). ■ Recurrent bacterial oral infections are not uncommon ■ Chronic oral candidosis has also been described where there is an associated immune defect.

Dental management

Risk assessment The danger of dental treatment in a patient with hypoadrenocorticism, especially when undertaking surgery under general anaesthesia, is of precipitating hypotensive collapse. Clinical findings suggestive of acute adrenal insufficiency include weakness, nausea, vomiting, headache and abdominal pain.

Acute adrenal insufficiency is managed as follows: ■ call for immediate help ■ lay patient flat with legs raised ■ give hydrocortisone 200 mg IM ■ oxygen 10 L/min ■ if IV access can be obtained, give 1 litre dextrose saline ■ check blood pressure.

Appropriate oral health care The need for patients on long-term steroid treatment to increase their dose of glucocorticoids when undergoing stressful procedures has been the subject of much controversy. In 1998, Nicholson et al reviewed all the available evidence and published new recommendations for steroid cover, where hydrocortisone supplementation is given intravenously. Patients who have taken steroids in excess of 10 mg prednisolone, or equivalent, within the last 3 months, should be considered to have some degree of hypothalamic–pituitary–adrenal (HPA) suppression and will require supplementation. Patients who have not received steroids for more than 3 months are considered to have full recovery of HPA axis and require no supplementation. These guidelines have been adopted by anaesthetists in the UK (see Steroids) and are increasingly used by other specialties, including dentists.

However, the implementation of Nicholson's guidelines is not universal amongst the dental profession. Some are still using regimens such as doubling the normal daily steroid dose on the day of procedure (Gibson & Ferguson 2004).

Preventive dentistry Oral hygiene and regular professional dental care are especially important, because increased susceptibility to infection has been described.

Pain and anxiety control Cortisol levels normally increase in the postoperative period following oral surgical procedures. This increase is blunted by the use of analgesics, strongly suggesting that the increased cortisol levels are a physiological response to pain. Hence in patients with Addison's disease, postoperative analgesia is extremely important. In view of this, if significant postoperative pain is expected, the patient's usual steroid dose may be doubled on the following day. **Local anaesthesia** Adrenocortical hypofunction does not affect the selection of local anaesthetic. **Conscious sedation** There are no contraindications regarding the use of conscious sedation. **General anaesthesia** The major determinant of secretion of ACTH and cortisol during surgery is recovery from general anaesthesia and extubation rather than the trauma of surgery itself. In these patients, steroid supplementation with 25 mg hydrocortisone at induction, followed by 100 mg/day for 48–72 h are recommended.

Patient access and positioning Patients with Addison's disease are best treated early in the day – when serum cortisol levels are highest.

Treatment modification Most patients undergoing routine dental procedures need no supplemental steroids. However steroid cover is advisable for those patients undergoing surgical procedures, including dental extractions, periodontal surgery and placement of implants. It may also be considered for those patients that are particularly anxious. The guidelines recommended by Nicholson et al in 1998 are outlined below:

Perioperative steroid supplementation Patients currently taking steroids (prednisolone)/stopped within last 3 months:

- < 10mg/day:
  - assume normal HPA response – additional steroid cover not required
- ≥ 10mg/day:
  - Minor surgery – 25mg hydrocortisone at induction
  - Moderate surgery – 25mg hydrocortisone at induction + 100mg/day for 24h
  - Major surgery – 25mg hydrocortisone at induction + 100mg/day for 48–72h.

Surgery Delayed healing has been observed after dentoalveolar surgery. Antibiotic prophylaxis is advised before any procedure causing significant

Table 3.2 **Key considerations for dental management in Addison's disease (see text)**

	Management modifications*	Comments/possible complications
Risk assessment	2	Acute adrenal insufficiency
Appropriate oral health care	2	Consider steroid cover
Preventive dentistry	1	Increased susceptibility to infection
Pain and anxiety control		
– Local anaesthesia	0	
– Conscious sedation	0	
– General anaesthesia	2/4	ACTH and cortisol secretion
Patient access and positioning		
– Access to dental office	0	
– Timing of treatment	1	Early morning
– Patient positioning	0	
Treatment modification		
– Oral surgery	1	Delayed healing
– Implantology	1	Delayed healing
– Conservative/Endodontics	0	
– Fixed prosthetics	0	
– Removable prosthetics	0	
– Non-surgical periodontology	0	
– Surgical periodontology	1	Delayed healing
Hazardous and contraindicated drugs	0	

*0 = No special considerations. 1 = Caution advised. 2 = Specialised medical advice recommended in some cases. 3 = Specialised medical advice mandatory. 4 = Only to be performed in hospital environment. 5 = Should be avoided.

bleeding, including oral surgery, implantology and periodontal surgery. Good postoperative pain control is essential. Steroid cover should be considered.

Drug use No local anaesthetics, analgesics, sedative drugs or antibiotics are contraindicated.

Further reading ● Bsoul S A, Terezhalmy G T, Moore W S 2003 Addison disease (adrenal insufficiency). Quintessence Int 34:784–785 ● Gibson N, Ferguson J W 2004 Steroid cover for dental patients on long-term steroid medication: proposed clinical guidelines based upon a critical review of the literature. Br Dent J 197:681–685 ● Nicholson G, Burrin J M, Hall G M 1998 Peri-operative steroid supplementation. Anaesthesia 53:1091–1104 ● Miller C S, Little J W, Falace D A 2001 Supplemental corticosteroids for dental patients with adrenal insufficiency: reconsideration of the problem. J Am Dent Assoc 132:1570–1579 ● Ziccardi V B, Abubaker A O, Sotereanos G C, Patterson G T 1992 Precipitation of an Addisonian crisis during dental surgery: recognition and management. Compendium 13:518–524.

ALCOHOLISM

Definition Alcohol, the most common drug of abuse, is a central nervous system (CNS) depressant. It initially releases inhibitions, impairs the capacity to reason, and interferes with the cerebellum, causing ataxia and motor incoordination. Eventually it interferes with higher centres, causing unconsciousness. Alcoholism is a psychological and usually also physical state, characterised by compulsive continuous or episodic consumption of alcohol (ethanol), with the objective of achieving some psychological effects or avoiding the unpleasantness related to alcohol withdrawal.

General aspects

Aetiopathogenesis Prolonged alcohol abuse causes malnutrition, anaemia, impairment of immune function and other effects, including: ■ CNS – memory loss, disinhibition ■ liver – fatty liver, alcoholic hepatitis, cirrhosis ■ GIT – gastritis, peptic ulcer, pancreatitis ■ heart – cardiomyopathy, hypertension.

Clinical presentation ■ Alcohol at blood levels above 35 mg/dL (35 mg/100 mL) impairs judgment, while signs of intoxication are clinically obvious at a blood alcohol level above 100 mg/dL, with slurred speech, loss of restraint and ataxia. At a blood alcohol level above 200 mg/dL some people become aggressive. ■ Thus the acute effects of alcohol are mainly on judgment, concentration and coordination, and are dose-related as shown in Table 3.3 ■ Earlier signs or symptoms of *chronic* excessive alcohol drinking include an evasive, truculent, over-boisterous or facetious manner, slurred speech, smell of alcohol on the breath, signs of self-neglect, gastric discomfort (particularly heartburn), anxiety (often with insomnia), or tremor ■ Later signs or symptoms of chronic excessive alcohol drinking include palpitations and tachycardia, cardiomyopathy, liver disease, malnutrition, peripheral neuropathy, amnesia and confabulation (in Wernicke's and Korsakoff's CNS syndromes), cerebellar degeneration with ataxia, or dementia (Fig. 3.3, Table 3.4) ■ Alcohol can interact with other drugs such as warfarin, paracetamol/acetaminophen, and CNS-active agents such as benzodiazepines.

Diagnosis ■ Gamma glutamyl transpeptidase increased ■ Complete blood count (macrocytosis often without anaemia) ■ Blood alcohol levels raised.

Table 3.3 Acute effects of alcohol

Blood alcohol level in mg/dL	Effect
<100	Dry and decent
100–200	Delighted and devilish
200–300	Delinquent and disgusting
300–400	Dizzy and delirious
400–500	Dazed and dejected
>500	Dead drunk

Table 3.4 Chronic effects of alcohol

	Possible effects	Biochemical changes
Cardiac	Cardiomyopathy, arrhythmias	
CNS	Intoxication Dementia Wernicke–Korsakoff syndrome	Raised blood alcohol Decreased thiamine levels
Gastric	Gastritis	
Haematological	Pancytopenia Immune defect	Reduced haemoglobin Reduced platelet count Leukopenia Macrocytosis Reduced blood clotting factors II, VII, IX, X
Hepatic	Hepatitis Fatty liver (steatosis) Cirrhosis	Raised gamma glutamyl transpeptidase Raised other liver enzymes Raised bilirubin Reduced albumin
Intestinal	Malabsorption of glucose and vitamins	Reduced folate, thiamine and vitamins B_{12}, A, D, E and K
Oesophageal	Gastro-oesophageal reflux disease Mallory–Weiss syndrome (tears from vomiting)	
Pancreatic	Pancreatitis	Raised serum amylase

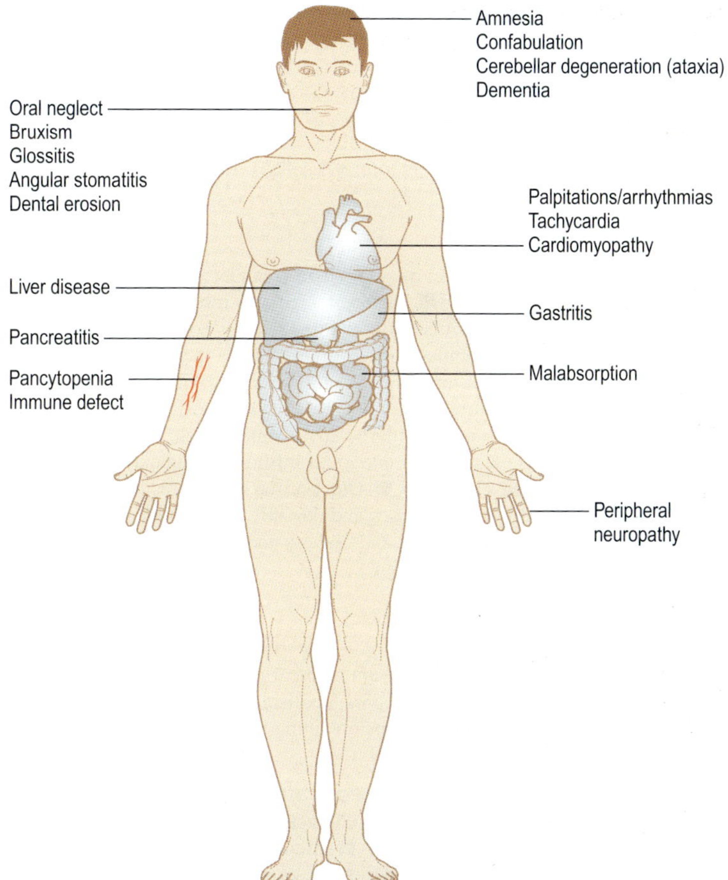

Figure 3.3 **Chronic effects of alcoholism**

Treatment ■ Cognitive therapy ■ Naltrexone ■ Acamprosate ■ High-protein, high-calorie and low-sodium diet (± vitamin supplementation).

Prognosis The high mortality rate in alcoholism is mainly as a result of road traffic accidents and assaults. After a large alcoholic binge, suppression of protective reflexes, such as the cough reflex, can result in inhalation of vomit, and death.

■ Mortality related to alcoholic hepatitis diagnosis is 10–25%, and life quality and expectancy can be affected by diseases including: ● liver disease, especially alcohol-induced hepatitis and cirrhosis ● nutritional defects ● pancreatitis ● gastritis and peptic ulcer ● immune defects leading to infections, especially pneumonia and tuberculosis, and impaired wound healing • cardiomyopathy • myopathy • brain damage and epilepsy.

■ Social difficulties from alcohol misuse can affect the six 'Ls': • law – breach of the criminal, civil and/or professional codes • learning – intellectual difficulties • livelihood – job problems • living – housing problems • lover – interpersonal difficulties of all kinds, husband/wife, partner, employer/employee etc. • lucre (Latin – lucrum = wealth) – money problems.

Oral findings

■ The most common oral effect of alcoholism is neglect, leading to advanced caries and periodontal disease ■ Dental erosion may result from regurgitation ■ Nocturnal bruxism by reticular system stimulation is common, and may predispose to temporomandibular joint disorders ■ If there is deficiency of folate or other B complex vitamins (niacin, piridoxine, riboflavine or thiamine), sore mouth, recurrent aphthae, glossitis, dysgeusia, tongue depapillation, dysaesthesia and angular stomatitis may result ■ Painless, bilateral, parotid gland enlargement due to fat infiltration (sialosis) is frequent in patients with alcoholic cirrhosis ■ Other orofacial features include a smell of alcohol on the breath, telangiectases and possibly rhinophyma (enlargement of the nose with dilation of follicles and redness and prominent vascularity of the skin, also known as 'grog blossom').

Dental management

Risk assessment The main relevant medical complications are related to liver cirrhosis, which may delay the metabolism of many drugs, and also result in a bleeding tendency. Problems obtaining valid consent may arise, particularly if the patient is intoxicated.

Preventive dentistry and patient education ■ Dentists should screen for alcohol abuse by recognising characteristic clinical and laboratory findings and behavioural disturbances ■ Alcohol is a known risk factor for oral cancer development, thus a periodical examination for detection of suspicious soft-tissue lesions is mandatory ■ Dentists should provide specific preventive information to patients with alcoholism and refer them to health care providers for assessment or treatment ■ Oral health care advice should be given ■ Diet counselling should be provided.

Pain and anxiety control **Local anaesthesia** Tolerance to local anaesthetics (LA) has been described, especially in long-term alcohol abusers. Even with larger than normal doses, the efficacy and duration of LA can be limited. **Conscious sedation** Sedatives (including benzodiazepines) or hypnotics generally have an additive effect with alcohol, although these interactions are not entirely predictable. Heavy drinkers, however, may become tolerant not only of alcohol but also of other sedatives. Once liver disease develops the position is reversed and drug metabolism is impaired – drugs then have a disproportionately greater effect. **General anaesthesia** Alcoholics are also notoriously resistant to general anaesthesia (GA). Heavy drinkers are especially prone to aspiration lung abscess.

GA may also be contraindicated in patients with alcoholic heart disease, hypoalbuminaemia or severe anaemia. In consequence, GA is best avoided.

Patient access and positioning Alcoholics are best given a morning appointment, when they are least likely to be under the influence of alcohol. Erratic attendance for dental treatment is not uncommon. Appointments should be for longer if local anaesthetic tolerance is anticipated.

Treatment modification Because of erratic attendance, and neglect of caries and periodontal disease, only simple restorative procedures should be planned. Consent issues may arise if the patient is intoxicated, particularly if Wernicke's encephalopathy or Korsakoff's syndrome is also present. Careful consideration of the patient's ability to understand and weigh up the information provided is needed, and consent may not be valid on subsequent appointments if the patient is unable to remember the discussion. If available, an escort is desirable as this may improve patient attendance and improve discharge arrangements and care. **Surgery** Two of the most important complications of excessive alcohol intake are maxillofacial trauma and head

Table 3.5 **Key considerations for dental management in alcoholism (see text)**

	Management modifications*	Comments/possible complications
Risk assessment	2	Liver cirrhosis, consent
Preventive dentistry and education	1	Alcoholism screening, oral cancer screening and diet counselling
Pain and anxiety control		
– Local anaesthesia	1	Tolerance
– Conscious sedation	1	Additive effect
– General anaesthesia	5	Resistance, aspiration
Patient access and positioning		
– Access to dental office	0	
– Timing of treatment	1	Morning
– Patient positioning	0	
Treatment modification		
– Oral surgery	1	Bleeding tendency
– Implantology	5	Poor risk group
– Conservative/Endodontics	1	Maintenance compromised
– Fixed prosthetics	1	Maintenance compromised
– Removable prosthetics	0	
– Non-surgical periodontology	1	Maintenance compromised
– Surgical periodontology	1	Bleeding tendency
Hazardous and contraindicated drugs	2	Sedatives, NSAIDs, metronidazole, cephalosporins

*0 = No special considerations. 1 = Caution advised. 2 = Specialised medical advice recommended in some cases. 3 = Specialised medical advice mandatory. 4 = Only to be performed in hospital environment. 5 = Should be avoided.

injuries. Care should be taken when surgery is contemplated, as liver disease causes a bleeding tendency due to a reduction in blood coagulation factors, and some patients may also have thrombocytopenia. Wound healing may be impaired in the severe chronic alcoholic. Indeed, in a series reported in the USA, alcoholism was found to be a common factor in patients with osteomyelitis following jaw fractures. Before providing treatment, laboratory tests including full blood cell count, liver enzyme levels and coagulation screening should be performed and a physician consulted. **Implantology** Although there is no direct evidence that alcoholism is a contraindication to implants, such patients may not be a good risk group, because of neglected oral health, tobacco smoking, bleeding problems, and osteoporosis. **Periodontology** It is important to avoid any alcohol-containing preparations, such as some antimicrobial and antiplaque mouthwashes. Maintenance by the patient will be often compromised and this has to be considered before planning periodontal treatment.

Drug use ■ Diazepam, lorazepam and other sedatives increase CNS depression ■ Aspirin should be avoided since it is more likely in the alcoholic patient to cause gastric erosions and bleeding, and to precipitate bleeding. The hepatotoxic effects of acetaminophen/paracetamol are enhanced, although it is still probably the safest analgesic in this group, and may be used in reduced dosage. ■ Metronidazole and cephalosporins can interact with alcohol to cause widespread vasodilatation, nausea, vomiting, sweating, headache and palpitations similar to the antabuse reaction (disulfiram effect). The effects are unpleasant or alarming but rarely dangerous.

Further reading ● van der Bijl P 2003 Substance abuse – concerns in dentistry: an overview. S Afr Dent J 58:382–385 ● Friedlander A H, Marder S R, Pisegna J R, Yagiela J A 2003 Alcohol abuse and dependence: psychopathology, medical management and dental implications. J Am Dent Assoc 134:731–740.

ALZHEIMER'S DISEASE

Definition Alzheimer's disease is a progressive neurodegenerative disorder, which causes loss of cognitive and motor functions. It represents the main cause of dementia, especially in patients over 65 years of age.

General aspects

■ Dementia is a chronic organic brain disease characterised by amnesia (especially for recent events), inability to concentrate, disorientation in time, place or person and intellectual impairment (including loss of normal social awareness) ■ It has many causes (Table 3.6), the most common being: ● Alzheimer's disease ● multi-infarct (vascular) dementia ● Lewy body dementia ■ Dementia is usually seen in old age, and may be mimicked by acute organic brain disease, confusional states, drug-induced disorders and psychiatric disease.

Aetiopathogenesis Cortical atrophy and consequent ventricular enlargement are present, probably related to deficiency of acetylcholine and other brain

Table 3.6 **Causes of dementia**

Common causes	Uncommon causes
Alcoholism	AIDS
Alzheimer's disease (>60% of all dementia)	Brain trauma, haemorrhage or infection
Cortical Lewy body dementia (10%)	Creutzfeldt–Jakob disease
Huntington's chorea	Metabolic causes (e.g. hypothyroidism)
Hydrocephalus	Pick's disease (frontal lobar atrophy)
Multi-infarct dementia (25%)	
Tumours	

neurotransmitters. Suggested risk factors include: ■ gene defects (20% of cases) ■ apolipoprotein-Epsilon 4 (apoE4) ■ insulin resistance ■ herpes virus infection ■ others (cerebral ischaemia, immunological disturbances, etc).

Clinical presentation ■ First stage: ● memory loss ● disorientation in time and place ● judgment impaired ● lack of spontaneity ● poor appearance ■ Second stage: ● loss of intellect ● aphasia ● inability to feed or clothe self ● acquired defects of visual–spatial skill ■ Third stage: ● apathy and mutism ● inability to communicate ● anxiety, depression, irritability ● hyperorality ● hyper-reflexia ● absolute dependence ● disruptive behaviour may be present.

Diagnosis A definitive diagnosis can only be made at autopsy. However the following allow a working diagnosis to be made: ■ History and clinical findings: ● development of multiple cognitive disturbances ● memory impairment ● problems with language (aphasia), motor activities (apraxia), recognition (agnosia), planning, organisation ■ Neuropsychiatric tests ■ Neuroimaging (cortical atrophy and ventricular enlargement).

Treatment ■ Rivastigmine ■ Donepezil ■ Galantamine ■ Aspirin and gingko biloba may delay onset.

Prognosis Patients need increasing support as they become progressively more helpless. At the end stage of their disease, they may become bed-ridden and require nasogastric feeding; they often succumb to aspiration pneumonia or secondary infection.

Oral findings

■ Oral hygiene neglect typically increases with Alzheimer's disease progression ■ Xerostomia, due to poor saliva production and drugs (phenothiazines), gives rise to candidosis, cervical caries and prosthesis intolerance ■ Periodontal disease is common, as is halitosis ■ Loss of taste ■ Depapillated, red, dry, fissured tongue ■ Trauma due to apraxia is not unusual, and may present with: ● maxillofacial injuries ● traumatic oral ulcers ● missing and broken teeth ● attrition ● severe alveolar ridge atrophy secondary to ill-fitting dentures ■ Oral dyskinesia due to antipsychotic medication.

Dental management

Studies have shown that about 75% of patients with Alzheimer's disease need dental attention. The stage of the Alzheimer's disease and the complexity of the dental treatment will decide if the patient can be treated in the dental clinic, at hospital or at home (bed-ridden). Comprehensive oral rehabilitation is best completed as early as possible since the patient's ability to cooperate during dental treatment diminishes with advancing disease. If long-term care is anticipated, full mouth diagnostic radiographs should be taken and kept for future use. In dentate patients, fabrication of custom mouthguards for fluoride treatment facilitates long-term fluoride therapy, but many people with advanced disease will not tolerate this. The best alternative is more frequent recall visits including prophylaxis and application of topical fluoride. Informed consent is a complex issue in all patients with dementia and requires consultation with the patient's physician.

Risk assessment The patient with Alzheimer's disease may be relatively healthy or may have accumulated a host of additional systemic diseases, but the chief problems are behavioural. Consultation with the patient's physician is recommended.

Preventive dentistry It is crucial to anticipate the future decline in oral hygiene due to progressive loss of motor and cognitive skills. When the patient is unable to undertake oral care effectively, it is important to involve and educate family, partners and care providers. Electric tooth brushing with use of chlorhexidine (mouthwash, gel or spray) may be helpful.

Pain and anxiety control **Local anaesthesia** The patient may accept treatment under local analgesia in the early stages of disease, but will need progressively more assistance. **Conscious sedation** Preoperative sedation with a short-acting benzodiazepine may be required. Nitrous oxide sedation may also be useful. **General anaesthesia** In patients with loss of ability to cooperate or those with hostile behaviour, general anaesthesia may be required.

Patient access and positioning **Access to dental surgery** With progressive disease, access may be significantly compromised. Escorts and/or domiciliary care are often required. Medications such as antidepressants administered to patients with Alzheimer's have been shown to increase the incidence of hip fracture, further restricting access. **Timing of treatment** Dental appointments and instructions are often forgotten unless a carer/family member is also involved. Treatment should, as far as possible, be carried out in the morning, when cooperation tends to be best. The usual carers should be present, and treatment undertaken in a familiar environment, with time allowed to explain every procedure before it is carried out. Time-consuming and complex treatments should be avoided. **Patient positioning** Particularly in the end stages of diseases, the patient should be treated sitting upright in the dental chair or slightly reclined, in order to avoid aspiration and postural hypotension.

Treatment modification Whilst it is still possible to provide dental treatment, it should be planned with the knowledge that the patient will

Table 3.7 **Key considerations for dental management in Alzheimer's disease (see text)**

	Management modifications*	Comments/possible complications
Risk assessment	2	Behaviour control; other systemic diseases; consent
Preventive dentistry	1	Electric toothbrushing; chlorhexidine
Pain and anxiety control		
– Local anaesthesia	1	Behaviour control;
– Conscious sedation	1	other systemic diseases
– General anaesthesia	3/4	
Patient access and positioning		
– Access to dental office	1	Hip fracture
– Timing of treatment	1	Morning; carer present
– Patient positioning	1	Sitting upright
Treatment modification		
– Oral surgery	1	
– Implantology	5	Poor oral hygiene
– Conservative/Endodontics	1	Single procedures
– Fixed prosthetics	1	Single procedures, early stages
– Removable prosthetics	1/5	Lost, broken, poorly tolerated
– Non-surgical periodontology	1	
– Surgical periodontology	1	
Hazardous and contraindicated drugs	2	Tolerance of sedatives

*0 = No special considerations. 1 = Caution advised. 2 = Specialised medical advice recommended in some cases. 3 = Specialised medical advice mandatory. 4 = Only to be performed in hospital environment. 5 = Should be avoided.

sooner or later become unmanageable for treatment under local analgesia. Later, there is progressive neglect of oral health as a result of forgetting the need or even how to brush the teeth or clean dentures. Dentures are also frequently lost or broken or cannot be inserted or tolerated. Complex dental treatment such as dental implants, which require follow-up and meticulous oral hygiene, are not indicated.

Drug use Regular use of sedatives can lead to tolerances, addiction, and cognitive impairment.

Further reading ● Henry R, Smith B 2004 Treating the Alzheimer's patient. A guide for dental professionals. J Mich Dent Assoc 86: 32–42 ● Frenkel H 2004 Alzheimer's disease and oral care. Dent Update 31:273–278 ● Kocaelli H, Yaltirik M, Yargic L I, Ozbas H 2002 Alzheimer's disease and dental management. Oral Surg Oral Med Oral Pathol Oral Radiol Endod 93:521–524.

AMPHETAMINE, LSD AND ECSTASY ABUSE

Definition Stimulants are drugs that enhance brain activity, increasing alertness and attention and heightening awareness.

General aspects

The most common drugs of misuse are amphetamines, LSD (lysergic acid diethylamide) and ecstasy (MDMA – 3,4-methylene-dioxymethamphetamine). ■ Dextroamphetamine (amphetamine) and methylphenidate are the most representative drugs. Stimulants are prescribed for treating only a few health conditions, including narcolepsy, attention-deficit hyperactivity disorder, and deep depression. Amphetamines are misused or abused for their euphoriant effect, to stave off fatigue in order to continue working and for slimming. ■ LSD (lysergic acid diethylamide), manufactured from lysergic acid (found in ergot, a fungus that grows on rye and other grains), is a major hallucinogen, considered one of the most potent mood-changing chemicals ■ MDMA (3,4-methylenedioxymethamphetamine), popularly known as 'ecstasy', is a synthetic, psychoactive drug with sympathomimetic properties, and both stimulant (amphetamine-like) and hallucinogenic (LSD-like) properties.

Pathogenesis **Amphetamines** ■ These are the main drugs in a group of central stimulants which also includes phenmetrazine, methylphenidate and, to a lesser extent, diethylpropion. They produce a range of effects by stimulating alpha- and beta-adrenergic receptors, increasing the levels of monoamines (which include norepinephrine and dopamine) and thus stimulating the CNS and peripheral nervous system. ■ Acute amphetamine toxicity causes dry mouth, dilated pupils, tachycardia, aggression, talkativeness, tachypnoea and hallucinations, leading to seizures, hypertension, hyperpyrexia, arrhythmias and collapse ■ Chronic amphetamine toxicity causes restlessness, hyperactivity, loss of appetite and weight, tremor, repetitive movements, bruxism and picking at the face and extremities ■ High doses of amphetamines can cause mood swings and psychoses (including hallucinations and paranoia), and can cause respiratory failure and death ■ Combining use with other drugs such as alcohol can result in nausea, difficulty breathing and unconsciousness. **LSD** ■ The effects of LSD are unpredictable but prolonged (~12h), depending on the amount taken, the user's personality, mood, and expectations, and the surroundings in which the drug is used ■ Typically, LSD produces several different emotions at once or users swing rapidly from one emotion to another within 30–90 minutes. Synaesthesia, the overflow from one sense to another when, for example, colours are heard, is common. There is often lability of mood, panic ('bad trip') and delusions of magical powers, such as being able to fly. If taken in a large enough dose, the drug produces delusions and visual hallucinations. The user's sense of time and self changes. ■ Many LSD users experience flashbacks, recurrence of certain aspects of a person's experience, without having taken the drug again. A flashback comes suddenly, often without warning, and may be within a few days or more than a year after LSD use. ■ The physical effects from LSD are similar to those of catecholamines and include: ● dilated pupils ● raised body temperature, heart rate and blood pressure ● sweating ● loss of appetite ● sleeplessness ● dry mouth ● tremors. ■ Severe adverse effects include terrifying thoughts and feelings and despair, occasionally leading to fatal accidents. **MDMA** ■ MDMA (ecstasy) affects dopamine-containing neurones that use the chemical serotonin to communicate with other neurones; a decrease in serotonin transporters has been recently demonstrated in the brain of MDMA users by positron emission tomography (PET) ■ Ecstasy, like amphetamines, produces euphoria and appetite suppression, but is more potently hallucinogenic, possibly because of chemical affinities with mescalin. ■ It is usually taken by mouth, producing effects after 20–60 minutes ■ Adverse effects of MDMA are not dose-related, and include: ● psychiatric sequelae such as agitation or paranoia ● neurological effects such as ataxia and seizures ● cardiovascular such as tachycardia, arrhythmias or infarction ● renal or hepatic failure ● other effects ■ MDMA users face risks similar to those found with the use of cocaine and amphetamines: ● psychological difficulties, including confusion, depression, sleep problems, drug craving, severe anxiety, and paranoia – during and sometimes weeks after taking MDMA ● physical symptoms such as muscle tension, involuntary teeth clenching, nausea, blurred vision, rapid eye movement, faintness, and chills or sweating ● raised heart rate and blood pressure, a special risk for people with circulatory or heart disease ■ There is evidence that people who develop a rash that looks like acne after using MDMA may be risking severe side effects, including liver damage, if they continue to use the drug.

Clinical presentation The most significant risks from drug abuse are behavioural disturbances and psychoses. Intravenous use of these drugs is further complicated by the risk of transmission of infections (HIV, hepatitis B), infective endocarditis or septicaemia.

Findings that may indicate a drug addiction problem include: ■ Work absenteeism, frequent disappearances from the workplace, making improbable excuses and taking frequent or long trips to the toilet or to the stockroom where drugs are kept ■ Personality change – mood swings, anxiety, depression, lack of impulse control, suicidal thoughts or gestures, and deteriorating interpersonal relations with colleagues and staff; the user rarely admits errors or accepts blame for errors or oversights ■ Unreliability in keeping appointments, meeting deadlines, and work performance – which alternates between periods of high and low productivity. Many suffer from mistakes made due to inattention, poor judgment, bad decisions, confusion, memory loss, and difficulty concentrating or recalling details and instructions. Ordinary tasks require greater effort and consume more time. ■ Progressive deterioration in personal appearance and hygiene, and uncharacteristic deterioration of handwriting and charting ■ Other common signs are: ● tachycardia (amphetamines) ● hyperpyrexia (ecstasy) ● bruxism – amphetamines or ecstasy ● drug-associated diseases ● psychosis.

Recognition of individuals who may be abusing drugs is critical. Behavioural problems or drug interactions may interfere with dental treatment. Intravenous drug use (IVDU) is associated with the risk of transmission of infections (HIV, hepatitis B), and complications such as infective endocarditis (which will require antibiotic prophylaxis).

Withdrawal and treatment ■ Amphetamines have no true withdrawal syndrome and, in this respect, amphetamine addiction is quite different from opioid or barbiturate dependence ■ LSD is not considered an addictive drug since it does not produce compulsive drug-seeking behaviour as do cocaine, amphetamine, heroin, alcohol, and nicotine; most users of LSD voluntarily limit or stop its use over time ■ After long-term use of ecstasy, tolerance develops but there is neither physical dependence nor withdrawal symptoms.

Oral findings

Amphetamines ■ Bruxism may result from chronic amphetamine use ■ There can be xerostomia and greater caries incidence.

MDMA ■ Jaw clenching appears to be common ■ Bruxism, TMJ dysfunction, dry mouth, attrition, erosion, mucosal burns or ulceration and periodontitis have been reported.

Ecstasy has been associated with significantly increased wear of the occlusal surfaces of the back teeth, which contrasts to the usual pattern of tooth wear affecting the front teeth. It has been suggested that ingestion of carbonated and acidic beverages during ecstasy use may contribute to this problem.

Dental management

Risk assessment Care should be taken with any patient who is a known IVDU or who: ■ has subjective symptoms of dental pain, with no objective evidence of the disorder ■ makes a self-diagnosis and requests a specific drug, especially a psychoactive agent ■ appears to have a dramatic but unexpected complaint such as trigeminal neuralgia ■ firmly rejects treatments that exclude psychoactive drugs ■ has no interest in the diagnosis or investigations or refuses a second opinion.

Pain and anxiety control **Local anaesthesia** Amphetamines enhance the sympathomimetic effects of epinephrine and thus vasoconstrictors are best avoided, since hypertension and cardiotoxicity can result.
Conscious sedation CS should be used with great caution due to the potential deleterious effects of amphetamine/LSD/MDMA use (cardiovascular, renal and hepatic). If CS is strongly indicated, it is important to ensure that the patient is not concurrently abusing drugs, and treatment may be best undertaken in a hospital environment. Opioids are contraindicated.
General anaesthesia Amphetamine addicts may be remarkably resistant to GA. Furthermore, if using intravenous drugs, patients may have problems with venous access and many of the infective problems of opioid addicts. Intravenous barbiturates should be avoided because they may induce convulsions, respiratory distress or coma. Opioids are also contraindicated.

Patient access and positioning Patients are best given a morning appointment, when they are least likely to be under the influence of drugs. Ideally, the patient should be instructed not to use drugs within 12 hours of the appointment. Erratic attendance for dental treatment is not uncommon.

Treatment modification Consent issues may arise if the patient is under the influence of drugs. If available, an escort is desirable as this may improve patient attendance and improve discharge arrangements and care. The considerations that need to be taken into account when treatment is undertaken depend on the degree of drug abuse and related social, medical

Table 3.8 **Key considerations for dental management in amphetamine, LSD or ecstasy abuse (see text)**

	Management modifications*	Comments/possible complications
Risk assessment	2	Drug abusers recognition; abnormal behaviour; drug interactions; infections with IVDU; consent issues
Pain and anxiety control		
– Local anaesthesia	2	Avoid epinephrine
– Conscious sedation	3/4	Avoid opioids
– General anaesthesia	3/4	Avoid halothane, ketamine, suxamethonium, barbiturates and opioids; resistance to GA
Patient access and positioning		
– Access to dental office	0	
– Timing of treatment	1	Morning appointment; 12 hours after last dose; failed appointments
– Patient positioning	0	
Treatment modification		
– Oral surgery	1	
– Implantology	1/5	Neglected oral hygiene; periodontitis; bruxism; xerostomia; heavy smokers
– Conservative/Endodontics	1	
– Fixed prosthetics	1/5	Neglected oral hygiene; heavy smokers
– Removable prosthetics	1	
– Non-surgical periodontology	1	
– Surgical periodontology	1/5	Neglected oral hygiene; heavy smokers
Hazardous and contraindicated drugs	1	Avoid opioids

*0 = No special considerations. 1 = Caution advised. 2 = Specialised medical advice recommended in some cases. 3 = Specialised medical advice mandatory. 4 = Only to be performed in hospital environment. 5 = Should be avoided.

and dental complications. Hence each patient must be assessed on an individual basis, as the necessary modification may vary from caution, to the planned procedure being contraindicated. Examples of factors that may compromise care for all types of dental treatment planned include: ■ social issues, such as availability of escorts, discharge arrangements, financial constraints ■ medical issues, such as related cardiac, renal or hepatic complications ■ dental issues, such as degree of dental neglect, degree of xerostomia, concurrent smoking.

Further reading ● van der Bijl P 2003 Substance abuse – concerns in dentistry: an overview. S Afr Dent J 58:382–385 ● Cornelius J R, Clark D B, Weyant R et al 2004 Dental abnormalities in children of fathers with substance use disorders. Addict Behav 29:979–982 ● Milosevic A, Agrawal N, Redfearn P, Mair L 1999 The occurrence of toothwear in users of Ecstasy (3,4-methylenedioxymethamphetamine). Community Dent Oral Epidemiol 27:283–287 ● Sandler N A 2001 Patients who abuse drugs. Oral Surg Oral Med Oral Pathol Oral Radiol Endod 91:12–14 ● Shaner J W 2002 Caries associated with methamphetamine abuse. J Mich Dent Assoc 84:42–47.

ANAEMIAS (DEFICIENCY)

Definition Anaemia is diagnosed when the haemoglobin level falls > 10% from normal concentrations established for age and sex.

General aspects

Aetiopathogenesis Anaemia is related to: ■ a decrease in the number of circulating red blood cells, due to: ● decreased production ● increased red blood cell loss (usually haemorrhage) ■ or an abnormality in the haemoglobin.

Anaemia is not a disease in itself but a feature of many diseases (Table 3.9). The most common cause of anaemia in developed countries is chronic blood loss and consequent iron deficiency. In women, this is normally caused by heavy menstruation, and in men, blood loss is via occult sources (gastrointestinal or genitourinary). Dietary deficiency and malabsorption (post-gastrectomy) may also cause iron deficiency anaemia. Folate and vitamin B_{12} (cobalamin) deficiency are the next most common causes of anaemia.

Clinical presentation Clinical findings are mainly influenced by the underlying cause, the severity of anaemia and the time it takes to develop (Fig. 3.4). In the early stages, anaemia is frequently asymptomatic. The effect of anaemia is to reduce the oxygen-carrying capacity of the blood and this may eventually lead to dyspnoea and increased cardiac output (palpitations, murmurs, cardiac failure). Most symptoms are thus the consequence of cardiovascular and ventilatory efforts to compensate for oxygen deficiency, and include the following. **General** Tiredness, anorexia and dyspnoea. **Skin and mucosa** Pallor of the oral mucosa, conjunctiva or palmar creases suggests severe anaemia, although skin colour can be misleading. Splitting and spooning of the nails (koilonychia) may be detected. Sickling disorders

Table 3.9 **Main causes and classification of anaemias**

Type of anaemia	Examples
Microcytic hypochromic	Iron deficiency Thalassaemia
Macrocytic	Vitamin B_{12} deficiency Folate deficiency Haemolysis Hypothyroidism Liver disease Aplastic anaemia
Normocytic	Chronic diseases Renal failure Hypothyroidism Haemolysis: – metabolic defects of red cells – red cell membrane defects – haemoglobin abnormalities, e.g. sickling disorders (disorders of structure), thalassaemia (disorders of chain number)

may be associated with jaundice. **Cardiovascular** Tachycardia and palpitations. Anaemia also exacerbates, or can cause, heart failure, angina, and the effects of pulmonary disease. Thrombosis occurs in sickling disorders. **Nervous system** Headache and behaviour changes may be seen, and in children there can be learning impairment. Paraesthesia of the fingers and toes and CNS damage (subacute combined degeneration of spinal cord causing loss of joint position and vibration sense and possibly paraplegia) are associated with pernicious anaemia.

Classification Anaemia is classified on the basis of erythrocyte size as microcytic (small), macrocytic (large) or normocytic (normal size erythrocytes) (Table 3.9). **Microcytic anaemia** (mean corpuscular [cell] volume [MCV] below 78 fL). This is the most common – usually due to iron deficiency, occasionally secondary to thalassaemia or chronic diseases. **Macrocytic anaemia** (MCV more than 99 fL). This is usually caused by vitamin B_{12} or folate deficiency (not infrequently in alcoholics), sometimes because folate and vitamin B_{12} are used up in chronic haemolysis, pregnancy or malignancy; and occasionally caused by drugs (methotrexate, azathioprine, cytosine or hydroxycarbamide [hydroxyurea]). **Normocytic anaemia** (MCV between 79 and 98 fL). This may result from a range of chronic diseases including leukaemia, liver disorders, renal failure, infection, malignancy or other causes, particularly sickle cell disease and thalassaemia. Sickle cell disease results from a single amino acid change on both beta chains of haemoglobin (HbSS). It is more common in Africa, followed by India, the Middle East and Southern Europe. Beta thalassaemia mainly occurs in Mediterraneans and reflects at least 100 different genetic defects that result in a deficiency in the number of beta chains of haemoglobin. Only beta thalassaemia major results in severe anaemia, requiring blood

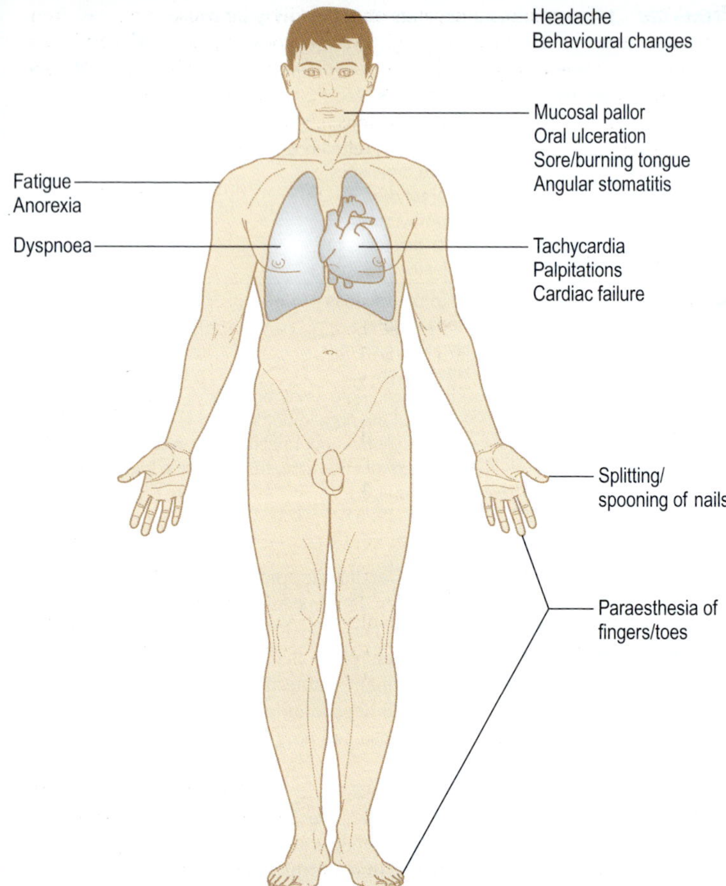

Figure 3.4 **Clinical presentation of anaemia**

transfusions. Alpha thalassaemia is caused by gene deletions on chromosome 11, resulting in a deficiency of one or more alpha chains of haemoglobin. It occurs predominantly in the Far East, Middle East and Africa, and rarely requires blood transfusions.

Diagnosis The diagnosis is made from a combination of clinical findings and special tests: ■ haemoglobin (Hb) assay/complete blood count ■ mean corpuscular volume (MCV), mean corpuscular haemoglobin (MCH) and haemoglobin concentration (MCHC) ■ serum iron and ferritin (iron deficiency anaemia) ■ serum vitamin B_{12} and autoantibodies (pernicious anaemia) ■ red cell folate assays ■ haemoglobin electrophoresis (haemoglobinopathies).

Treatment The treatment depends on the underlying cause, e.g.: ■ iron deficiency anaemia: treat cause and give oral ferrous sulphate ■ pernicious anaemia: give vitamin B_{12} by injection for life and/or oral folic acid ■ folic acid deficiency: give oral folic acid ■ sickle cell anaemia: splenectomy, folic acid, penicillin, exchange transfusions, chelating agents, pain control ■ thalassaemia: exchange transfusions, chelating agents, splenectomy.

Prognosis The prognosis is related to the severity of the underlying disease.

Oral findings

■ Deficiency anaemias can cause oral lesions such as ulcers, angular stomatitis, sore or burning tongue or glossitis ■ Hunter's and Moeller glossitis (depapillated sore tongues) and mouth ulcers are seen in pernicious anaemia; oral paraesthesia and dysgeusia are also related to pernicious anaemia ■ Features described in thalassaemia: ● enlargement of maxilla (chipmunk face), due to extramedullary haemopoiesis ● migration and spacing of upper anterior teeth ● oral ulceration (very rare) ● painful swelling of parotids and xerostomia (due to iron deposits) ● sore or burning tongue due to folate deficiency ● alveolar bone may have a 'chickenwire' like radiological appearance ● delayed pneumatisation of maxillary sinuses ■ Features described in sickle cell anaemia: ● trigeminal neuropathy due to osteomyelitis ● pain due to infarction ● radiological features may include: hypercementosis/dense lamina dura, possible hypomineralisation of permanent teeth, apparent mandibular osteoporosis due to bone marrow hyperplasia, skull/diploe thickening with hair-on-end appearance and radio-opacities due to previous infarcts.

Dental management

Risk assessment The haemoglobin assay/complete blood count should be determined before commencing any dental treatment. In patients with a haemoglobin level below 10 g/dL, caution is advised, and ideally only palliative dental treatment should be undertaken to stabilise the dentition, with perioperative nasal oxygen/pulse oximeter recommended.

In an emergency, anaemia can be corrected by whole blood transfusion, but this should only be given to a young and otherwise fit patient. Packed red cells avoid the risk of fluid overload and can be given in emergency to the elderly patient or those with incipient cardiac failure. A diuretic given at the same time further reduces the risk of congestive cardiac failure. The patient should be stabilised at least 24 hours preoperatively and it should be noted that haemoglobin estimations are unreliable for 12 hours post-transfusion or after acute blood loss.

Specific considerations for individuals with sickle cell anaemia include: ■ treat infections thoroughly to avoid crises ■ postoperative antibiotics for all surgical procedures ■ prophylactic antibiotics for post-splenectomy patients.

Specific considerations for individuals with thalassaemia, particularly beta thalassaemia major, include: ■ recurrent exchange transfusions, with the risk of carriage of hepatitis B, C, G viruses, possible HIV and TTV ■ cardiomyopathy ■ splenectomy implications.

Pain and anxiety control **Conscious sedation** Light sedation with benzodiazepines may be undertaken, although oxygen saturation must be carefully monitored. Nitrous oxide is contraindicated in vitamin B_{12} deficiency, since it interferes with B_{12} metabolism. **General anaesthesia** The main danger in anaemias is when a GA is given, as it is vital to ensure full oxygenation. Elective operations under GA should not usually be carried out when the haemoglobin is less than 10 g/dL (male).

Patient access and positioning Short appointments in the morning are recommended to ensure that the patient is not too fatigued. In those patients receiving regular exchange/blood transfusions, it is best to avoid treatment on the same day.

Treatment modification **Surgery** In patients with aplastic anaemia, elective surgery is contraindicated. In emergencies, platelets and antimicrobial cover may be required. **Removable prosthetics** In iron deficiency and

Table 3.10 **Key considerations for dental management in deficiency anaemias (see text)**

	Management modifications*	Comments/possible complications
Risk assessment	2	Haemoglobin assay Cardiac failure
Pain and anxiety control		
– Local anaesthesia	0	
– Conscious sedation	1	Avoid nitrous oxide in B_{12} deficiency
– General anaesthesia	3/4	Avoid if haemoglobin is less than 10 g/dL
Patient access and positioning		
– Access to dental office	0	
– Timing of treatment	1	If severe anaemia, morning; short appts
– Patient positioning	0	
Treatment modification		
– Oral surgery	2/4	Haemoglobin level
– Implantology	3/5	Avoid in aplastic anaemia; haemoglobin level
– Conservative/Endodontics	1	
– Fixed prosthetics	1	
– Removable prosthetics	1	May be poorly tolerated
– Non-surgical periodontology	1	
– Surgical periodontology	2/5	Avoid in aplastic anaemia
Hazardous and contraindicated drugs	1	Avoid drugs associated with haemolysis

*0 = No special considerations. 1 = Caution advised. 2 = Specialised medical advice recommended in some cases. 3 = Specialised medical advice mandatory. 4 = Only to be performed in hospital environment. 5 = Should be avoided.

pernicious anaemia patients with sore mouth, prostheses may not be tolerated. **Periodontology** In patients with aplastic anaemia, periodontal and mucogingival surgery are contraindicated.

Drug use Acetaminophen plus codeine is recommended for pain control. In individuals with sickle cell disease: ■ avoid prilocaine – causes methaemoglobinaemia ■ avoid drugs likely to cause haemolysis ■ avoid high dose aspirin (risk of inducing acidosis).

Further reading ● Terezhalmy G T, Moore W S 2003 Pallor. Quintessence Int 34:642–643.

ANKYLOSING SPONDYLITIS

Definition Ankylosing spondylitis is a seronegative spondyloarthropathy predominantly affecting the spine and sacroiliac joints, mainly in young males.

General aspects

Aetiopathogenesis ■ It is partly genetically determined: the family history may be positive, and over 90% of patients are HLA-B27 ■ Inflammation involves the insertions of ligaments and tendons and is followed by ossification forming bony bridges, which fuse adjacent vertebral bodies or other joints.

Clinical presentation ■ The onset is usually insidious, with low back pain (spondylitis) and stiffness followed by worsening pain and tenderness in the sacro-iliac region due to sacro-iliitis. Hip joints may also be involved ■ Slowly, the back becomes fixed in extreme flexion, chest expansion becomes limited and respiration impaired (Fig. 3.5) ■ About 25% of those affected develop eye lesions (uveitis or iridocyclitis) ■ About 10% develop cardiac disease (aortic incompetence or conduction defects).

Diagnosis There is no specific diagnostic test but the erythrocyte sedimentation rate (ESR) is raised and HLA-B27 is often positive. Radiography shows progressive squaring-off of vertebrae (which become rectangular), intervertebral ossification producing a bamboo spine appearance, calcification of tendon/ligament insertions (enthesitis) and obliteration of the sacro-iliac joints.

Treatment ■ Physiotherapy and exercises ■ Anti-inflammatory analgesics ■ Rarely, spine radiotherapy (carries the risk of leukaemia) ■ Surgery is a final option (rarely indicated).

Prognosis Patients with early diagnosis and adequate management have a good prognosis. In rare cases of severe and progressive disease, there can be joint deformity, refractory iritis and secondary amyloidosis.

Oral findings

The temporomandibular joints are involved in about 10% of cases, especially in those over 40 years of age with widespread disease. This results in restricted mandibular opening and muscle tenderness, but symptoms are usually mild.

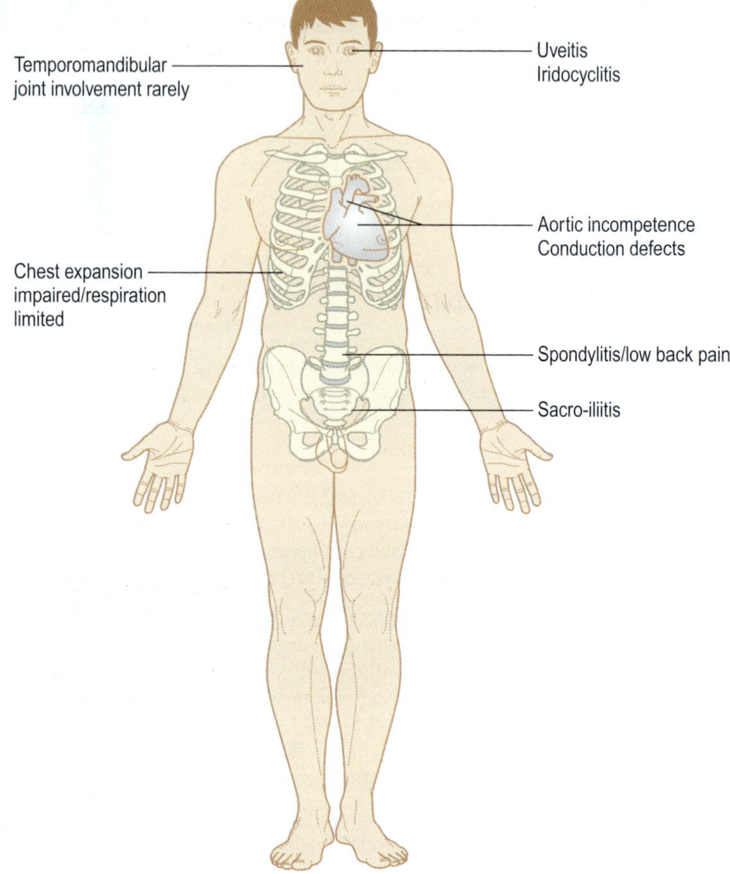

Figure 3.5 **Clinical presentation of ankylosing spondylitis**

Dental management

Risk assessment Patients may have aortic valve disease – when antibiotic prophylaxis against endocarditis should be considered. Chronic intake of anti-inflammatory drugs (e.g. indometacin or ibuprofen) may produce bone marrow depression, which can cause a bleeding tendency and immune defect and thus the need for antibiotic prophylaxis.

Pain and anxiety control Local anaesthesia Ankylosing spondylitis does not affect the selection of LA, although access may be compromised due to limited mouth opening. Conscious sedation There are no contraindications regarding the use of CS, although oxygen saturation should be carefully monitored where there is impaired respiratory exchange due to spinal deformity. **General anaesthesia** GA can be hazardous because of severely restricted opening of the mouth, impaired respiratory exchange associated with severe spinal deformity, or cardiac disease (aortic insufficiency).

Patient access and positioning Cushions and adapted head supports may be required if the patient's neck may be fixed in flexion. It may be best to keep the patient largely upright if the spinal deformity has resulted in breathing problems.

Treatment modification Surgical treatment may require antibiotic prophylaxis if there is any aortic valve disease. Furthermore, the extent and complexity of treatment offered may have to be limited if access may be compromised due to limited mouth opening and/or spinal deformity.

Further reading • Hill C M 1980 Death following dental clearance in a patient suffering from ankylosing spondylitis – a case report with discussion on management of such problems. Br J Oral Surg 18:73–76 • Wenneberg B, Kopp S 1982 Clinical findings in the stomatognathic system in ankylosing spondylitis. Scand J Dent Res 90:373–381.

Table 3.11 **Key considerations for dental management in ankylosing spondylitis (see text)**

	Management modifications*	Comments/possible complications
Risk assessment	2	Aortic valve disease; bone marrow depression
Pain and anxiety control		
– Local anaesthesia	1	
– Conscious sedation	1	
– General anaesthesia	3–5	Limited mouth opening; restricted chest expansion; cardiac disease
Patient access and positioning		
– Access to dental office	0	
– Timing of treatment	0	
– Patient positioning	1	Neck may be fixed in flexion
Treatment modification		
– Oral surgery	1	
– Implantology	1	
– Conservative/Endodontics	0	
– Fixed prosthetics	0	
– Removable prosthetics	0	
– Non-surgical periodontology	1	
– Surgical periodontology	1	
Hazardous and contraindicated drugs	0	

*0 = No special considerations. 1 = Caution advised. 2 = Specialised medical advice recommended in some cases. 3 = Specialised medical advice mandatory. 4 = Only to be performed in hospital environment. 5 = Should be avoided.

ANXIETY STATES

Definition Anxiety has been defined as emotional pain or a feeling of impending danger. Anxiety disorders are extremely common and have a common theme of excessive, irrational fear and dread.

General aspects

Anxiety is common in persons who are emotionally stressed, and may also be associated with systemic diseases (hyperthyroidism; mitral valve prolapse) or psychiatric disorders.

Aetiopathogenesis The aetiopathogenesis of anxiety remains unclear, but a role for the neurotransmitter gamma-aminobutyric acid (GABA) has been suggested. Benzodiazepines block GABA and have been found to be effective anxiolytics. Anxiety can be generated by dental or medical appointments, even amongst most normal patients. Indeed, 65% of all patients report some level of fear of dental treatment.

Clinical presentation Clinical findings are related to autonomic nervous system hyperactivity and include sweating, increased heart rate, dilated pupils, muscle tension, diarrhoea, polyuria and insomnia (Table 3.12).

Diagnosis Diagnosis is established by clinical findings. Typical signs of anxiety in the dental clinic include a fearful facial expression, agitation, moving eyes or fingers, continuously questioning and tremor.

Table 3.12 **Some possible effects of mild, acute and chronic stress**

	Mild	Acute	Chronic
CNS	Mood change	Increased concentration and clarity of thought	Anxiety, loss of sense of humour, depression, fatigue, headaches, migraines, tremor
Cardiovascular	Rise in pulse rate and blood pressure	Improved cardiac output and tissue perfusion	Hypertension Chest pain Ischaemic heart disease
Respiratory	Increased respiratory rate	Improved ventilation	Cough and asthma
Mouth	Slight dryness	Dry mouth	Dry mouth
Gastrointestinal	Increased bowel activity	Reduced digestion	Peptic ulceration Irritable bowel syndrome
Sexual	Male impotence and female irregular menstruation	Male impotence and female irregular menstruation	Male impotence and female amenorrhoea

Treatment In general, two types of treatment are available for anxiety disorders – psychotherapy ('talk therapy') and medication, either of which may be effective. Medications used for treating anxiety disorders include: ■ anti-anxiety medications such as buspirone or benzodiazepines, which relieve symptoms of anxiety quickly and with few adverse effects, except for drowsiness ■ beta-blockers, such as propranolol, help reduce physical effects such as tremor ■ antidepressants, which need to be taken for several weeks before symptoms of anxiety start to fade.

Prognosis Unlike the mild, brief anxiety caused by a stressful event, anxiety disorders are chronic, relentless, and can grow progressively worse if not treated.

Oral findings

Oral manifestations in chronically anxious people may include: ■ facial arthromyalgia ■ atypical facial pain ■ burning mouth syndrome ■ dry mouth ■ lip-chewing ■ bruxism ■ cancer phobia.

Other lesions that may develop or worsen in anxious patients include: ■ aphthae ■ geographic tongue ■ lichen planus ■ TMJ dysfunction.

Dental management

According to the General Dental Council (UK) all dentists have the duty to provide adequate pain and anxiety control. Various physical, chemical and psychological modalities may be used, including behavioural management and pharmacological agents, such as those used to provide effective local anaesthesia, conscious sedation and general anaesthesia. It is important to evaluate every patient on an individual basis to prescribe the appropriate measure. General measures in all anxious patients may include: ■ initial consultation with the patient in a non-clinical environment ■ explain the dental plan in detail ■ start with single simple procedures ■ provide very effective pain control ■ tell–show–do ■ give positive reinforcements.

Risk assessment Patients may have uncontrollable anxiety (often increased by the dental appointment) and can move or even get up unexpectedly during treatment.

Pain and anxiety control **Local anaesthesia** Some patients have a low pain tolerance. **Conscious sedation** Symptoms such as agitation, tachycardia and dry mouth (caused mainly by sympathetic overactivity), are usually controllable by reassurance and possibly a very mild anxiolytic or sedative such as a low dose of a beta-blocker, buspirone or a short-acting (temazepam) or moderate-acting (lorazepam or diazepam) benzodiazepine – provided the patient is not pregnant and does not drive, operate dangerous machinery or make important decisions for the following 24 hours. Intravenous or intranasal sedation with midazolam, or relative analgesia using nitrous oxide and oxygen, are also useful. Informed consent, written instructions and an escort with appropriate discharge arrangements are essential. **General anaesthesia** Patients requiring complex dental treatment and those uncontrolled with sedation may be treated under GA.

Patient access and positioning Cancellation of appointments and delay are common and precipitate neglect of oral health. To try and minimise this, the waiting time between visits should be short, and initial appointments made to try and acclimatise the patient.

Treatment modification Treatment planning may have to be modified depending on the patient's cooperation and the use of behavioural and pharmacological methods of anxiety control.

Drug use Benzodiazepine metabolism is impaired by azole antifungals and macrolide antibiotics such as erythromycin and clarithromycin. Alcohol, antihistamines and barbiturates have additive sedative effects with benzodiazepines.

Further reading • Bare L C, Dundes L 2004 Strategies for combating dental anxiety. J Dent Educ 68:1172–1177 • Smith T A, Heaton L J 2003 Fear of dental care: are we making any progress? J Am Dent Assoc 134:1101–1108.

Table 3.13 **Key considerations for dental management in anxiety states (see text)**

	Management modifications*	Comments/possible complications
Risk assessment	2	Unexpected movement
Pain and anxiety control		
– Local anaesthesia	1	Low pain tolerance
– Conscious sedation	1	Strongly recommended
– General anaesthesia	2–4	May be indicated
Patient access and positioning		
– Access to dental office	0	
– Timing of treatment	1	Appointment cancellation and delay are usual
– Patient positioning	0	
Treatment modification		
– Oral surgery	1	
– Implantology	1	
– Conservative/Endodontics	1	
– Fixed prosthetics	1	
– Removable prosthetics	1	
– Non-surgical periodontology	1	
– Surgical periodontology	1	
Hazardous and contraindicated drugs	1	Benzodiazepine interactions

*0 = No special considerations. 1 = Caution advised. 2 = Specialised medical advice recommended in some cases. 3 = Specialised medical advice mandatory. 4 = Only to be performed in hospital environment. 5 = Should be avoided.

AORTIC VALVE DISEASES

AORTIC STENOSIS

Definition Aortic stenosis (AS) is a narrowing of the aortic valve; this generates an increased pressure in the left ventricle to maintain the blood volume per beat.

General aspects

Aetiopathogenesis Causes include: ■ senile calcification ■ bicuspid valve (usually asymptomatic, even in athletes, but a high risk for infective endocarditis which may be the first clue to the defect) ■ hypertrophic cardiomyopathy ■ William's syndrome.

Clinical presentation Features include angina, dyspnoea, syncope and congestive cardiac failure.

Diagnosis AS is confirmed by echocardiography, ECG and cardiac catheterisation.

Treatment Endocarditis prophylaxis is the only requirement for asymptomatic patients. Severe AS necessitates surgical treatment such as percutaneous balloon valvotomy, or commissurotomy, or prosthetic valve replacement.

Prognosis In symptomatic patients, the mean survival is 5 years. In severe aortic stenosis, sudden death is not uncommon.

AORTIC REGURGITATION (INCOMPETENCE)

Definition The blood propelled to the aorta during systole returns to the left ventricle during diastole due to a defective aortic valve.

General aspects

Aetiopathogenesis Causes may include: ■ congenital defect ■ rheumatic carditis ■ infective endocarditis ■ collagen disorders (Marfan syndrome or Ehlers–Danlos syndrome) ■ hypertension ■ arthritides ■ tertiary syphilis ■ ankylosing spondylitis.

Clinical presentation Features may include: ■ dyspnoea ■ palpitations ■ cardiac failure.

Diagnosis Diagnosis is based on echocardiography, ECG, chest radiograph and cardiac catheterisation.

Treatment Heart valve replacement/surgical correction by valvotomy, grafts or prosthetic valves is the treatment of choice in moderate or severe regurgitation. Endocarditis prophylaxis should be administered when indicated.

Prognosis Long-term surgical results are usually successful but the perioperative mortality rate is high.

Dental management

Risk assessment All patients with aortic valve disease require antibiotic prophylaxis to prevent infective endocarditis when undergoing risky procedures. Patients with prosthetic valves are particularly susceptible to infective endocarditis, with an associated high mortality rate. Infection within the first 6 months is rarely of dental origin but usually involves *Staphylococcus aureus*, and has a mortality of around 60%. Replacement of the diseased valve while the infection is still active, together with vigorous antimicrobial treatment, frequently eradicates the disease.

Patient access and positioning Timing of treatment Patients scheduled for cardiac surgery should ideally have excellent oral health established before operation. Elective dental care should be avoided for the first 6 months after cardiac surgery.

Preventive dentistry Teeth with a reasonable prognosis (shallow caries and minimal periodontal pocketing) should be conserved but those with a poor pulpal or periodontal prognosis are best removed before cardiac surgery, particularly in patients who are to have valve replacement, major surgery for congenital anomalies, or a heart transplant.

Pain and anxiety control Local anaesthesia An aspirating syringe should be used to give a local anaesthetic, since epinephrine in the anaesthetic given intravenously may (theoretically) increase hypertension and precipitate arrhythmias. Blood pressure tends to rise during oral surgery under local anaesthesia, and epinephrine theoretically can contribute to this – but this is usually of little practical importance. Conscious sedation Conscious sedation requires special care and should be undertaken in a hospital setting. General anaesthesia General anaesthesia requires special care. It must be remembered that some patients having heart surgery may postoperatively have a residual lesion that makes them a poor risk for general anaesthesia and a high risk for endocarditis. They may also be on anticoagulants.

Treatment modification Careful monitoring of patients is required regardless of the procedure planned. A pulse and blood pressure determination before starting the dental procedure is mandatory to avoid false alarms. Patients with severe aortic stenosis have reduced pulse and systolic blood pressure. Patients with severe aortic regurgitation have increased differential blood pressure and high systolic blood pressure. Perioperative use of a cardiac monitor may be considered.

Drug use Most patients are on anticoagulant treatment; those who have received a heart transplant are taking immunosuppressant drugs.

Further reading
• Chu J, Wilkins G, Williams M 2004 Review of 65 cases of infective endocarditis in Dunedin Public Hospital. NZ Med J 117:1021 • Mackenzie W K 2002 Infective endocarditis. Aust Dent J 47:82 • Watkin R W, Baker N, Lang S, Ment J 2002 *Eikenella corrodens* infective endocarditis in a previously healthy non-drug user. Eur J Clin Microbiol Infect Dis 21:890–891.

Table 3.14 **Key considerations for dental management in aortic valve disease (see text)**

	Management modifications*	Comments/possible complications
Risk assessment	2	Infective endocarditis; antibiotic prophylaxis
Preventive dentistry and education		Thorough assessment; stabilisation essential to minimise risk of infective endocarditis
Pain and anxiety control		
– Local anaesthesia	1	Aspirating syringe
– Conscious sedation	3/4	
– General anaesthesia	3/4	
Patient access and positioning		
– Access to dental office	0	
– Timing of treatment	1	Delay 6 months after cardiac surgery
– Patient positioning	0	
Treatment modification		
– Oral surgery	1	Monitor pulse and blood pressure
– Implantology	1	
– Conservative/Endodontics	1	
– Fixed prosthetics	1	
– Removable prosthetics	0	
– Non-surgical periodontology	1	
– Surgical periodontology	1	
Hazardous and contraindicated drugs	2	Some patients are treated with anticoagulants

*0 = No special considerations. 1 = Caution advised. 2 = Specialised medical advice recommended in some cases. 3 = Specialised medical advice mandatory. 4 = Only to be performed in hospital environment. 5 = Should be avoided.

ASPLENIA

Definition Asplenia is defined as absence of a functional spleen.

General aspects

■ The spleen is essential for controlling the quality of erythrocytes and is the site of sequestration of effete erythrocytes ■ The spleen is also essential for the production of opsonins and thus has an important function in the phagocytosis of opsonised microorganisms and in T-cell-independent immune responses such as antibody production. Two splenic opsonins in particular, properdin and tuftsin, protect against bacteria such as pneumococci.

Aetiopathogenesis Asplenia may be caused by: ■ Congenital asplenia: ● very uncommon and usually related to polymalformative syndromes ■ Splenectomy: ● after serious splenic injuries in abdominal trauma ● in some haemolytic anaemias, hereditary spherocytosis, autoimmune haemolysis ● in idiopathic thrombocytopenic purpura ● in some lymphomas ■ The spleen becoming hypofunctional: ● infarction in sickle cell disease (auto-splenectomy), and other disorders.

Treatment and prognosis There is a lifetime risk from infection. Most infections occur within the first 2 years after splenectomy, and up to one-third may manifest at least 5 years later, but cases have occurred more than 20 years later. Children are 10 times more likely than adults to develop sepsis. ■ Infection after splenectomy: ● is almost invariably by encapsulated bacteria [*Streptococcus pneumoniae* (pneumococcus) is the most common pathogen and, together with *Haemophilus influenzae* and *Neisseria meningitidis* (meningococcus), accounts for 70–90% of cases; other infections include *Escherichia coli*, malaria, babesiosis, and *Capnocytophaga canimorsus* from

Table 3.15 **Key considerations in dental management in asplenia (see text)**

	Management modifications*	Comments/possible complications
Risk assessment	2	Antimicrobial prophylaxis is not indicated Thrombocytopenia Chlorhexidine mouthwash before dental treatment
Pain and anxiety control		
– Local anaesthesia	0	
– Conscious sedation	0	
– General anaesthesia	3/4	
Patient access and positioning		
– Access to dental office	0	
– Timing of treatment	0	
– Patient positioning	0	
Treatment modification		
– Oral surgery	1	Possible bleeding tendency
– Implantology	1	Possible bleeding tendency
– Conservative/Endodontics	0	
– Fixed prosthetics	0	
– Removable prosthetics	0	
– Non-surgical periodontology	1	
– Surgical periodontology	1	Possible bleeding tendency
Hazardous and contraindicated drugs	1	Some patients are treated with corticosteroids

*0 = No special considerations. 1 = Caution advised. 2 = Specialised medical advice recommended in some cases. 3 = Specialised medical advice mandatory. 4 = Only to be performed in hospital environment. 5 = Should be avoided.

dog bites] ● only rarely emanates from the oral flora ■ Splenectomised patients are predisposed to hepatitis C, and tuberculosis ■ Splenectomised patients are also predisposed to some malignant neoplasms.

Treatment Few asplenic patients are aware of the increased risk for serious infection and the appropriate health precautions required: ■ prophylaxis: oral phenoxymethylpenicillin is usually given (e.g. 250 mg daily) ■ antimicrobial prophylaxis is indicated for surgery (*not* oral surgery) ■ all infections should be handled with special care ■ if patients become acutely unwell, they should promptly be given further penicillin or alternative antibiotics.

Dental management

Oral infections should be treated rigorously and increased attention given to regular preventive measures, if necessary accompanied by more frequent review.

Risk assessment ■ There is no indication for antimicrobial prophylaxis before dental procedures and, in any event, any attempts at prophylaxis might fail since oral bacteria are only rarely involved, but it may be considered for major procedures ■ Thrombocytopenia (no store of platelets) may lead to a bleeding tendency ■ There may be infections such as tuberculosis to be considered.

Treatment modification A chlorhexidine mouthwash should be performed before any dental manipulation.

Drug use Concurrent corticosteroid therapy can affect care.

Further reading ● Da F, Hirsch A 2002 Dental care of the pediatric patient with splenic dysfunction. Pediatr Dent 24:57–63 ● De Rossi S S, Glick M 1996 Dental considerations in asplenic patients. J Am Dent Assoc 127:1359–1363.

ASTHMA

Definition Asthma is a chronic inflammatory lung disease. Large airway (bronchial) inflammation has long been recognised as a major factor but recent evidence suggests that small airways may also play a significant role. The characteristic features of asthma are: ■ reversible airway obstruction ■ airway inflammation ■ increased bronchial hyper-responsiveness.

General aspects

Classification The most common classifications divide asthma into allergic or extrinsic, and idiosyncratic or intrinsic types (Table 3.16).

Aetiopathogenesis Asthma has been related to hypersensitivity to either known precipitants (extrinsic asthma) or unknown stimuli (intrinsic asthma).

Airway obstruction is caused by: ■ smooth muscle contraction – due to histamine and leukotrienes ■ inflammation and oedema – due to IgE-mediated mast cell and basophil degranulation releasing inflammatory mediators ■ mucus production.

Table 3.16 **Types of asthma**

Type of asthma	Extrinsic	Intrinsic
	Allergic	Idiosyncratic
Frequency	Most common	Least common
Association with atopy	+ IgE-mediated mast cell degranulation	–
Age of onset	Child	Adult
Main precipitants	Allergens in house dust, animal dander, feathers, animal hairs, moulds, milk, eggs, fish, fruit, nuts, non-steroidal anti-inflammatory agents and antibiotics	Emotional stress, gastro-oesophageal reflux, vagally-mediated responses

Episodes of either type of asthma can sometimes be initiated by:
■ allergens from house dust mite, animal fur, pollen or foods such as nuts, shellfish, strawberries or milk ■ emotional stress ■ infections (especially viral, mycoplasmal or fungal) ■ irritating fumes including cigarette smoke ■ exercise ■ possibly due to the cold air temperature and climate changes ■ food additives such as tartrazine ■ drugs, particularly aspirin and other non-steroidal anti-inflammatory drugs, beta-blockers, antibiotics and ACE inhibitors.

Clinical presentation Features vary in severity but include wheeze, cough, dyspnoea, and use of accessory muscles in respiration (Table 3.17).

Diagnosis ■ Peak expiratory flow rate (PEFR) – lowered ■ Chest radiograph ■ Arterial blood gases.

Treatment ■ Inhaled beta-2-agonist (e.g. salbutamol) ■ Corticosteroids ■ Leukotriene receptor antagonists.

Table 3.17 **Severity of asthma**

Severity of asthma	Symptom duration	Attack frequency per week	Other comments	Typical therapy
Mild	<1 h	<2	Attacks follow exercise or exposure to trigger	Beta agonist as required
Moderate	days	>2	Activity restricted	Beta agonist plus steroid
Severe	persistent	persistent	Audible wheezing Tachypnoea Activity and sleep severely restricted	Beta agonist plus steroid plus theophylline

Prognosis Prognosis is usually good, especially when asthma appears first during childhood. In a few adults, asthma may progress to respiratory failure but the most serious complication is status asthmaticus – an asthmatic attack that persists for hours or even days, and represents a potentially lethal complication requiring emergency treatment.

Oral findings

■ Corticosteroid inhalers occasionally cause oral or pharyngeal thrush and, rarely, angina bullosa haemorrhagica ■ Beta-2-agonists and ipratropium bromide (isopropyl atropine) can cause a dry mouth ■ Anti-asthmatic drugs may lower the salivary pH, favouring caries development ■ Periodontal inflammation is greater in asthmatics than in those without respiratory disease ■ Gastro-oesophageal reflux is not uncommon, with occasional tooth erosion.

Dental management

Risk assessment ■ Asthmatic attacks may occasionally be precipitated by anxiety – it is important to attempt to lessen fear of dental treatment by sympathetic handling and reassurance ■ In approximately 15% of asthma sufferers even routine dental treatment can trigger a clinically significant decrease in lung function ■ Always remind patients to bring their medication to a dental appointment ■ Prophylactic use of the bronchodilator before starting the dental appointment is advisable; this should be kept at the chair-side in case it is required again ■ If the patient has an acute exacerbation of asthma during treatment: • stop treatment and remove all instruments/equipment from the mouth • remain calm as further anxiety will exacerbate the shortness of breath • sit the patient up • give the patient's usual medication such as a beta-2-agonist inhaler (salbutamol 400 μg), via a volumetric flask if available; a nebuliser unit is a helpful adjunct • if the attack resolves, monitor the patient closely before discharge as a further episode/intense bronchospasm may follow • if the attack does not resolve, give oxygen 10 L/min • if there is still no improvement, give salbutamol 400 μg every 2 minutes and call for an ambulance ■ If an asthmatic attack is severe, hydrocortisone 200 mg intravenously plus prednisolone 20 mg orally should also be given ■ Elective dental care in severe asthmatics should be deferred until they are in a better phase. However, for patients with severe intrinsic asthma who are not likely to improve, this may not be practical. Consider a steroid cover for patients on systemic steroids.

Patient education The use of aerosol-holding chambers and metered-dose inhalers, as well as mouth rinsing after their usage, can reduce the risk of developing oral mucosal lesions.

Pain and anxiety control **Local anaesthesia** Although local anaesthesia is generally safe, the following precautions are advisable: ■ occasional patients with asthma may react to the sulphites present as preservatives in some vasoconstrictor-containing local anaesthetics; therefore, it is better where possible to avoid solutions containing sulphites ■ if epinephrine-containing local analgesics are indicated, they should be given with an aspirating syringe since epinephrine may theoretically enhance the risk of arrhythmias with beta-2-agonists ■ epinephrine is contraindicated in patients using theophylline as it may precipitate arrhythmias.

Conscious sedation Relative analgesia with nitrous oxide and oxygen is preferable to intravenous sedation. Sedatives are also best avoided as they cause respiratory depression. Indeed, in an acute asthmatic attack, even benzodiazepines can precipitate respiratory failure.

General anaesthesia GA is best avoided. It may be complicated by hypoxia and hypercapnia – which can cause pulmonary oedema even if cardiac function is normal, and cardiac failure if there is cardiac disease. The risk of postoperative collapse of the lung or pneumothorax is also increased. Halothane, or better still, enflurane, isoflurane, desflurane or sevoflurane, are the preferred anaesthetics if GA is unavoidable, but ketamine may be useful in children. Drugs causing histamine release directly may precipitate an asthmatic attack – morphine and some other opioids, methohexitone, thiopentone, suxamethonium, tubocurarine and pancuronium should therefore be avoided.

Table 3.18 **Key considerations in dental management in asthma (see text)**

	Management modifications*	Comments/possible complications
Risk assessment	2	Asthmatic attack Prophylactic bronchodilators Consider steroid cover
Pain and anxiety control		
– Local anaesthesia	1	Avoid epinephrine (sulphites)
– Conscious sedation	1	Avoid sedatives
– General anaesthesia	3–5	Pulmonary complications; cardiac failure
Patient access and positioning		
– Access to dental office	0	
– Timing of treatment	1	Late morning
– Patient positioning	1	
Treatment modification		
– Oral surgery	1/4	Consider INR
– Implantology	1/4	
– Conservative/Endodontics	1	
– Fixed prosthetics	1	Materials selection
– Removable prosthetics	1	Materials selection
– Non-surgical periodontology	1	
– Surgical periodontology	1/4	
Hazardous and contraindicated drugs	2	Avoid aspirin, NSAIDs, sulphites, penicillin, and other erythromycin drugs interacting with theophylline

*0 = No special considerations. 1 = Caution advised. 2 = Specialised medical advice recommended in some cases. 3 = Specialised medical advice mandatory. 4 = Only to be performed in hospital environment. 5 = Should be avoided.

Patient access and positioning **Timing of treatment** Patients with nocturnal asthma attacks are better treated in the late morning.

Treatment modification **Surgery** In patients with frequent attacks, surgical procedures are best performed in hospital. **Prosthetics** Acrylic monomer, colophony and cyanoacrylates may occasionally precipitate an asthmatic attack. **Paediatric dentistry** An increased prevalence of caries has been described in children with asthma.

Drug use ■ Allergy to penicillin may be more frequent in asthmatic patients ■ Interactions of theophylline with drugs such as epinephrine, erythromycin, clindamycin, azithromycin, clarithromycin or ciprofloxacin may result in dangerously high levels of theophylline ■ Patients on leukotriene-modifying medications may have a prolonged INR and bleeding tendency, because of impaired liver metabolism ■ Systemic corticosteroid treatment brings with it the risks from steroid complications and operations can be hazardous on such patients without adequate preparation ■ Drugs to be avoided, since they may precipitate an attack, include particularly: ● aspirin ● NSAIDs ● sulphites in local anaesthetics.

Further reading ● Coke J M, Karaki D T 2002 The asthma patient and dental management. Gen Dent 50:504–507 ● Eloot A K, Vanobbergen J N, De Baets F, Martens L C 2004 Oral health and habits in children with asthma related to severity and duration of condition. Eur J Paediatr Dent 5:210–215 ● Marx J, Pretorius E 2004 Asthma – a risk factor for dental caries. S Afr Dent J 59:323–326.

ATTENTION DEFICIT HYPERACTIVITY DISORDER

Definition Attention deficit hyperactivity disorder (ADHD), once called *hyperkinesis* or *minimal brain dysfunction*, is one of the most common of childhood mental disorders, affecting 3–5% of children, and is twice as common in boys than girls. ADHD often continues into adolescence and adulthood.

General aspects

Parents not infrequently describe their badly behaved child as 'hyperactive.' However, the term should be limited to those who demonstrate gross behavioural abnormalities including: ■ uncontrolled activity ■ impulsiveness ■ impaired concentration ■ motor restlessness ■ extreme fidgeting.

These activities are seen particularly when orderliness is required, for example in the dental waiting room or surgery. True hyperactivity or overactivity are terms that apply to *gross* misbehaviour such as reckless escapes from parents while on public transport.

Aetiopathogenesis The aetiopathogenesis remains unclear, but minor head injuries or undetectable brain damage, or refined sugar and food additives make some children hyperactive and inattentive. Overactivity can also be caused by external factors, or factors affecting parents, the child or the child–parent relationship. There is also a familial predisposition.

Clinical presentation ADHD is characterised by inattention and hyperactivity and/or impulsivity that are excessive, long-term, and pervasive. Hyperactive children always seem to be in motion and seem unable to curb their immediate reactions or think before they act. Deficit in attention and motor control and perception (DAMP) may be a variant.

Signs of inattention include: ■ becoming easily distracted by irrelevant sights and sounds ■ failing to pay attention to details and making careless mistakes ■ rarely following instructions carefully and completely ■ losing or forgetting things such as toys, or pencils, books, and tools needed for a task.

Signs of hyperactivity and impulsivity include: ■ feeling restless, often fidgeting with hands or feet, or squirming ■ running, climbing, or leaving a seat, in situations where sitting or quiet behaviour is expected ■ blurting out answers before hearing the whole question ■ having difficulty waiting in line or for a turn.

Commonly associated disorders may include: ■ developmental language disorders ■ oppositional-defiant disorders affect nearly half of all children with ADHD, overreacting or lashing out when they feel bad about themselves ■ motor and coordination difficulties ■ Tourette's syndrome – an inherited, neurological disorder characterised by repeated and involuntary body movements (tics) and uncontrollable vocal sounds and words (coprolalia) ■ epilepsy – it has been estimated that 20% of epileptic children have ADHD.

Diagnosis Diagnosis is established by clinical findings. To make a diagnosis of ADHD, the behaviours must appear before age 7 years, and continue for at least 6 months.

Treatment ■ Specialised educational help, behavioural therapy, emotional counselling, and practical support are required ■ Stimulants seem to be the most effective treatment in both children and adults, and include methylphenidate, dextroamphetamine, and pemoline ■ Sedatives and tranquillisers should be avoided as they may impair learning ability, or cause paradoxical reactions such as aggressive behaviour ■ In some cases antidepressants and antihypertensive agents have also been successfully administered.

Oral findings

Individuals with ADHD are liable to caries and/or bruxism.

Dental management

Risk assessment The patient may show inappropriate behaviour with uncontrolled movements or self-directed aggression during dental treatment. It is advisable that some family member be present at all times to act as an escort. Patience and an empathetic approach are indispensable. Adequate behavioural control technique selection is the basis of dental treatment success. 'Training sessions' at home with the family, where the child can run through the process of visiting the dentist, ideally with visual aids such as pictures, can be of benefit. However, some overactive children are often almost impossible to manage in the dental surgery, and frequently succeed in frustrating all concerned. In view of this, dental treatment may be an exhausting experience.

Preventive health care Most patients need help to brush their teeth. Electric toothbrushes are often not well tolerated due to the bristle movement and the rotor sound.

Pain and anxiety control **Local anaesthesia** Patients may be manageable by reassurance. The 'tell–show–do' technique may be of value, especially when applied by a paediatric dentist trained in child psychology. However, if LA cannot be safely given, alternative approaches may need to be considered. **Conscious sedation** Orally administered agents such as diazepam should be avoided as they usually exacerbate rather than depress overactivity. Relative analgesia using nitrous oxide and oxygen may be useful. Although intravenous sedation may be used, the success of sedation is

Table 3.19 **Key considerations for dental management in ADHD (see text)**

	Management modifications*	Comments/possible complications
Risk assessment	2/4	Evaluate cooperation; individualised management; training at home
Pain and anxiety control		
– Local anaesthesia	1	Evaluate cooperation
– Conscious sedation	1	Unpredictable
– General anaesthesia	3/4	May be indicated
Patient access and positioning		
– Access to dental office	1	Short appointments; no waiting time
– Timing of treatment	0	
– Patient positioning	0	
Treatment modification		
– Oral surgery	1	
– Implantology	1	
– Conservative/Endodontics	1	
– Fixed prosthetics	1	
– Removable prosthetics	1	
– Non-surgical periodontology	1	
– Surgical periodontology	1	
Hazardous and contraindicated drugs	1	Diazepam and midazolam idiosyncratic reaction

*0 = No special considerations. 1 = Caution advised. 2 = Specialised medical advice recommended in some cases. 3 = Specialised medical advice mandatory. 4 = Only to be performed in hospital environment. 5 = Should be avoided.

unpredictable – the outcome of previous sedations being the best prognosis indicator. **General anaesthesia** Patients requiring complex dental treatment and those uncontrolled with sedation may be treated under GA, although admission to hospital may be problematic.

Patient access and positioning Appointments should be short, with no waiting time before the patient is seen.

Treatment modification It is important to assess each patient on an individual basis and determine the effectiveness of methods of pain and anxiety control. This will determine what treatments are feasible and can be undertaken without undue stress to the patient or the operator.

Drug use Idiosyncratic reactions to diazepam and midazolam have been observed.

Further reading • Broadbent J M, Ayers K M, Thomson W M 2004 Is attention-deficit hyperactivity disorder a risk factor for dental caries? A case-control study. Caries Res 38:29–33 • Friedlander A H, Yagiela J A, Paterno V I, Mahler M E 2003 The pathophysiology, medical management, and dental implications of children and young adults having attention-deficit hyperactivity disorder. J Calif Dent Assoc 31:669–678 • Malki G A, Zawawi K H, Melis M, Hughes C V 2004 Prevalence of bruxism in children receiving treatment for attention deficit hyperactivity disorder: a pilot study. J Clin Pediatr Dent 29:63–67 • Ramanathan G, White G E 2001 Attention-deficit/hyperactive disorder: making a case for multidisciplinary management. J Clin Pediatr Dent 25:249–253 • Waldman H B, Swerdloff M, Perlman S P 2000 You may be treating children with mental retardation and attention deficit hyperactive disorder in your dental practice. ASDC J Dent Child 67:231, 241–245.

AUTISM SPECTRUM DISORDER

Definition Autism spectrum disorder (Greek 'autos' = self), is a spectrum of pervasive developmental disorders that usually begins in the first 30 months of life, causing long-term disability characterised by poor social skills (inability to get along with people), lack of interpersonal relationships, abnormal speech and language, ritualistic or compulsive behaviour with repetitive stereotyped activities. The most well known of these disorders are autism and Asperger's syndrome. Asperger's syndrome is unlike classic autism in that language is usually intact, features typically appear later in childhood, and patients show a particularly high intelligence quotient (IQ).

General aspects

Aetiopathogenesis Aetiopathogenesis remains unclear, but autism is three to four times more common in boys than girls and there may be chromosome 15 changes.

Clinical presentation People with autism have no distinguishing physical features but live isolated in worlds of their own, appear indifferent and remote and may be unable to form emotional bonds with others, or understand other people's thoughts, feelings, and needs. Children with autism seem to have great difficulty learning to engage in the give-and-take of everyday human interaction. Some people with autism are highly intelligent, but 70% have an IQ below 70. Temporal lobe epilepsy develops in about 30%.

They often: ■ Avoid eye contact ■ Appear deaf ■ Start developing language, then abruptly stop talking altogether (they often have echolalia, omit words, misuse pronouns and indicate consent by repeating a question) ■ Act as if unaware of the coming and going of others. They seem to prefer being alone, and may resist attention and affection or passively accept hugs and cuddling. ■ Practice repetitive actions like rocking or hand-flapping. Most characteristic are finger flicking near the eyes. Facial grimaces, jumping and toe walking are also common and all mannerisms are exaggerated if the person with autism is distressed or excited. ■ Have an obsessional desire for maintaining an unchanging environment and rigidly following familiar patterns in their everyday routines. Many insist on eating the same foods, at the same time, sitting at precisely the same place at the table every day. They may get furious or wildly upset if their toothbrush has been moved even slightly. A minor change in their routine may be deeply upsetting. ■ Show no sensitivity to burns or bruises, and may engage in self-mutilation, such as eye gouging. On the other hand, some are painfully sensitive to sound, touch, sight, or smell. Some display a combination of lack of response to stimuli, including pain, with abnormal fearlessness. Some cover their ears and scream at the sound of a vacuum cleaner, a distant aircraft, a telephone ringing, or even the wind.

Diagnosis Diagnosis of autism is established by clinical findings, but it may remain undiagnosed until the age of 4 or 5 years. It is essential to rule out other disorders which can resemble autism, such as hearing loss, speech problems, learning disability, neurological problems, and Rett's syndrome – a progressive brain disease that affects only girls and causes repetitive hand movements, bruxism and loss of language and social skills.

Treatment There is only limited evidence that drug treatments for autism are effective: ■ medications used to treat anxiety and depression being explored as a way to relieve symptoms include clomipramine, and SSRIs such as fluoxetine ■ beta-blockers have also been administered in some cases ■ specialised educational help is required.

Oral findings

■ People with autism may prefer sweet foods, sometimes given as rewards, and may have poor oral hygiene (these factors may increase risk for dental caries and periodontal disease; however, some epidemiological studies developed in people with autism living in institutions have shown a caries rate similar to that of the general population) ■ They may have signs of bruxism ■ More than 20% of children with autism bite objects or introduce their fingers in the mouth routinely, resulting in traumatic lesions ■ Oral lesions may also be present due to auto-aggression or convulsive crisis.

Dental management

Risk assessment Dental treatment can be an exhausting experience but patience and an empathetic approach are indispensable. People with autism do not fit easily into mainstream or so-called 'normalised' services as they may show inappropriate behaviour with uncontrolled movements or self-directed aggression during dental treatment. Progressive desensitisation with the use of visual aids and a set routine are invaluable. Simple step-by-step instructions are valuable. Questions should be avoided.

Preventive health care Most patients need help to brush their teeth. Electric toothbrushes are often not well tolerated due to the bristle movement and the rotor sound. Pictures may be useful for oral hygiene education.

Pain and anxiety control Progressive desensitisation can be useful but it involves time and staff and, in some cases, patients will only permit oral examination and preventive care. Nevertheless this is critical as it allows assessment of the patient's needs without the aid of more invasive methods such as general anaesthesia. The 'tell–show–do' technique is not indicated in people with autism as eye contact is often not possible. **Local anaesthesia** Many patients have low tolerance and may not accept LA. **Conscious sedation** Patients are usually manageable by reassurance and possibly a very mild anxiolytic or sedative such as a low dose of a beta-blocker or a short-acting (temazepam) or moderate-acting (lorazepam or diazepam) benzodiazepine. Intravenous or intranasal sedation with midazolam, or relative analgesia using nitrous oxide and oxygen, are also useful. However the success of sedation is unpredictable – the outcome of previous attempts at sedation being the best prognostic indicator. **General anaesthesia** Patients requiring complex dental treatment and those uncontrollable with sedation must be treated under GA, although admission to hospital may be disturbing for them. It is estimated that about 25% of patients need a GA for dental treatment every 5 years.

Patient access and positioning Access for dental visits may be improved by the following measures: ■ Previous training at the school or at home with visual aids including pictures and instruments, simulation of procedures, and single and repeated orders such as 'hands down' or 'look at me' may be useful ■ It is essential to develop a routine in which the patient is not kept waiting, has a short quiet visit, with a routine, including always seeing the same dental staff – a 'step-by-step' technique may be useful and can be converted to pictures the patient can take away ■ Patients may be disturbed by noise such as a high-speed aspirator or air rotor and then it may be necessary to avoid their use ■ It is advisable that some family member, or a carer known to the patient, be present.

Treatment modification It is important to assess each patient on an individual basis to determine what treatments are feasible and can be undertaken without undue stress to the patient.

Further reading ● Chen L C T, King N M, O'Donnell D 2006 Autism: the aetiology, management and implications for treatment modalities from the dental perspective. Dent Update 33:70–83 ● Diz Dios P 2003 Espectro autista e odontoloxía. Maremagnum 7:75–80 ● Friedlander A H, Yagiela J A, Paterno V I, Mahler M E 2003 The pathophysiology, medical management, and dental implications of autism. J Calif Dent Assoc 31:681–691 ● Klein U, Nowak A J 1998 Autistic disorder: a review for the paediatric dentist. Pediatr Dent 20:312–317 ● Medina A C, Sogbe R, Gomez-Rey A M, Mata M 2003 Factitial oral lesions in an autistic paediatric patient. Int J Paediatr Dent 13:130–137 ● Peak J, Eveson J, Scully C 1992 Oral manifestations of Rett's syndrome. Br Dent J 172:248–249 ● Surabian S R 2001 Developmental disabilities: epilepsy, cerebral palsy, and autism. J Calif Dent Assoc 29:424–432.

Table 3.20 **Key considerations for dental management in autism (see text)**

	Management modifications*	Comments/possible complications
Risk assessment	2/4	Evaluate cooperation; individualised management; training at home; visual aids
Pain and anxiety control		
– Local anaesthesia	1	Low tolerance
– Conscious sedation	1	Useful
– General anaesthesia	3/4	May be indicated
Patient access and positioning		
– Access to dental office	1	Develop a routine
– Timing of treatment	1	Short appointments; minimise waiting time
– Patient positioning	0	
Treatment modification		
– Oral surgery	1	
– Implantology	1	
– Conservative/Endodontics	1	
– Fixed prosthetics	1	
– Removable prosthetics	1	
– Non-surgical periodontology	1	
– Surgical periodontology	1	
Hazardous and contraindicated drugs	0	

*0 = No special considerations. 1 = Caution advised. 2 = Specialised medical advice recommended in some cases. 3 = Specialised medical advice mandatory. 4 = Only to be performed in hospital environment. 5 = Should be avoided.

BEDBOUND PATIENTS

Definition To be bedbound is the most severe degree of dependence. Dependent patients are those with a weakness or a disability that makes it difficult for them to accomplish their own personal care routines independently or safely.

General aspects

Aetiopathogenesis Reasons for being house/bedbound are, in decreasing frequency: ■ physical disability ■ medical illness ■ mental health problems.

Clinical presentation Common findings (Fig. 3.6) are constipation, uncontrolled bladder, skin breakdown (bedsores) and gingivitis and periodontitis. Features of any underlying diseases such as neuropsychiatric disorders, osteoarthritis and cardiovascular illness, may also be present.

Classification Most are patients with American Society of Anesthesiologists (ASA) scores of III, IV and V.

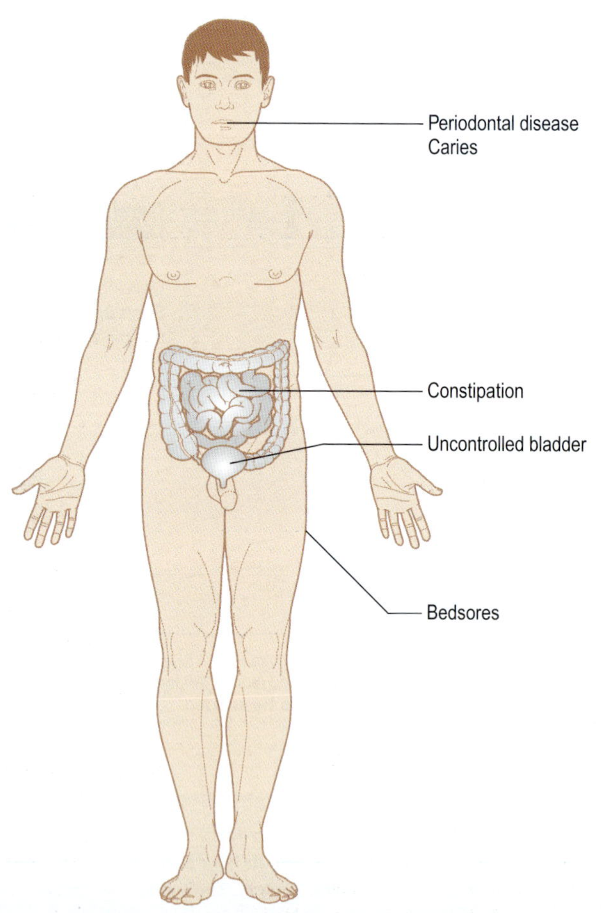

Figure 3.6 **Clinical presentation of bedbound patients**

Treatment Bedbound patients have basic personal-care needs including good skin care, adequate bowel and bladder function, and oral health care. Most patients take numerous drugs for their underlying medical problems.

Prognosis Prognosis is related to the underlying disease, but respiratory, infectious and vascular complications are common.

Oral findings

The main oral problems of these patients are: ■ toothache due to caries exacerbated by a soft cariogenic diet and limited access to toothbrushing ■ tooth loss due to progressive periodontal disease ■ uncomfortable dentures.

Table 3.21 **Key considerations for dental management in bedbound patients (see text)**

	Management modifications*	Comments/possible complications
Risk assessment	2/4	ASA score
Pain and anxiety control		
– Local anaesthesia	0	
– Conscious sedation	2	Grade of cooperation; avoid drug synergy
– General anaesthesia	3–5	Depends on underlying disease
Patient access and positioning		
– Access to dental office	2/4	
– Timing of treatment	0	
– Patient positioning	1	
Treatment modification		
– Oral surgery	2/4	Only simple, single procedures at home
– Implantology	5	
– Conservative/Endodontics	1/5	Individualised evaluation
– Fixed prosthetics	5	
– Removable prosthetics	1/5	Individualised evaluation
– Non-surgical periodontology	1/5	Individualised evaluation
– Surgical periodontology	5	
Hazardous and contraindicated drugs	2	Antibiotic selection; some patients receive anticoagulants or corticosteroids

*0 = No special considerations. 1 = Caution advised. 2 = Specialised medical advice recommended in some cases. 3 = Specialised medical advice mandatory. 4 = Only to be performed in hospital environment. 5 = Should be avoided.

Dental management

Risk assessment In patients with ASA scores of III, IV and V, any stressful procedure or one likely to cause significant bleeding should ideally be performed in a hospital environment. Only minimal manipulations should be undertaken with domiciliary care in the home.

Preventive dentistry Regular cleaning and antimicrobial rinses (chlorhexidine) may help in preserving oral hygiene and in reducing the prevalence of some infectious complications such as aspiration pneumonia. **Caregivers' education** ■ clean teeth at least once a day (sponge 'toothettes' or mouth swabs can be useful) ■ check dentures regularly for cleanliness and cracks ■ remove dentures for cleaning and soak for 10 minutes in an antiseptic liquid such as chlorhexidine or hypochlorite ■ remove dentures at night.

Pain and anxiety control The choice of the appropriate method of pain and anxiety control will be influenced by the degree of cooperation possible, and any underlying disease. Furthermore, some patients are taking neuroleptics that have synergy with sedative drugs.

Treatment modification **Surgery** Simple procedures such as anterior tooth extraction, or the extraction of mobile posterior teeth in cooperative patients can usually be performed at home. Dentoalveolar surgery needs a mobile dental unit (with vacuum aspiration). More extensive surgery should be undertaken in a hospital environment. **Prosthetics and conservation** These treatments are often difficult if not impossible in bedbound patients. They will be influenced by life expectancy, degree of cooperation, diet and oral function, oral health status, and risk of aspiration.

Drug use ■ Many bedbound patients are taking antibiotics long term (i.e. those with a vascular catheter or Foley catheter) – these may result in the emergence of resistant oral bacteria, which may not respond to routine antimicrobial therapy ■ Patients may have a bleeding tendency because of anticoagulants or platelet aggregation inhibitors ■ Corticosteroid treatment is not uncommon.

Further reading
● Lovel T 2000 Palliative care and head and neck cancer. Br J Oral Maxillofac Surg 38:253–254 ● http://www.bsdh.org.uk/guidelines/depend.pdf

BONE MARROW TRANSPLANTATION (BMT)

Definition Bone marrow transplantation (BMT) involves harvesting bone marrow cells from a donor and transplanting them into the recipient by injecting the cells intravenously. The transplant includes not only myeloid, erythroid and megakaryocyte cells but also lymphoid and macrophage cells. Although most haematopoietic stem cells are found in the bone marrow, some cells, called peripheral blood stem cells (PBSCs), are found in the bloodstream. Blood in the umbilical cord also contains haematopoietic stem cells. Cells from any of these sources can be used in transplants, and are known collectively as haematopoietic stem cell transplants (HSCT).

General aspects

Indications HCST is increasingly used in the treatment of: ■ aplastic anaemia ■ leukaemias and other haematological malignancies ■ some genetic defects.

Classification The donor cells are best harvested from an identical twin or a close relative who is also HLA-matched as much as possible to minimise graft rejection (Table 3.22). Most transplants are made between HLA-identical siblings, though other family members, or matched volunteers, may be used.

Treatment ■ Patients first must be prepared to reduce the chances of graft rejection by profoundly suppressing their immune response, often with cyclophosphamide (plus busulphan and total body irradiation [TBI] in leukaemia, to destroy the malignant cells) ■ The donor marrow is then mixed with heparin and infused intravenously, from where it colonises the recipient marrow and, over the next 2–4 weeks, starts to produce blood cells ■ Throughout this time and for the following 3 months or so, the patient is usually provided with an indwelling vascular catheter (Hickman line) to facilitate drug therapy and intravenous fluids.

Prognosis ■ The strong myeloablative treatment makes the recipient extremely immuno-incompetent and susceptible to infection ■ The recipient must therefore be isolated and protected from infections, and may require transfusions of granulocytes, platelets or red cells, granulocyte colony stimulating factors, and antimicrobials until the donor marrow is functioning fully ■ Prognosis is influenced by factors such as age, general health status, underlying disease or donor cell origin.

Oral findings

Mucositis ■ Mucositis affects up to 99% of patients receiving HSCT, typically beginning around 5 days post-HSCT infusion and persisting for 2–3 weeks; it is the most common symptom and distressing complication, and is particularly a problem after TBI in leukaemia, in allogeneic transplantation, and where neutrophil recovery is delayed ■ Oral mucositis

Table 3.22 **Donor cells used in HSCT**

Donor	Comments
Autologous	Cells readily available. Best for HSCT in non-malignant disease – no graft-versus-host disease (GVHD). In malignant disease, there is a risk of re-introducing malignant cells
Sibling: syngeneic (identical twin)	Best – no GVHD
Sibling (HLA-matched)	Minimal GVHD
Unrelated donor (HLA-matched)	Some GVHD

may be a predictor of gastrointestinal toxicity and the onset of hepatic veno-occlusive disease ■ Mucositis symptoms may be reduced by ● soft bland diet ● flavour-free/children's toothpastes ● soft toothbrush ● benzydamine HCl M/W 0.15% ● chlorhexidine aqueous rinse (0.12–0.2%) ● amifostine intravenously before each radiation ● potent opiate analgesia if the symptoms are very severe.

Infections ■ These may present as sinusitis, parotitis, pain or bleeding ■ Oral infections, particularly if bacterial, can be lethal and must be treated vigorously ■ Later (2–4 months after transplant), opportunist infections such as herpetic and fungal infections often develop.

Oral complications due to blood changes (anaemia, thrombocytopenia, neutropenia) ■ Mucosal pallor ■ Burning sensation ■ Oral ulceration ■ Spontaneous gingival/mucosal bleeding ■ Crusting of lips ■ Oral infections.

Graft-versus-host disease ■ This presents with lichenoid reactions or xerostomia.

Malignancies related to immunosuppressants ■ Lip and occasionally oral carcinomas ■ Kaposi's sarcoma ■ Lymphomas.

Dental management

Risk assessment Potential problems related to dental care include immunosuppression and bleeding tendency. Periapically involved teeth can become a medical emergency. Hence all HSCT candidates should be evaluated and receive dental treatment before immunosuppression to establish a rigorous oral hygiene programme, eliminate dental infections and stabilise carious lesions. This involves working as a part of the multidisciplinary team and coordinating care with the oncologists.

For 6 months after HSCT, elective dental care is best deferred. If surgical treatment is needed during that period, antibiotic prophylaxis is probably warranted after medical consultation. After a full recovery, a programme of periodic check-ups is needed.

Pain and anxiety control **Local anaesthesia** No specific modifications are required, although a preoperative chlorhexidine rinse is advisable. **Conscious sedation** Modification may be required depending on the patient's underlying disease. **General anaesthesia** Specific GA to facilitate dentistry should be avoided, as patients are at high risk of complications. However, it may be possible to undertake simple procedures, such as dental extractions, at the same time as a GA for other procedures (e.g. bone marrow harvest).

Preventive dentistry Oral hygiene should be closely monitored and maintained where possible. Significantly increased plaque and gingival inflammation scores have been recorded during the period of intense immunosuppression following allogeneic HSCT. Caries may be further prevented by sealant and fluoride application.

Patient access and positioning If dental extractions are required it may be possible to coordinate these with other concurrent general anaesthetic procedures, such as the bone marrow harvest, or placement of the central line. This is particularly advantageous for children who may not be able to cooperate for treatment under LA, and when time available prior to commencement of immunosuppression is limited.

Treatment modification **Surgery** The need for extraction of partially erupted permanent teeth should be evaluated, due to the risk of pericoronitis. **Implants** Although there is no evidence that immunosuppression is a contraindication to implants, such patients may not be a good risk group, and medical advice should be taken first. **Prosthesis** Complex dental prostheses are not indicated in patients with a poor prognosis. **Periodontology** Ciclosporin may induce gingival swelling. **Orthodontics** Orthodontic bands and appliances that contribute to poor

Table 3.23 **Key considerations in dental management in bone marrow transplantation (see text)**

	Management modifications*	Comments/possible complications
Risk assessment	3	Dental screening Delay elective dental treatment 6 months; Immunosuppression; Bleeding tendency
Pain and anxiety control		
– Local anaesthesia	0	
– Conscious sedation	0	
– General anaesthesia	3–5	
Patient access and positioning		
– Access to dental office	0	
– Timing of treatment	2	Coordinate with GA/other oncology treatment
– Patient positioning	0	
Treatment modification		
– Oral surgery	3	Evaluate partially erupted teeth
– Implantology	3	
– Conservative/Endodontics	2	Only simple procedures
– Fixed prosthetics	2	Only simple procedures
– Removable prosthetics	1	
– Non-surgical periodontology	3	
– Surgical periodontology	3	
Hazardous and contraindicated drugs	2	Immunosuppressants Steroid cover

*0 = No special considerations. 1 = Caution advised. 2 = Specialised medical advice recommended in some cases. 3 = Specialised medical advice mandatory. 4 = Only to be performed in hospital environment. 5 = Should be avoided.

oral hygiene or mucosal irritation should be removed.

Paediatric dentistry Mobile primary teeth and gingival operculum should be removed.

Drug use HSCT recipients may need immunosuppressive therapy with ciclosporin or methotrexate and corticosteroids for 6 months or more to prevent or ameliorate graft-versus-host disease. These drugs all have the potential to induce oral side effects and systemic complications. Furthermore, the need for steroid supplementation may need to be considered.

Further reading ● Elad S, Or R, Garfunkel A A, Shapira M Y 2003 Budesonide: a novel treatment for oral chronic graft versus host disease. Oral Surg Oral Med Oral Pathol Oral Radiol Endod 95:308–311 ● Majorana A, Schubert M M, Porta F, Ugazio A G, Sapelli P L 2000 Oral complications of pediatric hematopoietic cell transplantation: diagnosis and management. Support Care Cancer 8:353–365 ● Melkos A B, Massenkeil G, Arnold R, Reichart P A 2003 Dental treatment prior to stem cell transplantation and its influence on the posttransplantation outcome. Clin Oral Invest 7:113–115 ● Uderzo C, Fraschini D, Balduzzi A et al 1997 Long-term effects of bone marrow transplantation on dental status in children with leukaemia. Bone Marrow Transplant 20:865–869.

CANCER (HEAD AND NECK)

Definition Cancer is defined as an abnormal cell proliferation that invades the normal surrounding tissues and disseminates to distant organs. Head and neck cancer is usually squamous cell carcinoma (HNSCC). It is more common in males and with increasing age. High rates of HNSCC are seen particularly in India, Sri Lanka and Brazil, but there is a wide geographical variation in incidence. Worldwide more than 500000 new cases annually are projected.

General aspects

Aetiopathogenesis Several factors are predisposing causes for HNSCC including: ■ sun exposure ■ alcohol ■ tobacco ■ betel (areca nut) ■ genetic factors ■ infectious agents (i.e. chronic candidosis, syphilis and papillomaviruses) ■ immunosuppression ■ iron deficiency (i.e. Plummer–Vinson syndrome) ■ oral health status (i.e. mechanical injuries and edentulism).

Potentially malignant lesions include erythroplasia (erythroplakia) and particularly speckled leukoplakia or leukoplakias in the floor of the mouth.

Clinical presentation The clinical appearance of oral cancer is highly variable, including ulcers, red or white areas, lumps, or fissures. Common sites for oral SCC are the lips, lateral border of tongue and floor of mouth. There may be widespread dysplastic mucosa ('field change') or even a second primary neoplasm anywhere in the oral cavity, oropharynx or upper aerodigestive tract.

Classification The most common classifications are based on histological findings and the international tumour node metastases (TNM) system (Box 3.1). Several other classifications are available, e.g. STNM (S = site).

Box 3.1 TNM classification of malignant neoplasms

Primary tumour size (T)

Tx	No available information
T0	No evidence of primary tumour
Tis	Only carcinoma in situ
T1	Maximum diameter 2cm
T2	Maximum diameter of 4cm
T3	Maximum diameter over 4cm
T4	Massive tumour greater than 4cm diameter, with involvement of adjacent anatomical structures

Regional lymph node involvement (N)

Nx	Nodes could not be or were not assessed
N0	No clinically positive nodes
N1	Single ipsilateral node less than 3cm in diameter
N2a	Single ipsilateral nodes 3–6cm
N2b	Multiple ipsilateral nodes less than 6cm
N2c	Bilateral or contralateral nodes less than 6cm
N3	Any node greater than 6cm

Involvement by distant metastases (M)

Mx	Distant metastasis was not assessed
M0	No evidence of distant metastasis
M1	Distant metastasis is present

Diagnosis Diagnosis is still often delayed, even in developed countries. History, physical examination and lesional biopsy are essential for diagnosis. Features which suggest malignancy include: ■ erythroplasia ■ a granular appearance ■ abnormal blood vessels supplying a lump ■ induration ■ fixation of the lesion (or node) ■ cervical lymph node enlargement ■ non-healing ulcer or extraction socket.

Any lesion of dubious nature should be biopsied. Second primary tumours or metastases should be excluded by chest radiography and endoscopy.

Treatment ■ Patients with oral cancer are best managed by a team of specialists. Many early carcinomas can be treated by either surgery or radiotherapy but, in later stages, surgery is often the first option. Radical radiotherapy aimed at cure may be used as the sole treatment or in combination with surgery. ■ Chemotherapy is used primarily for palliative care in a patient with advanced SCC ■ Chemopreventive agents such as retinoids (synthetic vitamin A derivatives) and carotenoids (vitamin A precursors) show promise in the control of potentially malignant lesions such as leukoplakia ■ Bisphosphonates such as Pamidronate (Aredia) and Zoledronate (Zometal) may be used to treat cancer that has spread to the bones.

Prognosis Oral cancer is associated with significant morbidity and mortality, with a survival rate 5 years after diagnosis of about 50%. Major complications and death are often related to: ■ local obstruction of breathing and swallowing ■ infiltration into major vessels (e.g. carotid artery) ■ secondary infections ■ impaired function of distant organs (due to metastases) ■ wasting syndrome ■ complications of surgery or radiotherapy.

Dental management

See also Radiotherapy.

Risk assessment Patients with any cancer may have severe psychological disturbances in view of the nature of the illness. These problems are compounded in oral cancer since there are additional disabilities, particularly disfigurement, and interference with speech and swallowing. Bisphosphonates such as pamidronate (Aredia) and zoledronate (Zometal), in particular, can lead to painful refractory bone exposures in the jaws (sometimes termed osteochemonecrosis or osteonecrosis of the jaws: ONJ), typically following oral surgical procedures. Exodontia, periodontal surgery, endodontic surgery, and endosseous implants can be responsible. Most cases involve *intravenous* bisphosphonates used in metastatic disease in bone and after bisphosphonate therapy exceeding 6 months, so caution is especially warranted then. Pre-therapy dental care reduces this incidence, but only avoidance of surgical procedures can prevent new cases. FDA guidance issued at http://www.fda.gov/ohrms/dockets/ac/05/briefing/2005-4095B2 02 12-Novartis-Zometa-App-11.htm (accessed 22 May 2006) for prevention of ONJ is as follows:

Potential preventive measures prior to the initiation of IV bisphosphonate therapy ■ Avoid any elective jaw procedure that will require bone to heal ■ Recommend a routine clinical dental exam that may include a panoramic jaw radiograph to detect potential dental and periodontal infections ■ If bisphosphonate therapy can be briefly delayed without the risk of a skeletal-related complication, teeth with a poor prognosis or in need of extraction should be extracted and other dental surgeries should be completed prior to the initiation of bisphosphonate therapy. The benefit or risk of withholding bisphosphonate therapy has not been evaluated to date. Therefore, the decision to withhold bisphosphonate treatment must be made by the treating oncologist in consultation with an oral maxillofacial surgeon or another dental specialist. ■ Suggested preventive dentistry before initiation of chemotherapy, immunotherapy, and/or bisphosphonate therapy may include: ● Remove abscessed and non-restorable teeth and involved periodontal tissues ● Functional rehabilitation of salvageable dentition, including endodontic therapy ● Dental prophylaxis, caries control, and stabilising restorative dental care ● Examine dentures to ensure proper fit (remove dentures at night) ● Oral self-care hygiene education ● Prophylactic antibiotics are not indicated before routine dentistry unless otherwise required for prophylaxis of bacteraemia in those patients at risk (e.g. those with an indwelling catheter) ■ Educate patients regarding the importance of good dental hygiene and symptom reporting ● Suggest regularly scheduled hard- and soft-tissue oral assessments, possibly every 3 to 4 months, depending on risk ● Oncologists should perform a brief visual inspection of the oral cavity at baseline and at every follow-up visit.

Dental treatment for patients currently receiving bisphosphonate therapy ■ Maintain excellent oral hygiene to reduce the risk of dental and periodontal infections ■ Check and adjust removable dentures for potential soft-tissue injury, especially tissue overlying bone ■ Perform routine dental cleanings, being sure to avoid soft-tissue injury ■ Aggressively manage dental infections non-surgically with root canal treatment if possible or with minimal surgical intervention ■ Endodontic (root canal) therapy is preferable to extractions when possible. It may be necessary to carry out coronal amputation with subsequent root canal therapy on retained roots to avoid the need for tooth extraction and, therefore, the potential development of osteonecrosis.

Pain and anxiety control Caution is advisable when providing LA, CS or GA, as the anatomy of the oral cavity and pharynx may be altered by surgery, and may compromise the airway. Furthermore, surgery may also alter the position of nerve supply to the mouth, making the effectiveness of LA unpredictable. Radiotherapy may further compound these problems, particularly when associated with trismus (see Radiotherapy).

Patient access and positioning The patient may need to be kept in an upright position if the airway is compromised. Packs may be used to further protect the airway, providing there is no nasal obstruction.

Treatment modification Treatment should be provided in consultation with the multidisciplinary team involved in caring for the patient. All patients should receive: ■ a thorough preoperative assessment, including clinical evaluation of the structures that might remain after surgery, radiographs and functional silicone impressions ■ urgent dental treatment before tumour treatment (e.g. extractions) ■ stabilisation of the remaining dentition ■ patient education and details of help groups – advise the patient to stop smoking and drinking alcohol, and to maintain good oral hygiene to minimise the postoperative complications and the risk of a second primary cancer.

Patients receiving palliative therapy must be kept free of active dental disease, although it may not be possible to provide definitive care.

Removable maxillary prostheses In patients with maxillary resections, a surgical obturator is often recommended, because it minimises postoperative trauma, allowing tissues to heal, improves speech and swallowing and, sometimes, aesthetics. As much of the maxilla as possible should be conserved. In cases of posteriorly extended maxillectomy, the coronoid process is best removed. When possible, a surgical obturator constructed on preoperative casts can be intraoperatively adapted (with tissue conditioners or similar materials) and fixed to the unaffected palate bone using bone screws or transalveolar wires.

Intraoperative impressions will allow the construction of an interim prosthesis to be inserted 3 weeks after surgery and used for 4–6 months. The success of the definitive prosthesis depends on its fit and stability, which are influenced by the size and morphology of the surgical defect, presence and state of teeth, trismus and patient motivation and adaptability. Increased success has been reported with the use of light-cured hollow obturators and/or implants.

Removable mandibular prostheses The success of a mandibular prosthesis will be influenced by the extent and morphology of remaining bone, the degree of mandibular deviation and the number and state of

Table 3.24 **Key considerations in dental management in cancer (head and neck) (see text)**

	Management modifications*	Comments/possible complications
Risk assessment	2	Psychological disturbances Prognosis evaluation Osteochemonecrosis due to bisphosphonates
Pain and anxiety control		
– Local anaesthesia	1	Altered anatomy
– Conscious sedation	1	Compromised airway
– General anaesthesia	1	
Patient access and positioning		
– Access to dental office	0	
– Timing of treatment	0	
– Patient positioning	1	
Treatment modification		
– Oral surgery	2	Major indication Osteochemonecrosis due to bisphosphonates
– Implantology	2	Care if patient treated with bisphosphonates
– Conservative/Endodontics	1	
– Fixed prosthetics	1	
– Removable prosthetics	1	Maxillary obturator is recommended; mandibular reconstruction is mandatory
– Non-surgical periodontology	1	
– Surgical periodontology	2	Care if patient treated with bisphosphonates
Hazardous and contraindicated drugs	0	

*0 = No special considerations. 1 = Caution advised. 2 = Specialised medical advice recommended in some cases. 3 = Specialised medical advice mandatory. 4 = Only to be performed in hospital environment. 5 = Should be avoided.

remaining teeth. To achieve a functional prosthetic rehabilitation in patients with segmental mandibular resection, the defect has to be reconstructed using bone or a bone plate and a soft tissue flap (free or pedicle).

Implantology Osseointegrated dental implants provide retention and stability for prostheses, even in patients with extensive surgical defects. Implants may support obturators, overdentures, fixed bridges and facial prostheses. They can be inserted in normal bone, bone grafts, or even irradiated bone but, in the latter case, hyperbaric oxygen is recommended to enhance the success rate.

Further reading

● Bruins H H, Koole R, Jolly D E 1998 Pretherapy dental decisions in patients with head and neck cancer. A proposed model for dental decision support. Oral Surg Oral Med Oral Pathol Oral Radiol Endod 86:256–267 ● Diz Dios P, Castro Ferreiro M, Alvarez F J, Fernández Feijoo J 1994 Functional consequences of partial glossectomy. J Oral Maxillofac Surg 52:12–14 ● Diz Dios P, Wächter R, Fernández Feijoo J, Vázquez García E, Alvarez F J, Castro Ferreiro M 1998 The role of motivation in tumor patients with osseointegrated prosthesis. Cuidados Odontológicos Especiales 5:16–22 ● Frampton M 2001 Psychological distress in patients with head and neck cancer: review. Br J Oral Maxillofac Surg 39:67–70 ● McGuire D B 2003 Barriers and strategies in implementation of oral care standards for cancer patients. Support Care Cancer 11:435–441 ● Rankin K V 2000 Oral health in cancer therapy: evaluating and preventing oral complications. Dent Today 19:60–65 ● Wächter R, Diz Dios P, Einfluss B von 1993 Adaptation und Kompensationsmechanismen auf die postoperative Funktion bei Patienten mit Mundhölentumoren. Laryngo Rhino Otol 72:333–337.

CARDIAC ARRHYTHMIAS

Definition A cardiac arrhythmia is an alteration in the normal rhythm of the heartbeat.

General aspects

Aetiopathogenesis Most arrhythmias are the consequence of disorders in heart automaticity (impulse formation) or conductivity (block or delay). Causes include: ■ cardiac disease ■ drugs (caffeine, alcohol, smoking, beta-2-agonists, digoxin, dopa, tricyclics) ■ metabolic changes (hyperthyroidism) ■ electrolyte imbalance ■ chronic obstructive pulmonary disease ■ persistent vegetative neurological states.

Clinical presentation Palpitations are the most frequent symptom, followed by sickness, syncope, dyspnoea and anxiety.

Classification Disturbances of cardiac rhythm include: ■ bradycardia (slow rate) – causes include drugs (beta-blocker or digoxin), hypothyroidism, sinus dysfunction ■ tachycardia (fast rate) – may be narrow complex (supraventricular or atrial flutter/fibrillation) or broad complex (ventricular).

Diagnosis Diagnosis is usually made on electrocardiographic (ECG) findings. The electrode catheter technique for intracavitary monitoring may be especially useful in diagnosing conducting arrhythmias.

Treatment The treatment depends on type and severity of the arrhythmia (Table 3.25) and may include: ■ drugs ■ pacemaking (using a pacemaker or occasionally implantable cardioverter defibrillator, ICD) ■ external cardiac defibrillators, cardioversion or catheter ablation.

Drugs Drugs are used to control abnormal heart rhythms or treat related hypertension, coronary artery disease, and heart failure. Anticoagulants also may be given to reduce the risk of stroke in patients with some arrhythmias. Drugs used are mainly: ■ Class I drugs (act on sodium channels; disopyramide, flecainide, moracizine, procainamide, propafenone, quinidine) ■ Class II drugs (beta-blockers) ■ Class III drugs (act on potassium

Table 3.25 **Treatment of arrhythmias**

Heart rhythm changes	Treatment
Atrial fibrillation (AF)	Digoxin is the standard treatment Cardioversion Anticoagulants are advocated
Ventricular fibrillation (VF)	Defibrillation For acute VF, flecainide and disopyramide are indicated Lidocaine is the usual treatment but bretyllium, or mexilitine, may be required Implantable cardioverter defibrillators may be used
Extrasystoles	–
Sinus tachycardia	–
Atrial tachycardia	–
Ventricular tachycardia	Cardioversion Lidocaine
Paroxysmal supraventricular tachycardia	Vagal pressure or intravenous adenosine Cardiac glycosides or verapamil may be needed
Wolff–Parkinson–White syndrome	Medications or catheter ablation – to destroy the abnormal pathway
Torsades de pointes	Beta-blocker
Bradycardia (pathological)	Atropine may be indicated Bradycardia may need treatment with a pacemaker

channels; amiodarone, dofetilide, ibutilide, sotalol) ■ Class IV drugs (calcium channel blockers such as nifedipine, nicardipine or verapamil).

Pacemakers Pacemakers are small implanted electronic devices that stimulate the heart to beat, and 'pace' the rate when it is too slow (bradycardia). ■ Modern pacemakers are bipolar, implanted transvenously via the subclavian or cephalic vein, and typically located in the right ventricle or beneath the skin, on the chest wall or within the pectoral muscle, or in the abdominal wall ■ There is a wide variety of pacemakers; most modern ones work mainly on demand and are rate-adaptive, rather than continuous rate.

Implantable cardioverter defibrillators ICDs are electronic devices that are the most successful therapy to prevent ventricular fibrillation (99% effective in stopping life-threatening arrhythmias). Cardioversion is usually accomplished by a cardioverter device, which administers countershocks to the heart through electrodes placed on the chest wall or on or in the heart itself.

Catheter ablation Catheter ablation uses a burst of radiofrequency energy to destroy cardiac tissue that gives rise to the abnormal electrical signals causing arrhythmias.

Interference with pacemaking/defibrillation ■ High frequency, external electromagnetic radiation can interfere with the pacemaker sensing function of pacemakers and of implantable cardioverter defibrillators, and may induce fibrillation ■ Pacemakers can thus be disrupted by ionising radiation, ultrasonic, and electromagnetic interference (EMI) from a range of sources. The response of pacemakers to interference is varied, usually temporary and only seen while the patient remains within range of the source of interference. The response largely depends on the interference signal characteristics and includes a single beat inhibition (where the pacemaker may not pace the heart for a single cardiac cycle), total inhibition (where the pacemaker ceases to pace the heart), asynchronous pacing (where the pacemaker paces the heart at a fixed rate), rate rise, or erratic pacing. ■ Modern bipolar pacemakers have improved titanium-insulated interference-resistant circuitry, and thus the risk of electromagnetic interference is very small ■ The chief and real hazard to all pacemakers is with magnetic resonance imaging (MRI) because of static magnetic, alternating magnetic and radiofrequency (RF) fields produced by the MRI (Box 3.2) ■ Some dental electrical devices capable of generating electromagnetic radiation may pose a low-grade threat to dental patients but usually only if the devices are placed in close approximation to the pacemaker (Box 3.2) ■ Brief exposure of a pacemaker to electromagnetic anti-theft or surveillance devices, typically found in airports, shops and libraries, causes little, if any, disruption of function ■ An implanted ICD in contrast, will not only trigger airport security alarms but also, the use of strong magnets over the device may adversely affect its function and even render it non-operational ■ Digital mobile phones, and even television transmitters and faulty or badly earthed equipment, may cause interference – but the risk is very small and only when used in close proximity to the pacemaker ■ Domestic electrical appliances – remote controls, CB radios, electric blankets, heating pads, shavers, sewing machines, kitchen appliances, and microwave ovens – are safe ■ If a pacemaker does shut off, all possible sources of interference should be switched off and the patient given cardiopulmonary resuscitation in the supine position.

Prognosis Depends on type/severity of arrhythmia.

Oral findings

Several anti-arrhythmic drugs can cause oral lesions: ■ verapamil, enalapril and diltiazem may cause gingival swelling ■ some beta-blockers (e.g. propranolol) may rarely cause lichenoid ulceration and oral ulcers related

Box 3.2 Equipment used in oral health care and possible effects on cardiac pacemakers

May affect cardiac pacemakers
● Diathermy ● Electronic dental analgesia ● Electrosurgical units ● Ferromagnetic (magnetostrictive) scalers ● Lithotripsy ● Magnetic resonance imaging (MRI) ● Radiotherapy ● Transcutaneous electric nerve stimulation (TENS) ● Ultrasonography ● Ultrasonic instrument baths

Unlikely to affect cardiac pacemakers
● Electric toothbrushes ● Electronic apex locators ● Piezoelectric ultrasonic scalers ● Sonic scalers

to agranulocytosis ■ procainamide can cause a lupus-like reaction and mucosal ulcers due to agranulocytosis ■ disopyramide can produce xerostomia.

Dental management

Risk assessment Medical advice about type, severity and treatment of the arrhythmia is mandatory. High-risk patients with arrhythmias include those with: ■ symptoms ■ resting pulse >100 or <60 associated with any other arrhythmia ■ irregular pulse and bradycardia and wearing a pacemaker. High-risk patients and those with severe arrhythmias should have dental treatment in hospital.

The dental practitioner should evaluate the pulse, blood pressure and respiratory rate of all patients before starting any dental procedure. It is important to avoid stressful situations since they may trigger arrhythmias. Life-threatening cardiac arrhythmias are infrequent but, if it happens in the dental office, the dental practitioner should: ■ stop the dental procedure ■ evaluate vital signs ■ initiate cardiopulmonary resuscitation if indicated ■ administer oxygen ■ if there is chest pain, give sublingual nitroglycerine ■ call for medical assistance.

ICDs may activate without significant warning, potentially causing the patient to flinch, bite down, or perform other sudden movements that may result in injury to the patient or the clinician. Some patients with implanted defibrillators experience loss of consciousness when the device is activated. This is less likely to occur with newer devices that initially emit low level electrical bursts followed by stronger shocks if cardioversion does not occur immediately.

Pain and anxiety control **Local anaesthesia** ■ Adequate LA must be provided ■ Judicious use of local anaesthetics containing vasoconstrictors is desirable to obtain adequate anaesthesia for arrhythmic individuals, but the quantity of vasoconstrictor should be limited. Vasoconstrictors such as epinephrine or levonordefrin may increase blood pressure or lead to unanticipated atrial or ventricular arrhythmias, or even to fibrillation or asystole, and may adversely interact with digoxin, non-selective beta-adrenergic blocking drugs, antidepressants or cocaine. There appears to be no advantage or disadvantage to using levonordefrin as a substitute for epinephrine. ■ Epinephrine or other vasoconstrictors should be used with caution (reduced dose with careful monitoring) in patients with pacemakers and implanted cardioverter defibrillators ■ Mepivacaine 3% is preferable to lidocaine for use in patients taking beta-blockers ■ An aspirating syringe should be used to give the local anaesthetic ■ Intraosseous or intraligamentary injections with local anaesthetic agents containing vasoconstrictor should be avoided, in order to prevent excessive systemic absorption. **Conscious sedation** ■ Oral diazepam and nitrous oxide inhalation are useful to minimise stress ■ Oxygen saturation monitoring is recommended ■ In high-risk patients, anxious patients, and those where complex dental treatment has been planned, the dental treatment should be carried out in hospital. **General anaesthesia** Some general anaesthetic agents, especially halothane, may induce cardiac arrhythmias – particularly in the elderly (isoflurane is safer).

Patient access and positioning **Timing of treatment** Most sudden cardiac arrests occur during peak endogenous epinephrine levels in the early morning, and thus appointments are best made for late morning or early afternoon. **Patient positioning** Patients with pacemakers should be treated in the supine position, electrical equipment kept over 30 cm away, and repetitive switching of electrical instruments avoided.

Table 3.26 **Key considerations for dental management in cardiac arrhythmias (see text)**

	Management modifications*	Comments/possible complications
Risk assessment	3/4	Pulse, blood pressure and respiratory rate evaluation Avoid stress Emergency protocol Avoid electric devices in patients with a pacemaker
Pain and anxiety control		
– Local anaesthesia	1	Reduce epinephrine dose; epinephrine interacts with beta-blockers; avoid intraosseous and intraligamentary injections
– Conscious sedation	3/4	
– General anaesthesia	3/4	Avoid halothane
Patient access and positioning		
– Access to dental office	0	
– Timing of treatment	1	Late morning or early afternoon
– Patient positioning	1	Supine position; keep electrical equipment away
Treatment modification		
– Oral surgery	3	
– Implantology	3	
– Conservative/Endodontics	1	
– Fixed prosthetics	1	Avoid gingival retraction cords with epinephrine
– Removable prosthetics	1	
– Non-surgical periodontology	3	
– Surgical periodontology	3	
Imaging	1	MRI contraindicated in patients with a pacemaker
Hazardous and contraindicated drugs	1	Avoid erythromycin Some patients are anticoagulated

*0 = No special considerations. 1 = Caution advised. 2 = Specialised medical advice recommended in some cases. 3 = Specialised medical advice mandatory. 4 = Only to be performed in hospital environment. 5 = Should be avoided.

Treatment modification ■ Cardiac pacemakers these days usually have two (bipolar) electrode leads and present few problems for dental treatment ■ Unless a cardiac valve lesion is also present, patients with permanent pacemakers or implantable cardioverter defibrillators do not need antibiotic cover to prevent endocarditis. However, if a temporary transvenous pacemaker is present, the cardiologist or physician should be consulted. Diagnostic radiation and ultrasound have no effect on pacemakers – even with cumulative doses. ■ Some dental equipment may interfere with the pacemaker: ● electrosurgery, diathermy, transcutaneous nerve stimulation and magnetic resonance imaging are contraindicated ● the more modern piezoelectric scalers have no significant effect on pacemakers though activity rate responsive devices may exhibit increased pacing rates; dental equipment such as older piezoelectric ultrasonic scalers, ferromagnetic ultrasonic scalers, belt-driven motors in dental chairs, old X-ray machines and ultrasonic baths, pulp testers, electronic apex locators, and dental induction casting machines may occasionally cause pacemaker single beat inhibition of little consequence ● the only safe approach, however, is to avoid the use of all such equipment whenever a patient with a pacemaker is being treated, as it is difficult to assess the level of risk in any individual patient.

Fixed prosthetics and conservation Gingival retraction cords containing epinephrine should be avoided.

Imaging MRI is contraindicated in patients with cardiac pacemakers.

Drug use ■ Patients with atrial flutter may be treated with anticoagulants, which influence operative care ■ Erythromycin (but not clarithromycin) and azole antifungal drugs may induce arrhythmias, particularly in the elderly and patients with coronary artery disease or aortic stenosis taking pimozide, quinidine or terfenadine (or previously also cisapride or astemizole).

Further reading ● Rhodus N L, Little J W 2003 Dental management of the patient with cardiac arrhythmias: an update. Oral Surg Oral Med Oral Pathol Oral Radiol Endod 96:659–668 ● Scully, C, Roberts G, Shotts R 2001 The mouth in heart disease. Practitioner 245:432–437 ● Shibuya M, Kamekura N, Kimura Y, Fujisawa T, Fukushima K 2003 Clinical study of anesthetic management during dental treatment of 25 patients with cardiomyopathy. Spec Care Dentist 23:216–222.

CARDIAC FAILURE

Definition Cardiac failure manifests when the heart does not function efficiently as a pump, and cardiac output and blood pressure fail to meet the body's needs.

General aspects

Aetiopathogenesis ■ The main cause is myocardial disease (ischaemic heart disease, cardiomyopathy) (Box 3.3) ■ Other causes include: bradycardia, pulmonary disease, fluid overload or aortic stenosis.

Box 3.3 Main causes of heart failure

Left-sided mainly
• Ischaemic heart disease • Aortic valve disease • Mitral valve disease • Hypertension

Right-sided mainly
• Chronic obstructive pulmonary disease • Pulmonary embolism

Biventricular
• Ischaemic heart disease • Aortic valve disease • Mitral valve disease • Hypertension • Cardiomyopathies • Hyperthyroidism • Chronic anaemias • Arrhythmias

Clinical presentation ■ Features include: • left-sided heart failure results in damming of blood back from the left ventricle to the pulmonary circulation with consequent pulmonary hypertension and pulmonary oedema causing dyspnoea (orthopnoea), weakness, nocturnal cough and cold peripheries • right-sided heart failure manifests mainly with congestion of the systemic and portal venous systems affecting primarily the liver, gastrointestinal tract, kidneys and subcutaneous tissues and thus presenting with peripheral (dependent) oedema, ascites, nausea, anorexia and fatigue ■ Most patients eventually manifest biventricular failure since failure of one side of the heart usually leads to failure of the other.

Classification Heart failure has been graded (by the New York Heart Association; NYHA) as:

- Grade I: Asymptomatic
- Grade II: Slight limitation of physical activity
- Grade III: Marked limitation of physical activities
- Grade IV: Dyspnoea at rest.

Diagnosis Diagnosis is made based on clinical findings, echocardiography, ECG and chest radiography.

Treatment ■ Treat cause ■ Low salt diet ■ Diuretic (e.g. furosemide) ■ Angiotensin converting enzyme inhibitor (e.g. perindopril) ■ Beta-blocker (e.g. carvedilol).

Prognosis ■ Heart failure is usually progressive, but may cause few symptoms until activity becomes limited with breathlessness (dyspnoea), cyanosis and dependent oedema (usually swollen ankles) ■ Arrhythmias and sudden death may result.

Oral findings

■ ACE inhibitors can sometimes cause erythema multiforme, angioedema or burning mouth ■ Drugs used mainly in the past, which caused oral reactions, include procainamide (a lupus-like reaction) and acetazolamide (facial paraesthesia).

Dental management

Risk assessment ■ Dental treatment may precipitate arrhythmias or angina, or aggravate heart failure ■ Some drugs may complicate dental treatment, such as digitalis (causing vomiting) or ACE inhibitors (coughing) ■ Some patients may have liver dysfunction and thus a prolonged prothrombin time ■ Leucopenia is not unusual ■ Patients being treated with digoxin for atrial fibrillation or congestive heart failure are more prone to ECG changes such as ST segment depression during dental extractions under local anaesthesia than other cardiac patients ■ An episode of dyspnoea, anxiety, productive cough, or cyanosis may be indicative of acute pulmonary oedema – should this occur, the dental practitioner should: ● stop the dental procedure

Table 3.27 **Key considerations in dental management in cardiac failure (see text)**

	Management modifications*	Comments/possible complications
Risk assessment	3	Arrhythmias; angina; vomiting; coughing; leucopenia; bleeding tendency; emergency protocol
Appropriate dental care	3/4	
Pain and anxiety control		
– Local anaesthesia	1	Reduce epinephrine dose; epinephrine interacts with beta-blockers; avoid bupivacaine
– Conscious sedation	3/4	
– General anaesthesia	5	
Patient access and positioning		
– Access to dental office	0	
– Timing of treatment	1	Late morning
– Patient positioning	1	Upright position
Treatment modification		Grade of cardiac failure; cardiac monitoring
– Oral surgery	3	
– Implantology	3	
– Conservative/Endodontics	1	Avoid gingival retraction cords containing epinephrine
– Fixed prosthetics	1	
– Removable prosthetics	1	
– Non-surgical periodontology	3	
– Surgical periodontology	3	
Hazardous and contraindicated drugs	1	Avoid erythromycin, tetracycline, itraconazole, NSAIDs

*0 = No special considerations. 1 = Caution advised. 2 = Specialised medical advice recommended in some cases. 3 = Specialised medical advice mandatory. 4 = Only to be performed in hospital environment. 5 = Should be avoided.

● give oxygen ● maintain the dental chair in the erect position ● give 20 mg furosemide injection if available (hospital care only; medical assistance desirable) ● call for medical assistance.

Pain and anxiety control **Local anaesthesia** ■ An aspirating syringe should be used to give a local anaesthetic, since epinephrine in the anaesthetic given intravenously may (theoretically) increase hypertension and precipitate arrhythmias. Blood pressure tends to rise during oral surgery under local anaesthesia, and epinephrine theoretically can contribute to this – but this is usually of little practical importance. ■ Epinephrine-containing local anaesthetics should be avoided in patients taking beta-blockers. Interactions between epinephrine and the beta-blocking agent may induce hypertension and cardiovascular complications. ■ Bupivacaine should be avoided as it is cardiotoxic. **Conscious sedation** Conscious sedation can usually be used safely, providing that consideration is given to the underlying cause of the cardiac failure and the degree of failure. **General anaesthesia** General anaesthesia is contraindicated in cardiac failure until the failure is under control. Care should be taken after GA even in controlled patients, since there is a greater predisposition to venous thrombosis and pulmonary embolism.

Patient access and positioning **Timing of treatment** Appointments should be short. Recent evidence indicates that endogenous epinephrine levels peak during morning hours and adverse cardiac events are most likely in the early morning, so late morning appointments are recommended. **Patient positioning** It is dangerous to lay any patient with left-sided heart failure supine during dental treatment, since it may worsen dyspnoea. The dental chair should therefore be kept erect or in a partially reclining position. Drugs such as diuretics may cause orthostatic hypotension, and therefore the patient should be raised slowly to the upright position.

Treatment modification For all patients with cardiac failure: ■ Supplemental oxygen should be readily available ■ Cardiac monitoring may be desirable.

Dental care provision may need to be modified depending on the degree of compensation of the failure: ■ Mild controlled cardiac failure (Grades I or II): ● routine dental care can usually be provided with little modification apart from the need to minimise anxiety, and care to restrict use of vasoconstrictors ■ Poorly controlled or uncontrolled cardiac failure (increasing dyspnoea with minimal exertion, dyspnoea at rest, or nocturnal angina; Grades III or IV): ● medical advice should be obtained before any dental treatment ● elective dental treatment should be deferred until the condition has been stabilised with medical treatment ● emergency dental care should be conservative, principally consisting of the use of analgesics and antibiotics. **Fixed prosthetics and conservation** Gingival retraction cords containing epinephrine should be avoided.

Drug use ■ Erythromycin and tetracycline should be avoided in patients taking digitalis as they may induce toxicity by decreasing gut flora metabolism of the digitalis ■ Itraconazole may precipitate cardiac failure ■ NSAIDs other than aspirin should be avoided in patients taking ACE inhibitors since they increase the risk of renal damage.

Further reading ● Research, Science and Therapy Committee, American Academy of Periodontology 2002 Periodontal management of patients with cardiovascular diseases. J Periodontol 73:954–968 ● Rhodus N L, Falace D A 2002 Management of the dental patient with congestive heart failure. Gen Dent 50:260–265.

CEREBRAL PALSY

Definition Cerebral palsy (CP) is a generic term referring to abnormalities of motor control caused by damage to a child's brain early in the course of development, either in utero, during birth or in the first few months of infancy. It is the most common congenital physical handicap.

General aspects

Aetiopathogenesis The brain damage underlying CP is caused mainly by hypoxia, trauma, infection or hyperbilirubinaemia, but biochemical or genetic factors may be involved. Risk factors for CP include: ■ Antenatal: ● developmental abnormalities ● infections (CMV, rubella, toxoplasma, syphilis) ● hypoxaemia (placental haemorrhage, maternal hypotension) ● pre-eclamptic toxaemia ● irradiation ● maternal age < 20 or > 35 years ● twins ■ Natal: ● trauma ● breech delivery ● prolonged or precipitous delivery ● prematurity/postmaturity ■ Postnatal in preterm infants: ● cerebral ischaemia/haemorrhage ● hypoxaemia secondary to respiratory distress syndrome ● acidosis ● hypothermia ● hypoglycaemia ■ Postnatal in children with normal CNS at birth: ● encephalitis ● meningitis ● kernicterus ● trauma.

Clinical presentation ■ CP causes abnormalities of movement and posture (Table 3.28) ■ Up to 50% of patients with CP have additional disabilities: ● epilepsy ● defects of hearing ● defects of vision (accommodation defects, nystagmus or strabismus) ● defects of speech

Table 3.28 **Types of cerebral palsy**

Type	Subtype	Involves
Spastic	Monoplegic	Only one limb
	Paraplegic	Lower extremities
	Hemiplegic	One upper and lower limb on same side
	Double hemiplegic	All limbs, but mainly the arms
	Diplegic	All limbs, but mainly the legs
	Quadriplegic (tetraplegic)	All limbs equally
Athetoid	Athetosis	All limbs equally
	Chorea	
	Choreoathetosis	
Ataxic		
Rigid		
Mixed		

● emotional disturbances (depression) ● learning impairment; however, many patients with CP are highly intelligent (though severely impaired speech can mislead some unwary observers).

Classification CP types include (Table 3.28): ■ *Spastic* – the most common form (55%). It manifests with excessive muscle tone and contractures (Fig. 3.7), pathological reflexes and hyperactive tendon reflexes. ■ *Athetoid* – accounts for 20–25% of CP. It presents with smooth worm-like movements, which become exaggerated if the patient is anxious. ■ *Ataxic* – accounts for about 10% of all CP and is characterised by disturbance of balance.

Diagnosis Diagnosis is predominantly made from clinical signs such as: ■ delays in development of motor skills ■ weakness in one or more limbs

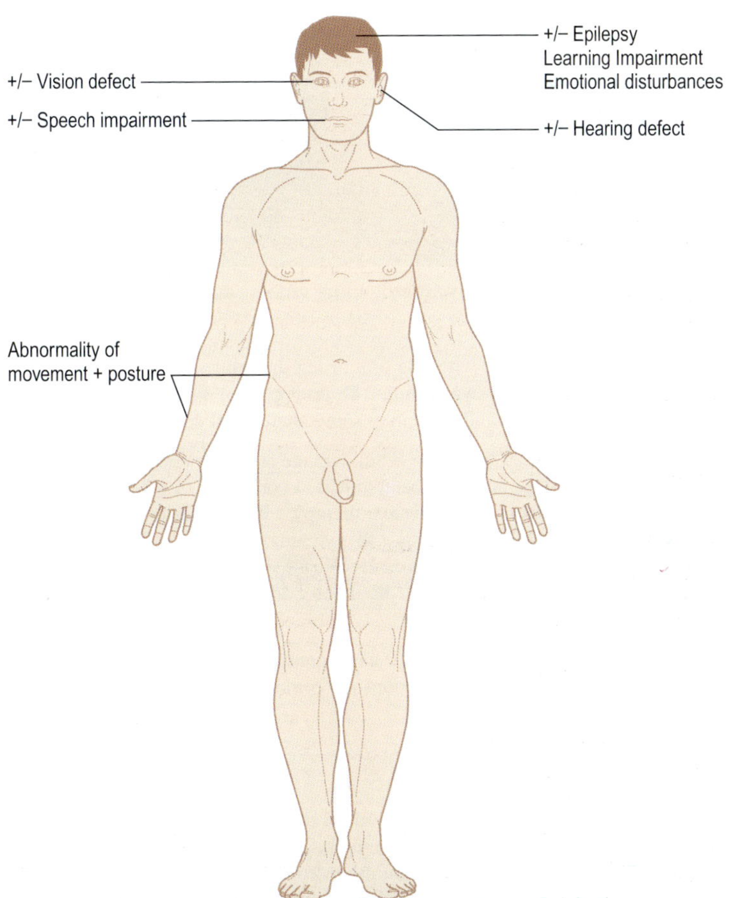

Figure 3.7 **Clinical presentation of cerebral palsy**

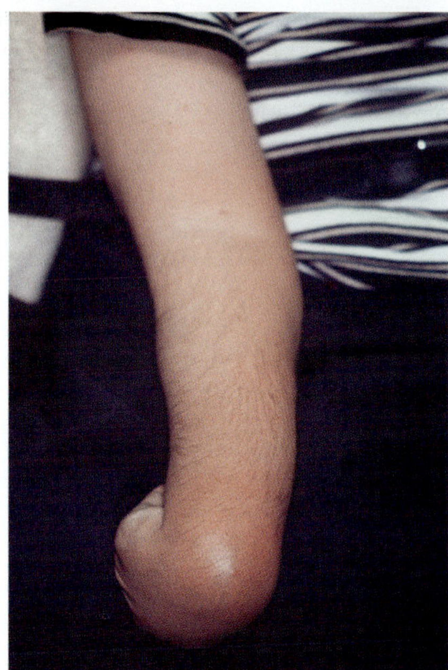

Figure 3.8 **Contracture in an individual with spastic cerebral palsy**

■ abnormal walking gait, with one foot or leg dragging ■ excessive drooling or difficulties in swallowing ■ poor control over hand and arm movement. Cerebral CT and MRI may show anatomical changes.

Treatment Although in CP the brain damage is irreversible, treatment involves a multidisciplinary approach aimed at correcting or stabilising some of the associated defects: ■ physical therapy ■ occupational therapy ■ speech therapy ■ hearing aids ■ eye aids or surgery ■ joint surgery ■ medications such as muscle relaxants to ease muscle stiffness and anticonvulsants to reduce seizures ■ dietary advice ■ special education/ equipment may be required.

Prognosis Life expectancy in CP has increased significantly in the last decades. However, respiratory infections are common, and aspiration pneumonia is a major cause of death.

Oral findings

■ Drooling, mainly caused by poor control of the oral tissues and head posture, although an impaired swallowing reflex has also been observed. Scopolamine patches can help to minimise drooling, as can Botox injections, and salivary duct repositioning. ■ Malocclusion is common and thought to be caused by abnormal muscle tone and behaviour. The maxillary arch is frequently tapered or ovoid, with a high palate. The upper teeth are often labially inclined, due to the pressure of the tongue against the anterior teeth during abnormal swallowing. Most, however, have skeletal patterns within normal limits, although there is an association of a Class II, division 2 skeletal pattern with spastic CP, and Class II, division 1 pattern with choreoathetoid CP. ■ Bruxism and abnormal attrition are common; spontaneous dislocation or subluxation of the temporomandibular joint may be seen ■ Periodontal disease is common, with extensive calculus deposits present, often exacerbated by a soft diet ■ There may be delayed eruption of the primary dentition and enamel hypoplasia is common.

Dental management

Risk assessment Dental management considerations include: ■ access difficulties (some individuals are wheelchair users) ■ uncontrollable movements, mainly in athetosis ■ communication difficulties, which may give a misleading impression of low intelligence ■ although some patients are very cooperative, in others who have learning disability cooperation may be very poor ■ epilepsy is not uncommon – a stressful situation may give rise to a seizure ■ abnormal biting reflex – inserting a mouth prop at the beginning of the procedure may help ■ abnormal swallowing and cough reflex present a hazard to the airway.

Preventive dentistry In cerebral palsy, preventive dental care is important. Parental counselling about diet, oral hygiene procedures and the use of fluorides should be started early.

Pain and anxiety control **Local anaesthesia** There are no contraindications regarding the use of local anaesthetic agents, although access may be limited in some patients. **Conscious sedation** Anxiety may worsen athetosis or spasticity, or precipitate an epileptic fit. Hence, anxiolytic and muscle relaxant drugs such as diazepam are useful as premedication. Sedation is also useful to reduce nausea and lingual dystonia. In patients taking neuroleptic drugs, and in those with respiratory difficulties, consultation with the patient's physician is recommended. **General anaesthesia** In some patients, because of uncontrollable movements or poor cooperation, dental treatment has to be carried out under general anaesthesia. During and after GA, special consideration should be taken of the: ■ propensity for gastro-oesophageal reflux ■ poor laryngeal and pharyngeal reflexes ■ liability to aspirate material into the lungs ■ increased risk of hypothermia.

Patient access and positioning **Access to dental surgery** Patients restricted to wheelchairs can sometimes be treated in their chair, particularly if there are facilities to tilt the wheelchair back slightly. Alternatively, the patient may be transferred to the dental chair by hoist, or by carrying them or by sliding them across a board placed between the wheelchair and dental chair. **Timing of treatment** Short appointments are advisable. **Patient positioning** Manual support is often required, although this must be provided with the patient's consent. Although some ataxic patients prefer to have the chair tilted backwards, others become apprehensive when this is done, resulting in increased movements.

Treatment modification Each patient must be assessed on an individual basis to ensure that treatment modifications are tailored to their needs. In particular: ■ treatment planning must consider the decreased control and function of the upper extremities and limited motor skills ■ the use of Makaton vocabulary or flip charts may improve communication with some patients ■ the preventive dental programme may require involvement of family member, partner or care provider ■ avoid preoperative mouthwashes (antimicrobials better administered as a gel or spray) ■ use rubber dam where possible (in view of drooling) ■ powerful aspiration is needed ■ the dental chair should be moved slowly to prevent spastic muscle responses; muscle relaxants can be of benefit.

Table 3.29 **Key considerations in dental management in cerebral palsy (see text)**

	Management modifications*	Comments/possible complications
Risk assessment	2/4	Uncontrollable movements; epilepsy; abnormal biting reflex and swallowing
Pain and anxiety control		
– Local anaesthesia	1	
– Conscious sedation	2	
– General anaesthesia	3/4	Gastro-oesophageal reflux; poor laryngeal reflex; aspiration possible; hypothermia.
Patient access and positioning		
– Access to dental office	1	Transfer to dental chair
– Timing of treatment	1	Short appointments
– Patient positioning	1	Manual support; tilt backwards
Treatment modification		
– Oral surgery	1/4	Possibly GA
– Implantology	1/4	Possibly GA
– Conservative/Endodontics	1/4	Possibly GA
– Fixed prosthetics	1/4	Possibly GA
– Removable prosthetics	1/5	Difficult to insert and stabilise
– Non-surgical periodontology	1/4	Possibly GA
– Surgical periodontology	1/4	Possibly GA
Hazardous and contraindicated drugs	0	

*0 = No special considerations. 1 = Caution advised. 2 = Specialised medical advice recommended in some cases. 3 = Specialised medical advice mandatory. 4 = Only to be performed in hospital environment. 5 = Should be avoided.

Preventive dentistry Manual dexterity is usually poor but favourable results are often achievable with an electric toothbrush or a modified handle to the normal brush. Most dental disease is more common when the arms are severely involved. In these cases, periodic professional tooth cleaning is mandatory. **Surgery** Surgical procedures may be dangerous if the patient has uncontrollable movements. In such cases, GA may be indicated. **Implantology** Dental implants may be useful, but the surgical phase usually has to be performed under GA. The success will be influenced by the ability to maintain adequate oral hygiene long term. **Fixed prosthetics and conservation** Removable prostheses can be difficult to insert and use. Thus, it is important to conserve the remaining natural teeth, and fixed prostheses are the treatments of choice. Epilepsy and ataxia are usually contraindications for removable prostheses. Tooth wear may need treatment. **Periodontology** Periodontal disease is common, because soft tissue movement is abnormal and oral cleansing is impaired. Mouth breathing worsens the periodontal state. A papillary hyperplastic gingivitis may be seen, even in the absence of treatment with phenytoin. Early treatment is then recommended. Antiseptics such as chlorhexidine can be applied more effectively as a gel or spray rather than a mouthwash. **Orthodontics** Abnormal muscle behaviour and oral breathing may produce malocclusion and impair the prognosis of orthodontic treatment. In a few cases, palatal expansion and retraction of anterior teeth are possible with fixed appliances, but recurrence is common. **Paediatric dentistry** There may be delayed eruption of the primary dentition and enamel hypoplasia is common. Caries activity is usually normal, but may remain untreated, particularly in primary teeth. This leads to premature loss of primary teeth, and earlier eruption of premolars and permanent canines.

Further reading • Griffiths J 2002 Guidelines for oral health care for people with a physical disability. J Disability Oral Health 3:51–58 • Loyola-Rodriguez J P, Aguilera-Morelos A A, Santos-Diaz M A et al 2004 Oral rehabilitation under dental general anesthesia, conscious sedation, and conventional techniques in patients affected by cerebral palsy. J Clin Pediatr Dent 28:279–284 • Rodrigues dos Santos M T, Masiero D, Novo N F, Simionato M R 2003 Oral conditions in children with cerebral palsy. J Dent Child (Chic) 70:40–46 • http://www.scope.org.uk/helpline/faq.shtml

CHEMOTHERAPY PATIENTS

Definition Cytotoxic chemotherapy drugs act mainly by interaction with the cancer cell DNA or RNA, to inhibit cell division and/or protein synthesis.

General aspects

Indications Chemotherapy is used especially in the treatment of lymphoproliferative diseases (leukaemias and lymphomas) and in conditioning for bone marrow (haematopoietic stem cell) transplantation.

Classification Cytotoxic agents include (Box 3.4): ■ Alkylating agents – DNA-damaging agents, such as chlorambucil, cyclophosphamide or melphalan, which damage DNA so severely that the cancer cell dies ■ Antibiotics (including anthracyclines) – these, such as daunorubicin, doxorubicin, idarubicin and mitoxantrone, insert themselves into the cancer cell DNA, prevent it from functioning normally and often kill the cancer cell ■ Enzyme inhibitors – camptothecin binds irreversibly to DNA–topoisomerase complex, inducing cell death ■ Antimetabolites – methotrexate, fludarabine, and cytarabine mimic substances that the cancer cell needs to synthesise normal DNA and RNA ■ Mitotic inhibitors – vincristine or vinblastine damage cancer cells by blocking mitosis; the taxanes, a group of drugs that includes paclitaxel and docetaxel, stop microtubules from breaking down and thus prevent cancer cells growing and dividing ■ DNA-repair enzyme inhibitors – etoposide or topotecan attack the DNA repair mechanisms.

Other cancer drugs: ■ Various hormones are used to control some tumours, especially in the case of breast (ethinyloestradiol, medroxyprogesterone, norethisterone or megestrol) and prostate cancers (diethylstilboestrol, fosfestrol) ■ Hormone antagonists are used in some tumours, such as breast (tamoxifen, toremifene, aminoglutethimide, anastrozole, letrozole, exemestane, trilostane, goserelin) and prostate cancers (buserelin, goserelin, leuprorelin, triptorelin, cyproterone acetate, flutamide, bicalutamide) ■ Antibodies made specifically to attach to cancer cells and linked to a toxin or radioactive substance can kill the cell ■ Gene therapy is being developed to replace damaged tumour suppressor genes, or otherwise influence cell activity.

Complications Most cytotoxic agents can cause complications by killing other rapidly dividing cells, particularly if treatment is prolonged or in high dosage, causing: ■ alopecia ■ bone marrow suppression (leading to a

Box 3.4 Drugs used in the treatment of malignant disease

Cytotoxic agents
● Alkylating agents ● Topoisomerase 1 inhibitors ● Cytotoxic antibiotics ● Antimetabolites ● Mitotic inhibitors

Sex hormones and antagonists
For breast carcinoma
● Tamoxifen ● Toremifene ● Progestogens

For prostate carcinoma
● Oestrogen ● Cyproterone ● Flutamide ● Bicalutamide ● Gonadotrophin releasing hormone analogues (buserelin, goserelin, leuprorelin, triptorelin)

Aromatase inhibitors
● Aminoglutethimide ● Anastrozole ● Formestan ● Letrozole

Somatostatin analogues
● Laureotide ● Octreotide

Recombinant interleukin-2
● Aldesleukin

bleeding tendency and liability to infections) and hyperuricaemia; allopurinol may be required ■ mucositis; approximately 90% of children and 50% of adults develop severely painful oral lesions (Table 3.30) ■ nausea and vomiting ■ reproductive function suppression, especially in males; alkylating drugs can cause permanent male sterility.

Oral findings

The most common findings are: ■ mucositis ■ infections ■ bleeding ■ xerostomia ■ craniofacial maldevelopment. When combined cytotoxic chemotherapy and radiotherapy are given, orofacial complications are especially likely.

Mucositis

- Chemotherapy-induced mucositis is characterised by erythema, ulceration and pain, which significantly affects quality of life. It is helpful to score the degree of mucositis in order to monitor progression and therapy (Box 3.5).
- Mucositis typically appears from 7 to 14 days after the initiation of drug therapy, is seen in most patients treated with fluorouracil and cisplatin, but also after use of many other agents.
- Mucositis may be a predictor of gastrointestinal toxicity and hepatic veno-occlusive disease and, in the presence of neutropenia, predisposes to septicaemia.
- There is benefit in prophylaxis and treatment of mucositis from use of: ● ice chips for 30 minutes before administration of 5-fluorouracil (5FU), methotrexate or melphalan ● folinic acid (as calcium folinate), levofolinic acid or disodium folinate before administration of methotrexate or fluorouracil.
- Other approaches include use of: ● biological response modifiers; various cytokines such as interleukin-1, interleukin-11, TGF-beta 3 and keratinocyte growth factor ● anti-inflammatory medications ● colony-stimulating factors – granulocyte macrophage (GM-CSF) and granulocyte (G-CSF) ● thalidomide – an angiogenesis-inhibiting drug ● cytoprotective agents (primarily free radical scavengers or antioxidants, such as amifostine, N-acetyl cysteine and vitamin E).
- Mucositis often necessitates the use of: ● opioid analgesics for pain control ● special diet (Box 3.6) or tube feeding ● good oral hygiene with twice-daily 0.2% aqueous chlorhexidine mouth rinses ● viscous 2% lidocaine or benzydamine rinse or spray can help lessen discomfort, and is particularly helpful before food ● prophylaxis for infectious complications.

Infections

- Oral candidosis is common, usually caused by *Candida albicans* or, less often, by other *Candida* species. Oral mucormycosis (phycomycosis) or aspergillosis are rare. Risk factors include leucopenia and the use of antibiotics. Nystatin suspension (100000U/mL) as a mouthwash or pastilles four to six times daily, may be given prophylactically. Avoid the

Table 3.30 **Main chemotherapeutic agents responsible for oral mucositis**

Alkylating agents	Anthracyclines	Antibiotics	Antimetabolites	Taxanes	Microtubule disassemblers
Busulphan	Daunorubicin	Actinomycin D	Cytosine arabinoside	Docetaxel	Etoposide
Cyclophosphamide	Doxorubicin	Amsacrine	5-Fluorouracil	Paclitaxel	Vinblastine
Mechlorethamine	Epirubicin	Bleomycin	Hydroxycarbamide		Vincristine
Melphalan		Dactinomycin	Methotrexate		Vinorelbine
Procarbazine		Daunorubicin	6-Mercaptopurine		
Thiotepa		Doxorubicin Mithromycin Mitomycin Mitoxantrone	Tioguanine		

Note: Oral ulceration can be a complication of virtually any cancer chemotherapeutic agent but is most common in these groups. Most of these agents also depress the bone marrow, leading to a tendency to infection and a bleeding state.

Box 3.5 WHO Mucositis scale (WHO 1979)

Grade	Clinical features
0	–
1	Soreness/erythema
2	Erythema, ulcers but able to eat solids
3	Ulcers but requires liquid diet
4	Oral alimentation not possible

Box 3.6 Diet in oral mucositis

Diet that is typically acceptable
● Liquids ● Purees ● Ice ● Custards ● Non-acidic fruits (banana, mango, melon, peach) ● Soft cheeses ● Eggs

Foods etc to avoid
● Rough food (potato chips, crisps, toast) ● Spices ● Salt ● Acidic fruit (grapefruit, lemon, orange)

Lifestyle habits to avoid
● Smoking ● Alcohol

use of pastilles or lozenges as these are not well tolerated when there is concurrent mucositis.

- Herpetic infections (herpes simplex or herpes zoster) are common and may cause chronic skin or oral ulcers. Aciclovir or valaciclovir prophylactically have lowered the incidence of herpes infections and mortality from zoster.
- Gram-negative oral infections due to *Pseudomonas*, *Klebsiella*, *Escherichia*, *Enterobacter*, *Serratia* or *Proteus* may develop and spread rapidly. Gram-negative infections may need treatment with gentamicin or carbenicillin as the oral lesions can be portals for systemic spread.

Bleeding Drug-induced thrombocytopenia may cause a bleeding tendency, presenting as gingival bleeding, mucosal petechiae or ecchymoses.

Xerostomia Xerostomia can follow chemotherapy (especially with doxorubicin), and can lead to caries and other oral infections.

Craniofacial maldevelopment In children, chemotherapy can delay development or cause abnormalities in craniofacial skeleton, jaws and dentition.

Dental management

Risk assessment Dental screening should be undertaken prior to commencement of chemotherapy and the patient's oral health stabilised. During chemotherapy, only emergency dental treatment should be performed. Precautions should be taken in relation to the type of blood cell deficit present (Table 3.31).

Table 3.31 **Dental treatment for patients on cytotoxic chemotherapy**

Blood cell type	Peripheral blood count	Precautions
Platelets	>50 × 10^9/L	Routine management, though desmopressin or platelets are required to cover surgery
	<50 × 10^9/L	Platelets needed for any invasive procedures*
Granulocytes	>2 × 10^9/L	Routine management
	<2 × 10^9/L	Prophylactic antimicrobials for surgery
Erythrocytes	>5 × 10^{12}/L	Routine management
	<5 × 10^{12}/L	Special care with general anaesthesia

*Any procedure where bleeding is possible.

In patients with herpes simplex antibodies, the prophylactic administration of aciclovir (200 mg three times a day) before any dental procedure has been suggested, to try to avoid any recurrence of the infection.

Pain and anxiety control **Local anaesthesia** There are no contraindications regarding the use of local anaesthetic agents, although the underlying disease process and side effects of therapy may need to be considered. **Conscious sedation** This should be used with caution, as the underlying disease process and side effects of therapy may need to be considered (e.g. anaemia, thrombocytopenia). **General anaesthesia** GA should be avoided in patients with severe anaemia.

Treatment modification Dental treatment preferably should be carried out in the day(s) before starting a new cytotoxic treatment cycle. Complex dental treatment is not indicated in patients with a poor prognosis (related to the underlying disease). **Preventive dentistry** There should be close attention to oral hygiene and preventive dentistry before, during and after chemotherapy. Caries prevention can be achieved by dietary control, sealant and fluoride application, and close review.

In patients with bleeding gingivae, aids such as interdental sticks, irrigating devices and dental floss should be avoided. During the acute phase, the toothbrush is better replaced by sponge-sticks/gauze soaked in chlorhexidine to clean the teeth.

Surgery Extractions and any other surgery should be completed before cytotoxic treatment. The need for extraction of partially erupted permanent teeth should be evaluated, as the risk of pericoronitis is increased. **Implantology** There is little evidence that cancer chemotherapy influences the success of implants in the long term. **Endodontics** Suspicious dental or periapical lesions should be treated early. Endodontics should be completed before chemotherapy. Where this is not possible, extractions may need to be considered. **Removable prostheses** Dentures should not be worn at night. Patients with moderate or severe mucositis should not wear their dental

Table 3.32 **Key considerations for dental management in chemotherapy (see text)**

	Management modifications*	Comments/possible complications
Risk assessment	3	Dental screening; bleeding tendency; infection
Pain and anxiety control		
– Local anaesthesia	1	
– Conscious sedation	1	
– General anaesthesia	3–5	Avoid in severe anaemia
Patient access and positioning		
– Access to dental office	0	
– Timing of treatment	0	
– Patient positioning	0	
Treatment modification		
– Oral surgery	2	Complete before starting a new cycle; single procedures; evaluate partially erupted teeth
– Implantology	2	Complete before chemotherapy; avoid during mucositis
– Conservative/Endodontics	1	
– Fixed prosthetics	1	
– Removable prosthetics	1	
– Non-surgical periodontology	2	Complete before chemotherapy
– Surgical periodontology	2	Complete before chemotherapy
Hazardous and contraindicated drugs	1	Avoid aspirin

*0 = No special considerations. 1 = Caution advised. 2 = Specialised medical advice recommended in some cases. 3 = Specialised medical advice mandatory. 4 = Only to be performed in hospital environment. 5 = Should be avoided.

prosthesis at all until the mucosa has healed. **Periodontology** Periodontal status should be evaluated and periodontal disease controlled before chemotherapy. Treatment has to be early and teeth of doubtful prognosis extracted. **Orthodontics** Orthodontic bands and appliances that contribute to poor oral hygiene or mucosal irritation should be removed before cytotoxic treatment. **Paediatric dentistry** Mobile primary teeth and any gingival operculum should be removed before starting chemotherapy.

Drug use Aspirin should not be given to patients on methotrexate as it may enhance toxicity.

Further reading

● Barker G J 1999 Current practices in the oral management of the patient undergoing chemotherapy or bone marrow transplantation. Support Care Cancer 7:17–20 ● Barker G J, Epstein J B, Williams K B, Gorsky M, Raber-Durlacher J E 2005 Current practice and knowledge of oral care for cancer patients: a survey of supportive health care providers. Support Care Cancer 13:32–41 ● Sonis S T 2004 Oral mucositis in cancer therapy. J Support Oncol 2:3–8.

CHRISTMAS DISEASE (HAEMOPHILIA B)

Definition ■ Christmas disease (so-called after the last name of the person first described with the disease) is a congenital bleeding disorder due to a defect in blood coagulation factor IX ■ Haemophilia B is about one-tenth as common as haemophilia A except in some Asian populations, where frequencies are almost equal ■ Female carriers of haemophilia B (unlike haemophilia A) often have a mild bleeding tendency.

General aspects (see also Haemophilia A)

Aetiopathogenesis Christmas disease is sex-linked inherited (the gene which expresses factor IX is located on chromosome 10).

Clinical presentation ■ Christmas disease is clinically identical to haemophilia A, with musculoskeletal problems arising from haemarthroses, and complications resulting from multiple transfusions (though the prevalence of HIV infection is lower than in patients with haemophilia A) ■ The severity of clinical findings depends on the degree of factor IX deficiency.

Classification The classification depends on the percentage of Factor IX present:

- Mild: > 5% of the normal value
- Moderate: between 1 and 5%
- Severe: < 1%.

Diagnosis ■ Prolonged partial thromboplastin time, with normal prothrombin and bleeding times ■ Factor IX deficit.

Treatment ■ Synthetic Factor IX is used for replacement therapy before interventive procedures; it is more stable than Factor VIII, with a half-life of 18 hours but often up to 2 days, so that replacement therapy can usually be given at longer intervals than in haemophilia A ■ Prothrombin complex (contains Factor II, VII, IX and X) may also be administered ■ Desmopressin (DDAVP) is not useful in Christmas disease.

Oral findings

Oral findings are similar to those observed in haemophilia A.

Dental management

■ Most comments on the dental management in haemophilia A apply equally to patients with haemophilia B ■ Consultation with the haematologist is mandatory ■ A dose of 20 units Factor IX per kg body weight is used intravenously 1 hour preoperatively prior to procedures associated with bleeding.

Table 3.33 **Key considerations for dental management in Christmas disease (see text)**

	Management modifications*	Comments/possible complications
Risk assessment	3	Haemorrhage; hazards of anaesthesia; hepatitis, liver disease, HIV infection; anxiety
Appropriate dental care	3/4	Factor replacement; tranexamic acid
Pain and anxiety control		
– Local anaesthesia	2	Avoid regional blocks and lingual infiltrations
– Conscious sedation	2	
– General anaesthesia	3/4	Avoid nasal intubation
Patient access and positioning		
– Access to dental office	1	Joint involvement
– Timing of treatment	1	1 h after
– Patient positioning	1	factor replacement
Treatment modification		
– Oral surgery	3/4	Factor replacement; minimal trauma; topical haemostatic agents; avoid catgut
– Implantology	4	Factor replacement; minimal trauma; topical haemostatic agents; avoid catgut
– Conservative/Endodontics	2	Local bleeding; intracanal LA with epinephrine
– Fixed prosthetics	2	Local bleeding
– Removable prosthetics	1	
– Non-surgical periodontology	2	Factor replacement; topical haemostatic agents
– Surgical periodontology	3/4	Factor replacement; minimal trauma; topical haemostatic agents; avoid catgut
Imaging	1	Do not rest radiographs on the floor of the mouth
Hazardous and contraindicated drugs	2	Avoid aspirin, indometacin and other NSAIDs; avoid intramuscular injections

*0 = No special considerations. 1 = Caution advised. 2 = Specialised medical advice recommended in some cases. 3 = Specialised medical advice mandatory. 4 = Only to be performed in hospital environment. 5 = Should be avoided.

Further reading ● Brewer A K, Roebuck E M, Donachie M et al 2003 The dental management of adult patients with hemophilia and other congenital bleeding disorders. Haemophilia 9:673–677 ● Ehl S, Severin T, Sutor A H 2000 DDAVP (desmopressin; 1-deamino-cys-8-D-arginine-vasopressin) treatment in children with haemophilia B.

Br J Haematol 111:1260–1262 ● Stubbs M, Lloyd J 2001 A protocol for the dental management of von Willebrand's disease, haemophilia A and haemophilia B. Aust Dent J 46:37–40.

CHRONIC OBSTRUCTIVE PULMONARY DISEASE (COPD)

Definition COPD is a chronic, progressive, essentially irreversible, airway obstruction. It consists of either or both: ■ *chronic bronchitis*, defined as a cough productive of sputum on most days for 3 months of 2 successive years ■ *emphysema*, defined as an enlargement of distal airspaces.

General aspects

Aetiopathogenesis ■ Caused mainly by smoking ■ Other factors such as environmental contamination, respiratory infections, and familial predisposition (e.g. alpha-1-antitrypsin deficit) may also be involved.

Clinical presentation Features include: ■ cough ■ sputum ■ dyspnoea ■ wheeze ■ possibly respiratory failure or cor pulmonale.

Diagnosis ■ Lung function tests (forced expiratory volume and forced vital capacity) impaired ■ Arterial blood gases – PaO_2 lowered.

Treatment ■ Controlled oxygen therapy ■ Bronchodilators (e.g. salbutamol, ipratropium and theophylline) ± antimicrobials ± corticosteroids.

Oral findings

■ Most patients are predisposed to tobacco-associated oral lesions ■ Xerostomia is common in mouth breathers ■ Ipratropium may cause dry mouth ■ Theophylline rarely produces erythema multiforme.

Dental management

Risk assessment Patients have been classified for dental treatment into ■ Low risk: ● dyspnoea on effort but with normal blood gases ● all dental treatment can be performed normally ■ Moderate risk: ● dyspnoea on effort, chronically treated with bronchodilators or recently with corticosteroids ● PaO_2 lowered ● medical consultation is advised before any dental treatment ■ High risk: ● symptomatic COPD with undiagnosed and untreated disease ● medical consultation is essential before any dental treatment.

Pain and anxiety control **Local anaesthesia** ■ Local anaesthesia is the preferred method for dental treatment ■ Avoid bilateral mandibular and palatal LA ■ In patients who also have coronary heart disease or hypertension the use of epinephrine should be limited.
Conscious sedation ■ In patients with chronic CO_2 retention, oxygen administration may produce respiratory depression; hence, nitrous oxide

Table 3.34 **Key considerations for dental management in chronic obstructive pulmonary disease (see text)**

	Management modifications*	Comments/possible complications
Risk assessment	1–3	Conditioned by severity of disease
Pain and anxiety control		
– Local anaesthesia	1	Reduce epinephrine dose; avoid bilateral mandibular and palatal anaesthesia
– Conscious sedation	3/4	Avoid benzodiazepines and nitrous oxide
– General anaesthesia	3–5	Stop smoking; eradicate infections; postoperative complications
Patient access and positioning		
– Access to dental office	0	
– Timing of treatment	1	Short appointments
– Patient positioning	1	Upright position
Treatment modification		
– Oral surgery	1	
– Implantology	1	
– Conservative/Endodontics	1	Rubber dam may not be tolerated
– Fixed prosthetics	1	
– Removable prosthetics	1	
– Non-surgical periodontology	1	
– Surgical periodontology	1	
Hazardous and contraindicated drugs	2	Antibiotic selection; avoid drugs interacting with theophylline; some patients receive corticosteroids

*0 = No special considerations. 1 = Caution advised. 2 = Specialised medical advice recommended in some cases. 3 = Specialised medical advice mandatory. 4 = Only to be performed in hospital environment. 5 = Should be avoided.

should be avoided in patients with emphysema and in those with moderate or severe COPD ■ Diazepam and midazolam are mild respiratory depressants and should not be used for intravenous sedation in COPD by the dentist ■ If intravenous sedation is absolutely necessary, it should only be undertaken in hospital, after full preoperative assessment by a specialist.
General anaesthesia ■ Patients with COPD should be given a GA only if absolutely necessary, and only after full preoperative assessment by an anaesthetist ■ Intravenous barbiturates, morphine and atropine are totally contraindicated ■ Many anaesthetists suggest that it is safest to avoid premedication ■ The most important single factor in preoperative care is cessation of smoking for at least 1 week preoperatively. Respiratory infections must also be eradicated. Thorough and frequent chest physiotherapy is

important preoperatively and, if there is congestive cardiac failure, diuretics are indicated ■ Secretions reduce airway patency, and if lightly anaesthetised the patient may cough and contaminate other areas of the lung ■ Postoperative respiratory complications are more prevalent in patients with pre-existing lung diseases, especially after prolonged operations ■ Pethidine can be used if the patient is in pain ■ Secondary polycythaemia may predispose to thromboses postoperatively.

Patient access and positioning **Timing of treatment** Short appointments are recommended. **Patient positioning** Patients with COPD are best treated in the upright position since they may become increasingly breathless if laid flat.

Treatment modification Treatment planning may need to be modified if there is a persistent cough and/or dyspnoea, as lengthy or complex procedures may not be practical. It may be difficult to use a rubber dam as patients with COPD may not tolerate the additional obstruction to breathing.

Drug use ■ Patients taking corticosteroids should be treated with appropriate precautions (see Steroids) ■ Interactions of theophylline with drugs such as epinephrine, erythromycin, clindamycin, azithromycin, clarithromycin or ciprofloxacin may result in dangerously high levels of theophylline ■ Antimicrobials should be carefully selected in patients on prolonged antibiotic therapy; antihistamines are contraindicated because they dry the respiratory mucosa and increase mucus adherence.

Further reading ● Foley N M 2000 Chronic obstructive pulmonary disease. SAAD Dig 17:3–12 ● Scannapieco F A, Bush R B, Paju S 2003 Associations between periodontal disease and risk for nosocomial bacterial pneumonia and chronic obstructive pulmonary disease. A systematic review. Ann Periodontol 8:54–69.

COCAINE ABUSE (SEE ALSO AMPHETAMINE, LSD & ECSTASY ABUSE)

Definition ■ Cocaine is a powerfully addictive drug of misuse derived from the plant *Erythroxylon coca*, considered the most potent stimulant of natural origin ■ Pure cocaine was first used in the 1880s in ophthalmology and dentistry because of its ability to provide anaesthesia as well as to constrict blood vessels and limit bleeding. These applications are now obsolete due to the development of safer drugs.

General aspects

Pathogenesis Cocaine has profound and almost immediate effects on the CNS, potentiates catecholamines and interferes with dopamine reabsorption.

Clinical presentation The most significant risks from drug abuse are behavioural disturbances and psychoses. Intravenous use of these drugs is further complicated by the risk of transmission of infections (HIV, hepatitis B, C, D and others), infective endocarditis, or septicaemia. ■ Findings that may indicate a drug addiction problem are as for amphetamine/LSD/MDMA abuse ■ Other common signs are: ● dilated pupils ● needle tracks or abscesses (wearing long sleeves when inappropriate) ■ Drug-abuse associated diseases: ● psychosis ● tachycardia (common with cocaine use).

Classification ■ 'Crack' is the street name given to cocaine that has been processed from cocaine with ammonia or sodium bicarbonate (baking soda) and water and heated to remove the hydrochloride to a free-base for smoking. The term 'crack' refers to the crackling sound heard when it is smoked (heated), presumably from the sodium bicarbonate. ■ The major routes of use of cocaine (including the hydrochloride and free-base or crack cocaine) are snorting, injecting or smoking ■ Immediate euphoric effects appear in less than 5 minutes and include hyperstimulation, reduced fatigue, and mental clarity. Cocaine misuse is characterised by feelings of wellbeing and heightened mental activity. ■ Large doses of cocaine cause paranoia, visual hallucinations (snowlights) and tactile hallucinations. The latter are typically of insects crawling over the skin ('cocaine bugs'). Smoking crack cocaine can produce a particularly aggressive paranoid behaviour in users. ■ Physical effects of cocaine use also mimic those of catecholamines, and include constricted peripheral blood vessels, dilated pupils, and raised temperature, pulse rate, and blood pressure.

Severe adverse effects ■ Toxic reactions to cocaine misuse include angina, coronary spasm, ventricular arrhythmias, myocardial infarction, cerebrovascular accidents, convulsions, respiratory depression and death ■ When people mix cocaine and alcohol consumption, the liver manufactures a third substance, cocaethylene, which intensifies cocaine's euphoric effects, and possibly raises the risk of sudden death ■ Some use cocaine plus heroin intravenously ('speedballing'), which is especially dangerous.

Withdrawal and treatment On stopping cocaine, symptoms proceed through a crash phase of depression and craving for sleep, a withdrawal phase of lack of energy and then an extinction phase of recurrence of craving evoked by various external stimuli but of lesser intensity. Depression, fatigue and bradycardia may be seen. Behavioural interventions, particularly cognitive behavioural therapy, can be effective in reducing cocaine misuse.

Oral findings

■ The main oral effects of cocaine addiction may be a dry mouth and bruxism or dental erosion ■ Caries and periodontal disease, especially acute necrotising gingivitis, are more frequent ■ Caries is particularly prevalent when sugar is mixed ('cut') with cocaine, and the mix placed in the labial/buccal sulcus (Fig. 3.9) ■ Oral use of cocaine temporarily numbs the lips and tongue and can cause gingival erosions ■ Prolonged cocaine snorting can result in ulceration of the nasal mucous membrane and can damage the nasal septum and cause it to collapse; snorting cocaine also predisposes to ulceration of the palate as a result of ischaemic necrosis, and to sphenoidal sinusitis, and occasionally leads to a brain abscess ■ Cocaine may precipitate cluster headaches, which can mimic atypical facial pain ■ Children born to cocaine-using mothers are more prone to have ankyloglossia.

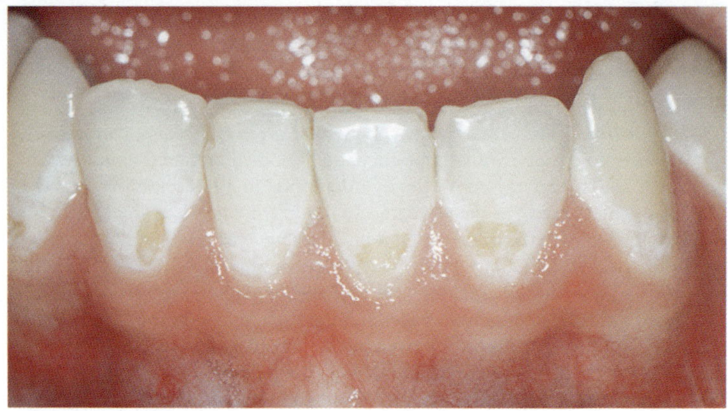

Figure 3.9 **Caries of the labial surface of the lower teeth in a cocaine user**

Dental management

Risk assessment Recognition of individuals who may be abusing drugs is critical. Behavioural problems or drug interactions may interfere with dental treatment. Intravenous drug use is associated with the risk of transmission of infections (HIV, hepatitis B), and complications such as infective endocarditis (which will require antibiotic prophylaxis). Care should be taken with any patient who makes suspicious requests for medication (as detailed for amphetamine/LSD/MDMA abuse).

Pain and anxiety control Local anaesthesia It is important to avoid epinephrine-containing local anaesthetics until at least 6 hours have elapsed after the last dose of cocaine, because of enhanced sympathomimetic action and subsequent arrhythmias, acute hypertension or cardiac failure. Ester-type local anaesthetics are best avoided since IV cocaine users may be allergic to benzoic acid. Conscious sedation Conscious sedation should be used with great caution due to the sympathomimetic effects of cocaine. If CS is strongly indicated, it is important to ensure that the patient is not concurrently abusing drugs, and treatment should be undertaken in a hospital environment. Opioids are contraindicated. General anaesthesia In cocaine users where GA is needed, isoflurane or sevoflurane are preferred to halothane as the latter may induce arrhythmias. Ketamine and suxamethonium are best avoided. Occasionally patients may be resistant to GA. Some cases of cocaine-induced hyperthermia during GA have been described.

Patient access and positioning Timing of treatment Dental treatment should not be given until 6 hours after the last dose of cocaine has been taken. Treatment modification Consent issues may arise if the patient is under the influence of drugs. If available, an escort is

Table 3.35 **Key considerations for dental management in cocaine abuse (see text)**

	Management modifications*	Comments/possible complications
Risk assessment	2	Drug abusers recognition; abnormal behaviour; blood-borne infections; others (cardiac lesions, drug interactions, etc); appropriate analgesia; consent issues; escort
Pain and anxiety control		
– Local anaesthesia	2	Avoid ester type and epinephrine
– Conscious sedation	3/4	Avoid opioids
– General anaesthesia	3/4	Avoid halothane, ketamine, suxamethonium, barbiturates and opioids; resistance to GA; hyperthermia
Patient access and positioning		
– Access to dental office	0	
– Timing of treatment	1	6 h after cocaine use; failed appointments
– Patient positioning	0	
Treatment modification		
– Oral surgery	1	
– Implantology	1/5	Neglected oral hygiene; periodontitis, xerostomia; heavy smokers
– Conservative/Endodontics	1	
– Fixed prosthetics	1/5	Neglected oral hygiene; heavy smokers
– Removable prosthetics	1	
– Non-surgical periodontology	1	
– Surgical periodontology	1/5	Neglected oral hygiene; heavy smokers
Hazardous and contraindicated drugs	1	Avoid opioids

*0 = No special considerations. 1 = Caution advised. 2 = Specialised medical advice recommended in some cases. 3 = Specialised medical advice mandatory. 4 = Only to be performed in hospital environment. 5 = Should be avoided.

desirable as this may improve patient attendance and improve discharge arrangements and care. The considerations that are needed when treatment is undertaken depend on the degree of drug abuse and related social, medical and dental complications. Hence each patient must be assessed on an individual basis, as the necessary modification may vary from caution, to the planned procedure being contraindicated. Examples of factors that may compromise care for all types of dental treatment are detailed in amphetamine abuse.

Further reading ● van der Bijl P 2003 Substance abuse – concerns in dentistry: an overview. S Afr Dent J 58:382–385 ● Cornelius J R, Clark D B, Weyant R et al 2004 Dental abnormalities in children of fathers with substance use disorders. Addict Behav 29:979–982 ● Mari A, Arranz C, Gimeno X et al 2002 Nasal cocaine abuse and centrofacial destructive process: report of three cases including treatment. Oral Surg Oral Med Oral Pathol Oral Radiol Endod 93:435–439 ● Sandler N A 2001 Patients who abuse drugs. Oral Surg Oral Med Oral Pathol Oral Radiol Endod 91:12–14.

CONGENITAL HEART DISEASE (CHD)

Definition CHD is any congenital structural defect of the heart or adjacent great vessels. Some 20% of patients have additional anomalies elsewhere. CHD represents the most common type of heart disease among children and, in developed countries, is considerably more prevalent than rheumatic heart disease.

General aspects

Aetiopathogenesis The causes of CHD are unknown in most cases, but may involve multifactorial, genetic and environmental factors. The best-known acquired causes are congenital rubella or cytomegalovirus infection and maternal drug misuse. The best-known genetic cause is Down syndrome.

Clinical presentation ■ The most striking feature of some types of CHD is cyanosis (seen when there is > 5 g reduced haemoglobin per dL of blood). It is caused by shunting deoxygenated blood from the right ventricle directly into the left side of the heart and the systemic circulation (*right to left shunt*), leading to chronic hypoxaemia. ■ Chronic hypoxaemia severely impairs development and causes gross clubbing of fingers and toes. Patients may crouch in an effort to increase venous return, and when polycythaemia develops, this can cause haemorrhages or thromboses.

Classification CHD has been anatomically classified as: ■ intracardiac shunting ■ obstruction to blood outflow ■ valvular malformation. However, a more practical classification based on clinical criteria, grouping CHD into cyanotic or acyanotic, has classically been applied as follows:

Cyanotic congenital heart defects Cyanotic congenital heart defects are those where there is shunting of blood from right-to-left sides of the heart and are, in general, the more severe types of CHD ('blue babies'). Cyanotic CHD includes the following:

- *Transposition of the great vessels* – reversal of the origins of the pulmonary artery and aorta. Causes cyanosis and breathlessness from birth, and early congestive cardiac failure.
- *Tetralogy of Fallot* – comprises: ● ventricular septal defect ● pulmonary stenosis ● straddling of the interventricular septum by the aorta

- compensatory right ventricular hypertrophy. Among the most obvious clinical features are severe cyanosis, loud cardiac murmurs and effects from chronic hypoxaemia. Paroxysms of cyanosis and breathlessness, which typically cause cerebral hypoxia and syncope, often supervene for no apparent reason. In the absence of treatment there is typically heart failure, respiratory infection or, less often, infective endocarditis or brain abscess.

- *Eisenmenger's syndrome* – refers to cyanosis from any reversal of a left-to-right shunt, usually through a ventricular septal defect.
- *Tricuspid atresia* – absence of the tricuspid valve, right ventricle and pulmonary valve. The pulmonary circulation is maintained through a patent ductus arteriosus.
- *Pulmonary atresia* – there is a three-chambered heart but the tricuspid valve is patent.

Acyanotic congenital heart defects Acyanotic congenital heart defects include:

- *Ventricular septal defect*. This is one of the most common congenital defects. It ranges from pinholes compatible with survival into middle age, to defects so large as to cause death in infancy if untreated. There is a left-to-right shunt. Right ventricular hypertrophy, right ventricular failure, reversal of the shunt and late onset cyanosis may develop. The jet of blood hitting the endocardium of the right ventricle causes it to thicken (jet lesion) and it may later be the site of infective endocarditis. Ninety per cent of patients with ventricular septal defect have an additional cardiac defect. Repair is by primary closure, or a patch of pericardium or Dacron®.
- *Atrial septal defect*. This is often located near the foramen ovale, and termed a secundum defect and, in 10–20%, is associated with mitral valve prolapse. It has little effect on cardiac function, though right ventricular failure usually develops. It is therefore the most common CHD presenting in adults. An embolus from a vein can pass from the right ventricle into the left and therefore directly into the systemic circulation and can occasionally cause a stroke and be fatal (paradoxical embolism). Atrial septal defect is repaired by primary closure, or a pericardial or Dacron® patch.
- *Patent ductus arteriosus*. This is a persistent opening (normally closed by the third month of life) between the aorta and pulmonary artery. It causes loud and continuous sawing, systolic and diastolic murmurs. Shunt is from left to right, initially acyanotic, and the typical complication is right ventricular failure. If patency of the ductus is not necessary to maintain the systemic circulation, its closure can be promoted in infancy by giving indometacin, a prostaglandin inhibitor. Alternatively, it is ligated.
- *Coarctation of the aorta*. This is aortic narrowing, usually sited beyond the origin of the subclavian arteries – therefore the blood supply to the head, neck and upper body is unobstructed and only the supply to the lower part of the body is restricted. As a consequence, there is severe hypertension in the upper body and a low blood pressure below with strong radial pulses but weak or absent femoral pulses (radio-femoral delay). Secondary changes are enlargement of collateral arteries (such as the intercostal) and degenerative changes in the aorta, which can lead to a fatal aneurysm.

Infective endocarditis or left ventricular failure are other possible causes of death. A bicuspid aortic valve is associated in over 50%. Coarctation is repaired by aortoplasty, or sometimes a Dacron® vascular prosthesis.

- *Pulmonary stenosis* – narrowing of the pulmonary valve. The main symptoms are breathlessness and right ventricular failure, often in childhood. It is usually treated by percutaneous balloon valvotomy, or commissurotomy, or prosthetic valve replacement.
- *Aortic stenosis.*
- *Mitral valve prolapse.*
- *Bicuspid aortic valve.*

Diagnosis ■ Auscultation (heart murmur) ■ Chest radiograph ■ ECG ■ Echocardiography ■ Arterial blood gases ■ Cardiac catheterisation ■ Angiocardiography.

Treatment ■ Surgical management of the anatomic defects is often the treatment of choice ■ Digitalis, diuretics and anticoagulants are often administered to control complications.

Prognosis The prognosis for patients with CHD has been enormously improved by surgery but up to 40% of children die during the first year of life, and residual defects can still predispose to infective endocarditis. Possible complications in CHD include: ■ pulmonary oedema ■ cardiac failure ■ cyanosis ■ polycythaemia ■ bleeding tendency ■ growth retardation ■ fatigue ■ infective endocarditis ■ brain abscess.

Oral findings

Oral abnormalities associated with congenital heart disease may include: ■ delayed eruption of both dentitions ■ an increased frequency of positional anomalies ■ greater caries and periodontal disease activity, probably because of poor oral hygiene and lack of dental attention ■ enamel hypoplasia; the teeth often have a bluish-white 'skimmed milk' appearance and there is gross vasodilatation in the pulps (especially in coarctation of the aorta) ■ cleft palate (associated mainly with ventricular septal defects) ■ fissured tongue (in tetralogy of Fallot) ■ after cardiotomy, transient small white, non-ulcerated mucosal lesions of unknown aetiology may be seen.

Dental management

Risk assessment Congenital heart lesions are susceptible to infective endocarditis, and have occasionally been discovered only as a result of the development of this. Antibiotic cover may therefore be required for dental treatment. A special hazard in some types of CHD, such as the tetralogy of Fallot, is the development of cerebral abscesses – very occasionally due to oral bacteria. Leucopenia may be a factor in some right-to-left shunts. Associated complications in CHDs must also be considered (e.g. polycythaemia, bleeding tendency).

Appropriate health care **Preventive dentistry** Poor oral hygiene and oral health status are frequent in children with CHD. It is important to

Table 3.36 Key considerations for dental management in congenital heart disease (see text)

	Management modifications*	Comments/possible complications
Risk assessment	2/3	Infective endocarditis; cerebral abscesses; bleeding tendency
Pain and anxiety control		
– Local anaesthesia	1	Reduce epinephrine dose
– Conscious sedation	3/4	
– General anaesthesia	3/4	
Patient access and positioning		
– Access to dental office	0	
– Timing of treatment	0	
– Patient positioning	0	
Treatment modification		
– Oral surgery	2	Bleeding tendency
– Implantology	2	Bleeding tendency
– Conservative/Endodontics	1	
– Fixed prosthetics	1	Avoid retraction cords containing epinephrine
– Removable prosthetics	1	
– Non-surgical periodontology	2	Bleeding tendency
– Surgical periodontology	2	Bleeding tendency
– Paediatric dentistry	1	Pulpotomy is contraindicated
Hazardous and contraindicated drugs	2	Some patients are treated with anticoagulants

*0 = No special considerations. 1 = Caution advised. 2 = Specialised medical advice recommended in some cases. 3 = Specialised medical advice mandatory. 4 = Only to be performed in hospital environment. 5 = Should be avoided.

apply preventive programmes and educate patients and parents in hygiene habits to minimise the risk of infections of oral origin.

Pain and anxiety control **Local anaesthesia** An aspirating syringe should be used to give a local anaesthetic, since epinephrine in the anaesthetic given intravenously may (theoretically) increase hypertension and precipitate arrhythmias. Blood pressure tends to rise during oral surgery under local anaesthesia – but this is usually of little practical importance. **Conscious sedation** Conscious sedation requires special sedation care, in hospital. **General anaesthesia** General anaesthesia requires special anaesthetic care, in hospital.

Treatment modification Treatment modifications may be required in relation to: ■ antibiotic prophylaxis of bacterial endocarditis before starting any invasive dental procedure ■ medical treatment may be needed before oral health care for patients with complications such as cardiac failure, polycythaemia, infective complications or emotional disturbances

■ defective platelet function and increased fibrinolytic activity in patients with CHD may cause bleeding tendencies; anticoagulants may also be used if there is a thrombotic tendency ■ associated problems which may also affect dental management include congestive cardiac failure, cleft palate, or syndromes such as Down syndrome, Turner syndrome, or idiopathic hypercalcaemia (William syndrome) ■ routine dental treatment may be performed in controlled patients without signs or symptoms of heart disease ■ in patients with pulmonary oedema, pulmonary hypertension or heart failure, dental care should be limited to emergency treatment (analgesics and antibiotics). **Surgery** Patients with polycythaemia may have a bleeding tendency and thus should be evaluated before any surgical procedure. **Fixed prosthetics and conservation** Gingival retraction cords containing epinephrine should be avoided. **Periodontology** Bleeding tendency should be evaluated before dental scaling or periodontal surgery. **Paediatric dentistry** Pulpotomy is contraindicated in children with CHD, because incomplete caries removal could result in bacteraemia. Extraction of primary teeth with deep caries involving the pulp is then recommended.

Drug use Some patients receive anticoagulants to avoid thromboses related to polycythaemia.

Further reading

● Balmer R, Bu'Lock F A 2003 The experiences with oral health and dental prevention of children with congenital heart disease. Cardiol Young 13:439–443 ● Knirsch W, Hassberg D, Beyer A et al 2003 Knowledge, compliance and practice of antibiotic endocarditis prophylaxis of patients with congenital heart disease. Pediatr Cardiol 24:344–349 ● Sirois D A, Fatahzadeh M 2001 Valvular heart disease. Oral Surg Oral Med Oral Pathol Oral Radiol Endod 91:15–19.

CREUTZFELDT–JAKOB DISEASE (CJD)

Definition ■ Creutzfeldt–Jakob disease (CJD) is a progressive brain disease, a transmissible spongiform encephalopathy (TSE) ■ TSEs are a group of lethal degenerative brain diseases (encephalopathies) characterised by the appearance of microscopic vacuoles in the brain grey matter, giving a sponge-like (spongiform) appearance ■ Several animal TSEs are known, including bovine spongiform encephalopathy (BSE; also known as 'mad cow disease') in cattle, and scrapie in sheep and goats ■ Some TSEs are transmissible from animal to man; BSE appears to be responsible for variant CJD in man.

General aspects

Aetiopathogenesis ■ TSEs were originally termed slow virus infections – although no virus has ever been associated with the disease ■ TSEs appear to be associated with an abnormal form of a host-encoded protein termed a prion (proteinaceous infectious particle) ■ Prions are composed of a cell surface glycoprotein ■ In prion diseases a protease resistant isoform (PrP^{sc} or PrP^{TSE}) accumulates in the brain ■ Prions do not evoke a protective immune response ■ CNS and posterior orbit are the tissues most likely to be infected ■ Transfusions of whole blood, component blood or blood derivatives have not been shown to transmit the classical CJD agent, but, to avoid the theoretical possibility of transmission, recipients of human growth hormone were excluded from blood donation in 1989, and recipients of other human-derived pituitary hormones have been excluded since 1993 in the UK ■ Cases of variant CJD have been reported in blood transfusion product recipients ■ Concern has been expressed over the use of human dura mater grafts and bovine products for periodontal reconstruction since theoretically they might be the source of prions ■ There may also be other potential but unproven sources of infection, such as products produced from cell lines grown in the presence of fetal bovine serum, some vaccines, and bovine products such as collagen.

Clinical presentation Persons with CJD display psychiatric symptoms (severe depression) and behavioural manifestations, together with persistent paraesthesias and dysaesthesias, followed by dementia, cerebellar and other neurological signs, myoclonus or other involuntary movements, and finally akinetic mutism.

Treatment There is no effective treatment yet for CJD.

Prognosis All TSEs have prolonged incubation periods of months to years, gradually increase in severity and lead to death over months or years.

Classification The human TSEs exist in inherited, acquired or sporadic forms (Table 3.37) and are frequently referred to collectively as Creutzfeldt–Jakob disease or CJD. **Sporadic CJD** ■ Sporadic CJD (sCJD), where no source is identifiable, accounts for about 85% of all cases of CJD ■ sCJD commonly develops in middle to late life with a peak age of onset between 60 and 65 years of age, presenting as a rapidly progressive multifocal dementia. **Familial CJD** ■ The inherited or familial forms of CJD (fCJD) account for around 10% of cases. These are rare autosomal dominant disorders that do not manifest until early to middle adult life: ● Fatal Familial Insomnia is characterised by progressive insomnia, dysautonomia, disruption of circadian rhythms, motor dysfunction and deterioration in cognition ● Gerstmann–Straussler–Scheinker syndrome is an autosomal dominant illness in which neuropathological findings are distinct, with many PrP^{sc} positive plaques throughout the brain. **Kuru** ■ Kuru is an acquired

Table 3.37 **Types of Creutzfeldt–Jakob disease**

Type	Abbreviation	Comments
Sporadic	sCJD	–
Familial	fCJD	Autosomal dominant
Kuru	–	Ritualistic cannibalism
Iatrogenic	iCJD	Contaminated surgical instruments Dura mater grafts or pituitary hormones
Variant	vCJD Sometimes termed nvCJD	Consumption of BSE-infected material

spongiform encephalopathy first described in the 1950s, which was endemic among the Fore ethnic group in the eastern highlands of Papua New Guinea and spread by cannibalism. **Iatrogenic CJD** ■ Iatrogenic CJD (iCJD), which ranges from a sCJD-like disease to a more slow-onset disease reminiscent of kuru, can be transmitted mainly by exposure to: ● cadaver-derived growth hormone ● pituitary gonadotropins ● dura mater homografting ● corneal grafts ● inadequately sterilised neurosurgical equipment. **Variant CJD (vCJD)** ■ Bovine spongiform encephalopathy (BSE) was first recognised in UK cattle in 1986 ■ It was recognised that the infective agent of BSE was spread by the use of meat and bonemeal in cattle food ■ In 1996, a variant of sporadic CJD (variant or vCJD) was first observed in humans in the UK, and linked with the consumption of bovine offal infected with BSE ■ The clinical course of vCJD is much longer than that of sCJD; also, affected patients do not have the same typical electroencephalogram (EEG) changes ■ It presents in a younger age group.

Diagnosis of vCJD Diagnosis is suggested by clinical presentation. Tests and investigations that can contribute to a diagnosis include: ■ MRI scans, which show characteristic bilateral symmetrical high signal in the thalamic pulvinar nuclei ■ EEG ■ blood tests for genetic mutations predisposing to vCJD ■ cerebrospinal fluid analysis ■ psychometric tests ■ tonsillar biopsy.

Oral findings

Orofacial manifestations of CJD comprise dysphagia and dysarthria (due to pseudobulbar palsy). In vCJD patients there may be orofacial dysaesthesia or paraesthesia or abnormal taste sensation, nausea or vomiting leading to dental erosion.

Dental management

Risk assessment

- A unique feature of PrP^{sc} is its remarkable capacity to bind to steel and its resistance to inactivation by conventional methods: heat, most disinfectants, ionising, ultraviolet and microwave radiations have little effect.
- This presents significant infection control problems when patients with CJD undergo medical or dental interventions.
- Details of the classification of patients with symptomatic CJD and patients who are considered 'at risk' of CJD while asymptomatic can be found in the guidance developed by the Advisory Committee on Dangerous Pathogens (ACDP) Transmissible Spongiform Encephalopathy (TSE) Working Group: *Transmissible spongiform encephalopathy agents: safe working and the prevention of infection.*
- Infectivity is highest in brain tissue, and is also present in some peripheral tissues, but appears generally absent from most body fluids, including saliva.
- In *sporadic* (and familial) CJD, significant infectivity is assumed to exist in the central nervous system, olfactory epithelium and eye.

- In *variant* CJD, significant infectivity is assumed to exist in these same tissues and also in gastrointestinal lymphoid tissue and peripheral lymphoid tissue.
- Animal studies showed prions in the trigeminal nerve, tooth pulp, gingiva and salivary glands and the potential for prion transmission via the dental route.
- To date, conventional dental treatment has no proven association with transmission of any form of CJD. The risks of transmission of infection from dental instruments are thought to be very low, provided optimal standards of infection control and decontamination are maintained. General advice on the decontamination of dental instruments can be found in guidance prepared by the British Dental Association (BDA) on 'Infection control in dentistry'. This document (known as the 'A12') is available from the BDA and can be accessed on their website at *www.bda-dentistry.org.uk*. Dental instruments used on patients defined in Box 3.7 can be handled in the same way as those used in any other low risk surgery,

Box 3.7 TSE Infection Control Guidelines: categorisation of patients by risk

1. Symptomatic patients
   1.1 Patients who fulfil the diagnostic criteria for definite, probable or possible CJD or vCJD (see text for diagnostic criteria).
   1.2 Patients with neurological disease of unknown aetiology who do not fit the criteria for possible CJD or vCJD, but where the diagnosis of CJD is being actively considered.
2. Asymptomatic patients at risk from familial forms of CJD linked to genetic mutations
   2.1 Individuals who have or have had two or more blood relatives affected by CJD or other prion disease, or a relative known to have a genetic mutation indicative of familial CJD.
   2.2 Individuals who have been shown by specific genetic testing to be at significant risk of developing CJD or other prion disease.
3. Asymptomatic patients potentially at risk from iatrogenic exposure*
   3.1 Recipients of hormone derived from human pituitary glands, e.g. growth hormone, gonadotrophin.
   3.2 Individuals who have received a graft of dura mater (people who underwent neurosurgical procedures or operations for a tumour or cyst of the spine before August 1992 may have received a graft of dura mater, and should be treated as at risk, unless evidence can be provided that dura mater was not used).
   3.3 Patients who have been contacted as potentially 'at risk' because of exposure to instruments used on, or receipt of blood, plasma derivatives, organs or tissues donated by, a patient who went on to develop CJD or vCJD**.

*A decision on the inclusion of corneal graft recipients in the 'iatrogenic at risk' category is pending completion of a risk assessment.
**The CJD Incidents Panel, which gives advice to the local team on what action needs to be taken when a patient who is diagnosed as having CJD or vCJD underwent surgery or donated blood, organs or tissues before CJD/vCJD was identified, will identify contacts who are potentially at risk.

i.e. these instruments can be reprocessed according to best practice and returned to use. Optimal reprocessing standards must be observed. Additionally, dentists are reminded that any instruments labelled by the manufacturer as 'single use' should not be re-used under any circumstances.

- *There is no reason why any of the categories of patients defined in Box 3.7 or their relatives should be refused routine dental treatment. They can be treated in the same way as any member of the general public.*
- When patients 'at risk' of CJD/vCJD undergo maxillofacial surgery that may disrupt certain cranial nerves, CNS, orbit or lymphoid tissues of the head and neck, special infection control precautions may need to be taken, as described in the TSE Infection Control Guidance.
- There are several groups of patients who are identified as being at an additional risk of CJD (i.e. a risk over and above the risk in the general UK population that is around 1 in a million for sporadic CJD and is currently unknown for vCJD). These patients are considered 'at risk' of CJD for public health purposes.
- There has been a considerable increase in the number of patients classified as 'at risk' of vCJD due to the notification of patients considered at risk due to receipt of UK blood products. This number may increase further if more blood donors develop vCJD.
- Patients identified as 'at risk' of CJD (including vCJD) for public health purposes are asked to take the following precautions to reduce any possible risk of spreading CJD: • not to donate blood, organs or tissues • to inform health care staff before they undergo medical, surgical or dental treatment • to inform their families in case they need emergency surgery in the future.
- The health care professionals who notify these patients of their 'at risk' status have been asked to arrange for the information to be recorded in patients' hospital medical records and/or primary care notes.
- The responsibility for informing Primary Dental Carers lies with the patients themselves.
- When treating a patient with CJD, or a patient who informs you that he/she has been identified as 'at risk' of CJD, you should **ensure that satisfactory standards of decontamination are observed**. Under these conditions, routine dentistry is understood to be low risk, and therefore no special infection control precautions are advised for the instruments used on symptomatic or 'at risk' patients. Primary Dental Carers should also ensure information about patients' CJD status is included in any referrals for head and neck surgery.
- Dental health care staff infected or potentially infected with prion disease should not practise invasive clinical procedures if there is a risk of motor and cognitive dysfunction.

Appropriate health care It has been recommended for the management of patients with confirmed CJD:

- Clinicians must be vigilant in their care.
- Standard infection control should be used, but with extra precautions on instruments if there is no access to Central Sterile Supply Department or other validated automated cleaning/sterilisation processes.
- Single-use instruments should be used, and then incinerated.

Table 3.38 **Key considerations for dental management in Creutzfeldt–Jakob disease (see text)**

	Management modifications*	Comments/possible complications
Risk assessment	2	Prions detected in dental tissue
Appropriate dental care	3/4	Evaluate risk group and record in notes and in referrals for surgery Standard infection control: single-use instruments; air and water supplies and suction device independent; concentrated bleach for cleaning
Pain and anxiety control		
– Local anaesthesia	0	
– Conscious sedation	0	
– General anaesthesia	3/4	
Patient access and positioning		
– Access to dental office	0	
– Timing of treatment	1	At the end of the working day
– Patient positioning	0	
Treatment modification		
– Oral surgery	2	Risk of the use of some grafts
– Implantology	2	
– Conservative/Endodontics	1	
– Fixed prosthetics	1	
– Removable prosthetics	1	
– Non-surgical periodontology	2	
– Surgical periodontology	2	Risk of the use of some grafts
Hazardous and contraindicated drugs	0	

*0 = No special considerations. 1 = Caution advised. 2 = Specialised medical advice recommended in some cases. 3 = Specialised medical advice mandatory. 4 = Only to be performed in hospital environment. 5 = Should be avoided.

- Concentrated bleach does appear to achieve inactivation of all strains and 20000 ppm available chlorine of sodium hypochlorite for 1 hour or 2M sodium hydroxide for 1 hour is considered effective.
- Effective cleaning (to remove adherent tissue) coupled with autoclaving (reduction of infectivity levels by several log fold) produces a significant reduction in infectivity levels on contaminated instruments if a non-porous load steam steriliser is used at 134–137°C for a single cycle of 18 minutes, or six successive cycles of 3 minutes each.
- All instruments used on CJD patients must be traceable from every operative procedure. Instruments used for procedures involving low risk tissues for CJD/vCJD – i.e., most dental interventions – except biopsy of lymphoid material (e.g. posterior third of the tongue)-do not need to be traced to

individual patients but a quality assurance system must trace the instrument through the decontamination process to prove that the said device has been appropriately cleaned and sterilised. According to current ACDP/SEAC guidelines, if instruments are only used on low risk tissues then they can be re-processed 'according to best practice and returned to use'.

- Dental equipment should be cleaned with detergent impregnated wipes ± disinfectant wipes.

Treatment modification **Surgery** There is no evidence to suggest that any patients who have received dura mater allografts for the management of maxillofacial defects have developed iCJD. Concerns exist, however, about the theoretical risk of the use of non-human animal-derived graft materials and heterologous human graft materials in oral or periodontal surgery.

Further reading • Hamilton K, Brewer A, Smith A 2004 Dental treatment of a patient in the new 'at-risk' category for CJD. J Hosp Infect 57:184–185 • Lumley J S P 2004 Creutzfeldt–Jakob disease (CJD) in surgical practice. RCS Bulletin 85:86–88 • Porter S, Scully C, Ridgway G L, Bell J 2000 The human transmissible spongiform encephalopathies (TSEs): implications for dental practitioners. Br Dent J 188:432–436 • Scully, C, Smith A, Bagg J 2003 Prions and the human transmissible encephalopathies. In: Glick M (ed) Infectious diseases and dentistry. Dent Clin N Amer 47:493–516 • Smith A J, Bagg J, Ironside J W, Will R G, Scully C 2003 Prions and the oral cavity. J Dent Res 82:769–775 • http://www.hpa.org.uk/infections/topics_az/cjd/menu.htm. • http://www.bda-dentistry.org.uk/advice/docs/A12.pdf • http://www.advisorybodies.doh.gov.uk/acdp/tseguidance/ • http://www.dh.gov.uk/PolicyAndGuidance/HealthAndSocialCareTopics/CJD/CJDGeneralInformation/CJDGeneralArticle/fs/en?CONTENT_ID=4032409&chk=a%2BL/hP

CROHN'S DISEASE

Definition Crohn's disease is a chronic granulomatous inflammation mainly affecting the terminal ileum (regional ileitis) and proximal colon.

General aspects

Aetiopathogenesis Despite wide-ranging hypotheses, the cause remains unknown. The onset of the disease is often in the second or third decade of life, although a second peak in patients over 60 years has been related to NSAID intake.

Clinical presentation Crohn's disease (Fig. 3.10) presents mainly with: ■ diarrhoea and abdominal pain ■ weight loss ■ anorexia, fever and fatigue ■ Other clinical features which may be present include: • mouth (ulcers) • lip/oral mucosa (swellings) • skin (pyoderma, erythema nodosum) • joints (arthritis, sacroiliitis) • eyes (conjunctivitis, episcleritis, iritis) • liver (various).

Diagnosis ■ Iron, folate and/or vitamin B_{12} defect ■ Barium enema radiography ■ Sigmoidoscopy ■ Rectal biopsy.

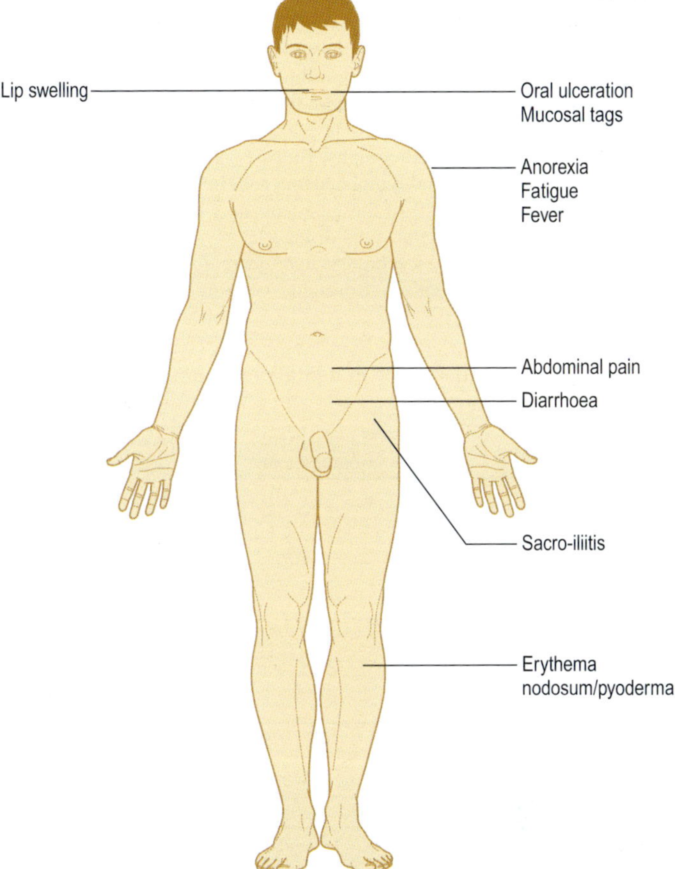

Figure 3.10 **Clinical presentation of Crohn's disease**

Treatment ■ Elemental diets ■ Immunosuppressive drugs (corticosteroids, sulfasalazine, 6-mercaptopurine, azathioprine, infliximab) ■ ± Surgery.

Prognosis Early recognition of oral lesions and initiation of treatment for Crohn's disease may improve the prognosis. Although no treatment is curative, periods of spontaneous remission may occur. Over a 20-year period, about 80% of patients need surgical intervention. An increased prevalence of intestinal cancer has been described in patients with Crohn's disease.

Oral findings

■ Ulcers ■ Facial or labial swelling ■ Mucosal tags or 'cobblestone' proliferation of the mucosa ■ Oral effects of malabsorption such as angular stomatitis may also be seen ■ A high prevalence of caries and periodontitis has also been reported.

Patients with atypical ulcers (especially when they are large, linear and ragged) or those with recurrent facial swellings, should have biopsy of the mucosa in addition to other investigations, particularly chest radiography, serum angiotensin-converting enzyme levels, serum ferritin and vitamin B_{12}, red cell folate and intestinal radiography. Biopsies in oral Crohn's disease typically show granulomas and lymphoedema and, in their absence, diagnosis is somewhat speculative. Some of these patients may have asymptomatic intestinal disease, or develop intestinal disease later.

Orofacial granulomatosis, sarcoidosis and tuberculosis are the main differential diagnoses. Melkersson–Rosenthal syndrome (facial swelling,

Table 3.39 **Key considerations in dental management in Crohn's disease (see text)**

	Management modifications*	Comments/possible complications
Risk assessment	1	Problems associated with drug therapy and malabsorption
Appropriate dental care	1	Avoid elective dental care during acute episodes
Pain and anxiety control		
– Local anaesthesia	0	
– Conscious sedation	0	
– General anaesthesia	1	Check for anaemia
Patient access and positioning		
– Access to dental office	0	
– Timing of treatment	1	Morning
– Patient positioning	0	
Treatment modification		Delay treatment during acute episodes or if ulceration is present
– Oral surgery	1	
– Implantology	1	
– Conservative/Endodontics	1	
– Fixed prosthetics	1	
– Removable prosthetics	1	
– Non-surgical periodontology	1	
– Surgical periodontology	1	
Hazardous and contraindicated drugs	2	Avoid NSAIDs, amoxicillin-clavulanate and clindamycin; some patients are on corticosteroids

*0 = No special considerations. 1 = Caution advised. 2 = Specialised medical advice recommended in some cases. 3 = Specialised medical advice mandatory. 4 = Only to be performed in hospital environment. 5 = Should be avoided.

facial palsy and fissured tongue) and cheilitis granulomatosa may possibly also be incomplete manifestations of Crohn's disease.

Dental management

Risk assessment Dental management may be complicated by any of the problems associated with malabsorption or by corticosteroid or other immunosuppressive treatment. Sulfasalazine can produce anaemia, leucopenia and thrombocytopenia.

Pain and anxiety control **Local anaesthesia** Local anaesthesia may be used safely in Crohn's disease. **Conscious sedation** Sedation for dental management may be useful because stress may exacerbate Crohn's disease. No technique is contraindicated. **General anaesthesia** The patient must undergo a full preoperative assessment, complete with blood tests to check for anaemia/other deficiencies (due to chronic blood loss/malabsorption).

Patient access and positioning Short appointments, preferably in the morning, are desirable.

Treatment modification During acute episodes of Crohn's disease, only emergency dental care should be provided. The oral cavity may be uncomfortable if ulceration or swelling is present. It may be best to delay treatment until these are stable.

Drug use ■ NSAIDs should be avoided; acetaminophen is the analgesic of choice ■ Some patients are treated with corticosteroids or other immunosuppressant drugs ■ Antibiotics that could aggravate diarrhoea should be avoided; these include amoxicillin-clavulanate and clindamycin.

Further reading ● Kalmar J R 1994 Crohn's disease: orofacial considerations and disease pathogenesis. Periodontol 2000 6:101–115 ● Leão J C, Hodgson T, Scully, C , Porter S R 2004 Review article: orofacial granulomatosis. Aliment Pharmacol Therap 20:1019–1027 ● Scheper H J, Brand H S 2002 Oral aspects of Crohn's disease. Int Dent J 52:163–172. ● Siegel M A, Jacobson J J 1999 Inflammatory bowel diseases and the oral cavity. Oral Surg Oral Med Oral Pathol Oral Radiol Endod 87:12–14

CUSHING'S SYNDROME

Definition Cushing's syndrome is the clinical picture resulting from the persistently increased adrenal cortex production of hormones, especially cortisol and androgens.

General aspects

Aetiopathogenesis ■ The main cause is Cushing's disease, usually caused by a pituitary microadenoma which produces excess ACTH, which then stimulates the adrenal glands ■ Other causes include: ● ACTH production by other tumours ● ACTH administration ● adrenal tumours ● corticosteroid therapy.

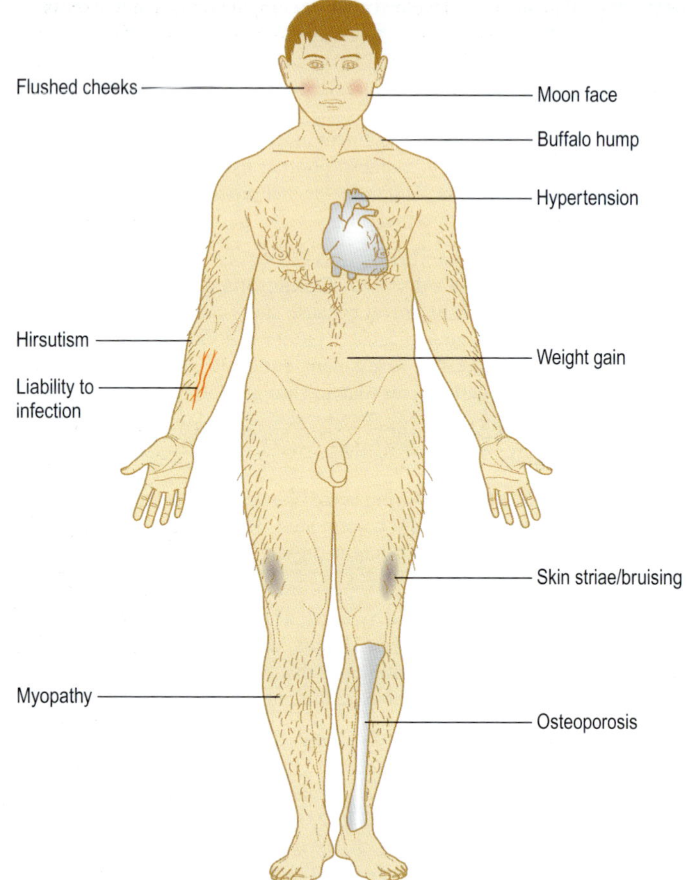

Figure 3.11 **Clinical presentation of Cushing's syndrome**

Clinical presentation ■ Weight gain ■ Hypertension ■ Fat redistribution with facial swelling ('moon face') and swelling over back of neck ('buffalo hump') ■ Protein breakdown (skin striae, bruising, myopathy and osteoporosis) ■ Hyperglycaemia (from gluconeogenesis) ■ Liability to infection ■ Hirsutism ■ Amenorrhoea.

Diagnosis ■ Plasma cortisol – raised ■ Urinary cortisol excretion – raised ■ Circadian rhythm of plasma cortisol – lost ■ Overnight dexamethasone suppression (of cortisol) test – reduced ■ CT/MRI – to locate any responsible tumour.

Treatment ■ Trans-sphenoidal surgery, or irradiation, of the pituitary tumour ■ Surgical resection of any adrenal tumour ■ Steroid antagonists.

Prognosis Patients may develop medical complications due to excess cortisol levels: ■ hypertension ■ cardiovascular disease ■ diabetes mellitus ■ psychosis ■ vertebral collapse or myopathy causing limited mobility ■ multiple endocrine adenomatosis.

Oral findings

There are no specific oral manifestations of Cushing's syndrome or disease. However the following have been described: ■ patients show a round plethoric 'moon face' with prominent and flushed cheeks ■ in children –

Table 3.40 **Key considerations for dental management in Cushing's syndrome (see text)**

	Management modifications*	Comments/possible complications
Risk assessment	2	Adrenal crisis; hypertension, cardiovascular disease, diabetes; poor wound healing
Appropriate dental care	1	Avoid elective dental care until disease is controlled; preoperative hydrocortisone
Pain and anxiety control		
– Local anaesthesia	0	
– Conscious sedation	1	Avoid drugs compromising ventilation
– General anaesthesia	3/4	Consider associated medical complications
Patient access and positioning		
– Access to dental office	0	
– Timing of treatment	0	
– Patient positioning	0	
Treatment modification		
– Oral surgery	1	Infections; poor wound healing
– Implantology	1	
– Conservative/Endodontics	0	
– Fixed prosthetics	0	
– Removable prosthetics	0	
– Non-surgical periodontology	0	
– Surgical periodontology	1	Infections; poor wound healing
Hazardous and contraindicated drugs	0	

*0 = No special considerations. 1 = Caution advised. 2 = Specialised medical advice recommended in some cases. 3 = Specialised medical advice mandatory. 4 = Only to be performed in hospital environment. 5 = Should be avoided.

delayed teeth eruption and crowding ■ loss of oral sensibility (discriminative capacity and stereognosis).

Dental management

Risk assessment Patients with Cushing's syndrome have an increased susceptibility to infection and poor wound healing. The medical complications that may be present due to excess cortisol levels also need to be considered. Patients are at risk from an adrenal crisis if subjected to surgery, anaesthesia or trauma. They should be maintained on corticosteroid replacement therapy and the physician consulted to confirm the correct dose of supplementation required for the planned procedure (see Nicholson et al 1998).

Preventive dentistry Since there is increased susceptibility to infections, oral hygiene and preventive dental care are major goals in these patients.

Pain and anxiety control **Local anaesthesia** Local anaesthesia can be carried out with normal precautions. **Conscious sedation** Conscious sedation can be carried out with normal precautions, but drugs that compromise ventilation should be avoided, because of respiratory muscle weakness. **General anaesthesia** General anaesthesia can be carried out with normal precautions, although perioperative steroid supplementation may be required. Furthermore, any medical complications associated with excess cortisol levels need to be considered.

Treatment modification Definitive dental treatment should be avoided until the condition is controlled.

Further reading ● Bain S, Hamburger J 2004 Physical signs for the general dental practitioner. Case 13. Cushing's disease. Dent Update 31:180 ● Huber M A, Drake A J 3rd 1996 Pharmacology of the endocrine pancreas, adrenal cortex, and female reproductive organ. Dent Clin North Am 40:753–777 ● Nicholson G, Burrin J M, Hall G M 1998 Peri-operative steroid supplementation. Anaesthesia 53:1091–1104.

CYSTIC FIBROSIS

Definition Cystic fibrosis is a defect in chloride and sodium transport, which results in an increased viscosity of mucus secreted by exocrine glands, especially the pancreas and lungs.

General aspects

Aetiopathogenesis Cystic fibrosis is an autosomal recessive condition. The gene responsible is on the long arm of chromosome 7. It occurs predominantly in individuals of Caucasian origin. Most carriers are asymptomatic.

Clinical presentation ■ Lung – cough, wheeze, recurrent infection, and possibly bronchiectasis ■ Gastrointestinal insufficiency (resulting in malabsorption) ■ Pancreatic insufficiency (leading to diabetes)

■ Liver cirrhosis (due to viscous bile production and portal hypertension) ■ Hepatic steatosis (secondary to malnutrition) ■ Nasal polyps ■ Sinusitis ■ Infertility.

Diagnosis ■ Sweat or salivary sodium and chloride – increased ■ Faecal elastase – increased.

Treatment ■ Physiotherapy and postural drainage ■ Diet – high-protein, high-calorie and low-fat diet, plus fat-soluble vitamins and pancreatic enzymes ■ Bronchodilators ■ Antimicrobials.

Prognosis The disease is progressive and finally fatal, mostly as a consequence of pulmonary complications and cor pulmonale. Lung transplantation may be indicated. Over 30% of patients now survive beyond 18 years of age.

Oral findings

■ Nasal polyps and recurrent sinusitis are common ■ Most patients have a high salivary sodium concentration ■ The major salivary glands may become enlarged, with associated xerostomia ■ Halitosis is common ■ The lower lip may become dry, enlarged and everted ■ The low-fat, high-carbohydrate diet and dry mouth predispose to caries but some studies have shown reduced caries – probably due to a high salivary pH ■ Enamel hypoplasia may be seen ■ Both dental development and eruption are delayed ■ Tetracycline staining of the teeth was common, but should rarely be seen now ■ Pancreatic enzymes may cause oral ulceration if held in the mouth.

Dental management

Risk assessment Reduced respiratory function, liver disease (that may result in a bleeding tendency) and diabetes may complicate treatment.

Pain and anxiety control **Local anaesthesia** This is the preferred method for dental treatment. **Conscious sedation** Diazepam and midazolam are mild respiratory depressants and should not be used for intravenous sedation in cystic fibrosis by the dentist. If intravenous sedation is absolutely necessary, it should only be undertaken in hospital, after full preoperative assessment by an anaesthetist. **General anaesthesia** General anaesthesia should be avoided in patients with cystic fibrosis. If a GA is absolutely necessary, an anaesthetist should undertake a full preoperative assessment, and the chest physician consulted. Chest physiotherapy, prophylactic antibiotics and extended hospital admission should be arranged.

Patient access and positioning **Timing of treatment** Short appointments are recommended. Mucus accumulation may increase at night when movements and postural drainage are reduced and thus early morning coughing is common. In consequence, early morning appointments are not recommended. **Patient positioning** Patients with cystic fibrosis are best treated in the upright position since they may become increasingly breathless if laid flat.

Table 3.41 **Key considerations for dental management in cystic fibrosis (see text)**

	Management modifications*	Comments/possible complications
Risk assessment	2/4	Reduced respiratory function; liver disease (bleeding tendency); diabetes
Pain and anxiety control		
– Local anaesthesia	0	
– Conscious sedation	2/4	May cause respiratory depression
– General anaesthesia	5	Avoid; if unavoidable requires careful planning
Patient access and positioning		
– Access to dental office	0	
– Timing of treatment	1	Avoid early morning
– Patient positioning	1	Upright position
Treatment modification		
– Oral surgery	1	
– Implantology	3	Depends on disease prognosis
– Conservative/Endodontics	1	
– Fixed prosthetics	1	
– Removable prosthetics	3	May impede airway
– Non-surgical periodontology	1	
– Surgical periodontology	1	
Hazardous and contraindicated drugs	1	Antibiotic selection

*0 = No special considerations. 1 = Caution advised. 2 = Specialised medical advice recommended in some cases. 3 = Specialised medical advice mandatory. 4 = Only to be performed in hospital environment. 5 = Should be avoided.

Drug use Antimicrobials for oral infections should be carefully selected because patients often have *Staphylococcus aureus* and *Pseudomonas aeruginosa* infections, and are already on prolonged antibiotic therapy.

Further reading

● da Costa C C, Cardoso L, de Carvalho Rocha M J 2003 Holistic approach of a child with cystic fibrosis: a case report. J Dent Child (Chic) 70:86–90
● Narang A, Maguire A, Nunn J H, Bush A 2003 Oral health and related factors in cystic fibrosis and other chronic respiratory disorders. Arch Dis Child 88:702–707.

DEPRESSION

Definition A depressive disorder is an illness that affects mood (the affect), and thoughts, which in turn affects the way one eats and sleeps, feels about oneself, and thinks about things.

General aspects

Aetiopathogenesis Some types of depression run in families, and episodes can be triggered by life events such as a serious loss, difficult relationship, financial problem, or any stressful (unwelcome or desired) change in life patterns. Depression may also accompany: ■ other mental diseases – such as schizophrenia ■ viral infections such as influenza, viral hepatitis, HIV/AIDS or infectious mononucleosis ■ use of drugs such as ibuprofen, indometacin, prednisone, benzodiazepines, levodopa, reserpine, methyldopa, fenfluramine, corticosteroids or oral contraceptives ■ withdrawal of psychoactive drugs such as amphetamines, benzodiazepines, or antidepressants ■ serious medical conditions (as a psychogenic reaction to these) e.g. ● Parkinsonism or stroke ● myocardial infarction ● malignant diseases ● HIV/AIDS ● endocrinopathies such as diabetes.

Women experience depression about twice as often as men. Hormonal factors may contribute to this, particularly such factors as menstrual cycle changes, pregnancy, miscarriage, postpartum period, premenopause and menopause. Men are also less likely to admit to depression, and doctors are less likely to suspect it, but it is often masked by manifesting as irritability, or anger, and may be suppressed by alcohol or drugs, or by the socially acceptable habit of working excessively long hours.

The main effects of depression appear related to changes in the hypothalamic centres that govern food intake, libido, and circadian rhythms. There are depleted cerebral amine levels, particularly of serotonin and norepinephrine, and hypercortisolism is common.

Clinical presentation Features of *major* depression include: ■ persistent feelings of: ● sadness, anxiety, or 'empty' mood ● hopelessness, pessimism ● guilt, worthlessness, helplessness, irritability ■ loss of interest or pleasure in hobbies and activities that were once enjoyed, including sex ■ a decrease in: ● energy ● concentration, ability to remember, and make decisions ● sleep (insomnia, early-morning awakening, or oversleeping) ■ altered appetite (weight loss or overeating and weight gain) ■ thoughts of death/ suicide or actual suicide attempts ■ chronic pain or other persistent bodily symptoms that are not caused by physical illness or injury.

Classification In addition to major depression, other types of depressive disorders have been defined including: ■ dysthymic disorder – a chronic, less intense form of depression which may progress to major depression ■ seasonal affective disorder – a chronic cyclic form of depression which appears as daylight hours shorten, is related to melatonin production, and is characterised by winter somnolence and craving for carbohydrates ■ involutional melancholia – characterised by severe anxiety and hypochondriasis, beginning in later life and mainly affecting women.

Diagnosis A depressive episode is diagnosed if five or more of the symptoms detailed in 'clinical presentation' last most of the day, nearly every day, for a period of 2 weeks or longer.

Treatment ■ Psychotherapy involves talking with a mental health professional, such as a psychiatrist, psychologist, social worker, or counsellor to learn how to deal with problems ■ Conventional antidepressant treatment has routinely been the use of medications that raise levels of brain serotonin and norepinephrine (Table 3.42). Serotonin is the 'feel good' hormone that encourages relaxation and enjoyment of life. Norepinephrine is a stimulant.

Antidepressants include mainly the monoamine oxidase inhibitors (MAOIs) that act by inhibiting the enzyme MAO that normally breaks down norepinephrine and serotonin, the tricyclics (TCAs) that work by preventing serotonin and norepinephrine from returning to the nerve cells that released them, and the selective serotonin reuptake inhibitors (SSRIs) that increase serotonin in the brain.

Monoamine oxidase inhibitors The most common adverse effects of MAOIs are: ■ xerostomia ■ hypotension ■ anorexia ■ nausea ■ constipation ■ sexual dysfunction. The most severe adverse effects are drug or food interactions. Hypertensive crises have resulted from interaction of these MAOIs with foods containing tyramine (particularly cheese) and also with yeast products, chocolate, bananas, broad beans, some red wines and beer, pickled herring or caviar.

Table 3.42 **Most commonly used antidepressants**

Class	Abbreviation	Mechanism of action	Drug	Side effects
Monoamine oxidase inhibitors	MAOI	Inhibit MAO-A	Moclobemide	
Tricyclic antidepressants	TCA	Block reuptake of Nor & 5HT	Amitriptyline Dolesupin Doxepin Lomipramine Lofepramine Nortriptyline Protriptyline	Sedation
Selective serotonin reuptake inhibitors	SSRI	Block reuptake of 5HT	Citalopram Fluoxetine Fluvoxamine Peroxetine Sertraline	Fewer adverse effects
Selective norepinephrine reuptake inhibitors	SNRI	Block reuptake of Nor & 5HT	Venlafaxine	
Noradrenaline reuptake inhibitor	NARI	Block reuptake of Nor	Reboxetine	
Noradrenergic and specific serotonergic antidepressant	NASSA	Block reuptake of Nor, 5HT2 & 5HT3	Mirtazapine	
Serotonin (5-hydroxytryptamine) antagonists	5HT	5HT antagonists	Nefazodone	

Interactions of MAOIs with pethidine and other opioids are dangerous and have sometimes been fatal. Interactions with tricyclics are also dangerous. Ephedrine and similar drugs often present in nasal decongestants or cold remedies may cause severe hypertension. Interactions with SSRIs have produced the serotonin syndrome of CNS irritability, hyper-reflexia and myoclonus.

Tricyclic antidepressants Tricyclic antidepressants are probably the most effective antidepressants. The onset of action of TCAs is, however, slow and they may take 4 weeks to exert their full effect. The action is dose-dependent and lack of effect is often the result of failure to achieve adequate plasma levels. Their most common undesirable side effects include: ■ dry mouth ■ constipation ■ bladder problems ■ sexual dysfunction ■ blurred vision ■ dizziness ■ drowsiness.

Tricyclics are contraindicated in patients with cardiac problems (arrhythmias, heart block, cardiac failure) and tricyclics are absolutely contraindicated if the patient has had a recent myocardial infarct. Epilepsy, liver dysfunction, blood dyscrasias, glaucoma and urinary obstruction (e.g. prostatic hypertrophy) are other contraindications. Adverse effects of the tricyclics are more serious in the elderly. Tricyclics should therefore only be given after a full blood count, liver function tests and, if the patient is over 45, an ECG should be undertaken, to ensure the patient is fit. They should not be used within 2 weeks of the use of MAOIs.

Selective serotonin reuptake inhibitors Though no more effective than older antidepressants, SSRIs have the advantage of fewer adverse effects, especially lower anticholinergic activity, weight gain or cardiac conduction effects. However, gastrointestinal effects are common. Common adverse effects of SSRIs include: ■ anorexia ■ nausea ■ anxiety ■ diarrhoea ■ sexual dysfunction ■ rarely mania, paranoia or extrapyramidal features. Other described undesirable effects such as arrhythmia if the patient is using terfenadine, headache, xerostomia and insomnia (trouble falling asleep or waking often during the night) may occur during the first few weeks; dosage reductions or time will usually resolve these.

SSRIs should not be used with tricyclics, carbamazepine or lithium, or within 2 weeks of MAOIs, since this may produce the serotonin syndrome of CNS irritability, hyper-reflexia and myoclonus, which may be lethal. SSRIs can inhibit cytochrome p450 enzymes and thus inhibit the metabolism of benzodiazepines, carbamazepine, codeine and erythromycin and are contraindicated in epilepsy, cardiac disease, diabetes, glaucoma, bleeding tendencies, pregnancy, liver or renal disease.

Prognosis The danger in depression is of suicide – the rate in men is four times that in women, though more women attempt it.

Oral findings

Dry mouth This is the most common oral complaint of depressed patients under treatment, especially as a result of the use of TCAs or lithium. It may predispose to oral candidosis and increased caries, especially since taste sensation may be disturbed, and patients tend to increase their dietary sugar. Xerostomia can occasionally lead to ascending suppurative parotitis. The most effective treatment is to change the antidepressant to another that has little anticholinergic activity but, if this is not acceptable, the dry mouth should be managed as in Sjögren's syndrome. Smoking and other drugs that may add to the xerostomia, such as antihistamines, hyoscine or other atropine-like drugs, or SSRIs, should be avoided.

Facial dyskinesias/tardive dyskinesia Both MAOIs and TCAs have been reported occasionally to cause facial dyskinesias and prolonged use of flupentixol can lead to intractable tardive dyskinesia.

Bodily complaints Often related to the mouth, these are common in depression and the dental surgeon should appreciate the possibility of a mental basis for such oral complaints. Depression is associated especially with the following disorders: ■ atypical facial pain ■ burning mouth or sore tongue (oral dysaesthesia) ■ temporomandibular pain-dysfunction syndrome (occasionally) ■ other complaints not confirmed by clinical examination or investigations: ● discharges (of fluid, slime or powder coming into the mouth) ● dry mouth ● sialorrhoea ● spots or lumps ● halitosis ● disturbed taste sensation.

Dental management

Risk assessment The features aiding recognition of depression have been suggested above and dental staff should be alert to this possibility particularly where the patient appears withdrawn, difficult or aggressive, or where there are oral complaints of the types described.

Appropriate health care ■ Great tact, patience and a sympathetic but unpatronising manner are needed in handling depressed patients ■ Dental treatment is preferably deferred until the depression is under control but preventive programmes should be instituted at an early stage.

Preventive dentistry Oral hygiene may be neglected. Professional dental cleaning, supplementary fluorides and chlorhexidine varnish applications have been recommended.

Pain and anxiety control **Local anaesthesia** There is no clinical evidence of interactions between tricyclic antidepressants and epinephrine in local anaesthetic agents used in dentistry causing either hypertension or significant arrhythmias. Nevertheless, aspirating syringes should always be used and the dose of epinephrine should not exceed 0.05 mg.
Conscious sedation Any CNS depressant, especially opioids and phenothiazines, given to patients on MAOIs (or within 21 days of their withdrawal) may precipitate coma. Pethidine is particularly dangerous. Benzodiazepines may be potentiated in patients on SSRIs.
General anaesthesia Patients on MAOIs are at risk from GA, since prolonged respiratory depression may result.

Patient access and positioning **Patient positioning** TCAs and MAOIs can cause postural hypotension and a patient should not be stood

Table 3.43 **Key considerations for dental management in depression (see text)**

	Management modifications*	Comments/possible complications
Risk assessment	2	Recognition of depression
Appropriate dental care	2	Sympathetic handling; avoid elective dental care until disease is controlled
Pain and anxiety control		
– Local anaesthesia	1	Reduce epinephrine dose
– Conscious sedation	2	Avoid benzodiazepines and opioids
– General anaesthesia	3–5	Respiratory depression
Patient access and positioning		
– Access to dental office	0	
– Timing of treatment	0	
– Patient positioning	1	Postural hypotension
Treatment modification		
– Oral surgery	1	
– Implantology	1/5	Xerostomia; neglected oral hygiene
– Conservative/Endodontics	1	
– Fixed prosthetics	1	Avoid gingival retraction cord with epinephrine
– Removable prosthetics	0	
– Non-surgical periodontology	1	
– Surgical periodontology	1	
Hazardous and contraindicated drugs	1	Avoid acetaminophen and erythromycin

*0 = No special considerations. 1 = Caution advised. 2 = Specialised medical advice recommended in some cases. 3 = Specialised medical advice mandatory. 4 = Only to be performed in hospital environment. 5 = Should be avoided.

immediately upright if they have been lying flat during dental treatment; the chair should slowly be brought upright.

Treatment modification **Implantology** Although cases have been successful, there have been no systematic studies on implant-retained prostheses in xerostomic patients. Neglected oral hygiene may lead to a poorer prognosis. **Fixed prosthetics and conservation** Gingival retraction cords containing epinephrine should be avoided.

Drug use Acetaminophen/paracetamol can inhibit the metabolism of TCAs. Erythromycin may be potentiated in patients on SSRIs.

Further reading • George S, Saksena A, Oyebode F 2004 An update on psychiatric disorders in relation to dental treatment. Dent Update 31:488–494 • Little J W 2004 Dental implications of mood disorders. Gen Dent 52:442–450.

DIABETES INSIPIDUS

Definition Diabetes insipidus (DI) is a disorder characterised by increased water intake and elimination, due to low posterior pituitary secretion of antidiuretic hormone (ADH) (Cranial or Central DI), or renal resistance to ADH (Nephrogenic DI).

General aspects

Aetiopathogenesis Although idiopathic and hereditary types have been recognised, most cases are: ■ cranial DI, caused by: ● head injury or trauma ● meningitis ● sarcoidosis ● autoimmune ● vascular ● tumours (craniopharyngioma) ■ nephrogenic DI, caused by: ● renal disease ● hypokalaemia ● hypercalcaemia ● drugs (lithium, demeclocycline).

Clinical presentation ■ Sudden onset of polydipsia and polyuria, with normal levels of urinary and blood glucose ■ Weakness, fever and psychiatric disorders are common in cases of dehydration.

Table 3.44 **Key considerations in dental management in diabetes insipidus (see text)**

	Management modifications*	Comments/possible complications
Risk assessment	0	Xerostomia
Appropriate dental care	1	Sips of water
Pain and anxiety control		
– Local anaesthesia	0	
– Conscious sedation	0	
– General anaesthesia	3/4	Dehydration
Patient access and positioning		
– Access to dental office	0	
– Timing of treatment	0	
– Patient positioning	1	Short appointments
Treatment modification		
– Oral surgery	0	
– Implantology	1	Dryness
– Conservative/Endodontics	0	
– Fixed prosthetics	0	
– Removable prosthetics	1	Dryness
– Non-surgical periodontology	0	
– Surgical periodontology	0	
Hazardous and contraindicated drugs	1	Avoid carbamazepine

*0 = No special considerations. 1 = Caution advised. 2 = Specialised medical advice recommended in some cases. 3 = Specialised medical advice mandatory. 4 = Only to be performed in hospital environment. 5 = Should be avoided.

Diagnosis ■ Clinical findings ■ Plasma osmolality – high ■ Urine osmolality – low ■ Water deprivation test – fails to significantly alter plasma osmolality.

Treatment ■ Treat the cause ■ Desmopressin.

Prognosis Severe dehydration can lead to death.

Dental management

Risk assessment Dentistry is usually uncomplicated by this disorder except for dryness of the mouth. Drinking water during dental treatment may be necessary.

Pain and anxiety control **Local anaesthesia** LA may be used safely with the usual routine precautions. **Conscious sedation** CS may be used safely with the usual routine precautions. **General anaesthesia** The risk of dehydration increases during GA. Monitoring liquid intake and excretion (bladder catheter) is then mandatory.

Patient access and positioning **Timing of treatment** Short appointments to avoid dehydration are recommended.

Drug use Carbamazepine used in the treatment of trigeminal neuralgia may have an additive effect with other drugs used to treat diabetes insipidus.

Further reading ● Seow W K, Thomsett M J 1994 Dental fluorosis as a complication of hereditary diabetes insipidus: studies of six affected patients. Pediatr Dent16:128–132.

DIABETES MELLITUS

Definition Diabetes is a chronic metabolic disorder characterised by a relative or absolute lack of insulin.

General aspects

Aetiopathogenesis It is estimated that diabetes affects approximately 2% of populations, but only 50% is recognised. It is more common in Indian and Pakistani populations. The origin of diabetes is multifactorial, with the following implicated: ■ genetic predisposition (e.g. HLA-B8, B15, DR3, DR4) ■ primary destruction of the pancreatic islets of Langerhans (e.g. pancreatitis or neoplasm) ■ endocrine anomalies (e.g. hyperthyroidism) ■ iatrogenic factors (e.g. corticosteroid therapy) ■ infectious agents (e.g. Coxsackie viruses).

Clinical presentation ■ Polyuria, polydipsia, polyphagia, weight loss and fatigue are common ■ Long-term complications include: ● angina pectoris, myocardial infarction, cerebral infarction and claudication due to macroangiopathy ● retinopathy and renal disease due to microangiopathy ● autonomic and peripheral polyneuropathy ● recurrent infections ● delayed healing (Fig. 3.12).

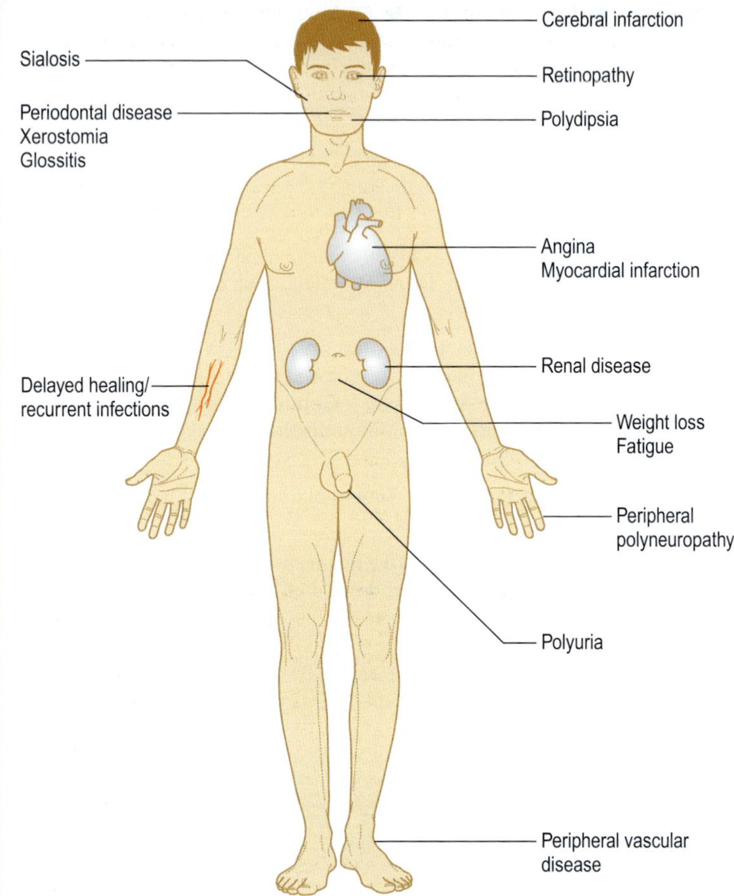

Figure 3.12 **Clinical presentation of diabetes mellitus**

Classification This has changed in recent years and is no longer based on insulin requirements (i.e. the terms IDDM/NIDDM are obsolete), but rather the aetiology: ■ *primary diabetes* may be: ● type I (absolute insulin deficiency) – this is associated with liability to ketosis and weight loss, associated with antibodies to pancreatic islet cells ● type II (relative deficiency; can reflect an insulin deficiency state or a peripheral resistance to insulin) ■ *secondary diabetes* can be caused by endocrinopathies (e.g. acromegaly, Cushing's disease), drugs (e.g. corticosteroids) or pancreatic disease (surgery, tumour or inflammation).

Diagnosis ■ Fasting venous plasma glucose – increased > 7 mmol/L ■ 2-hour oral glucose tolerance test – abnormal > 11.1 mmol/L ■ Plasma glycosylated haemoglobin (HbA_{1c}) – raised > 7%.

Treatment ■ Diet ■ Insulin ■ Oral hypoglycaemics ● sulphonylureas such as chlorpropramide and gliclazide stimulate insulin release ● biguanides such as metformin, alpha glucosidase inhibitor or thiazolidinedione reduce hepatic glucose output, modulate glucose absorption and stimulate muscle glucose uptake.

Prognosis Some diabetes-related complications, such as visual impairment, renal failure, gangrene, stroke or myocardial infarction, significantly affect the quality of life. When compared with the general population, diabetics also have a decreased life expectancy.

Oral findings

There are no specific oral manifestations of diabetes mellitus. However the following features have been observed: ■ Diabetics, even if well controlled, have more severe periodontal disease than controls ■ Initially tooth development appears to be accelerated but, after the age of 10 years, is delayed ■ A dry mouth may result from dehydration and occasionally there is swelling of the salivary glands (sialosis), due to autonomic neuropathy ■ Severe dentoalveolar abscess with fascial space involvement in a seemingly healthy individual may arise in diabetes, and therefore such patients should be investigated to exclude diabetes; orofacial infections should be vigorously treated as they may precipitate ketosis ■ The tongue may show glossitis and alterations in filiform papillae ■ There may be burning mouth sensations in the absence of physical changes ■ If control is poor, oral candidosis may develop and presents, for example, with angular stomatitis ■ Severe diabetics with ketoacidosis are predisposed to mucormycosis in the paranasal sinuses and nose (indeed, this is the main cause of mucormycoses) ■ In patients with insulin-treated diabetes, circumoral paraesthesia is a common and an important sign of impending hypoglycaemia ■ Oral mucosal lichenoid reactions may result from the use of chlorpropamide and some other antidiabetic agents; however, the 'Grinspan syndrome' (diabetes, lichen planus and hypertension) may be purely the coincidental associations of common disorders probably related to drug use ■ Chlorpropamide may cause facial flushing.

Dental management

Risk assessment ■ Patients with findings that suggest diabetes should be referred to a physician for advice ■ The main hazard during dental treatment is of hypoglycaemia: dental disease and treatment may disrupt the normal pattern of food intake. Hypoglycaemia is avoidable by appropriate planning, such as to give oral glucose just before the appointment, and ensure patients take their normal meals. Patients should be asked to inform the dentist if they feel a hypoglycaemic episode starting. ■ Management of hypoglycaemia in a known diabetic patient involves: ● if the patient is conscious and able to swallow, give a glucose drink, or 150 mL carbonated drink, or two teaspoons sugar in water/orange squash ● if the patient is drowsy, give a sublingual carbohydrate gel, such as Gluco Gel ● if the patient is unconscious, give glucagon 1 mg intramuscularly, and follow, when conscious, with a drink containing sugar/glucose ● if the patient remains unconscious, with no response to glucagon in 2–3 minutes, call for an ambulance and continue to monitor the airway and pulse ■ The long-term complications of diabetes may require management (e.g. angina, hypotension, cardiac arrest).

Appropriate health care ■ Poorly controlled diabetics (whether Type I or II), with fasting glucose levels above 14 mmol/L (250 mg/dL): ● these patients should be referred for improved control of their blood sugar before non-emergency surgery is performed ● if emergency surgery is needed, then prophylactic antibiotics are prudent, using the accepted principles of such use ■ Infections in diabetic patients: ● regardless of the patient's diabetic control levels, infections should be managed aggressively, including possible early referral to oral and maxillofacial surgeon ■ Routine non-surgical procedures: ● routine dental treatment or short minor surgical procedures under local anaesthesia can be carried out with no special precautions apart from ensuring that treatment does not interfere with eating ■ Surgical procedures: ● the essential requirement is to avoid hypoglycaemia and also keep hyperglycaemia below levels which may be harmful because of delayed wound healing or phagocyte dysfunction; the desired whole blood glucose level is therefore ~5 mmol/L ● special management considerations apply to the diabetic who is to undergo anything more than simple dentoalveolar procedures under GA (Table 3.45); the effects of stress and trauma may raise insulin requirements and precipitate ketosis ● precautions required during oral surgery in diabetics depend mainly on: the type and severity of the diabetes and complications such as autonomic neuropathy that may predispose to hypotension or cardiac arrest, the type of anaesthetic, the extent of surgery, the extent of interference with normal feeding postoperatively ■ Many different management regimens have been suggested and each patient requires individual handling: the following therefore provides only general guidelines and the diabetic consultant should always decide the final regimen.

Diabetics controlled by diet alone ■ These diabetics are often obese or elderly with little liability to ketosis and, if they are well controlled, many can tolerate minor surgical procedures, such as single extractions under local anaesthetic, without problems. A brief general anaesthetic can be given without special precautions apart from monitoring the urine sugar before the operation and on recovery, at 2-hourly intervals. However, such patients must have the anaesthetic in hospital, so that if ketonuria develops, blood sugar levels can be rapidly estimated. ■ Not all such patients are necessarily well controlled. In this case, or if more major surgery is planned, the patient should be admitted to hospital preoperatively for assessment and possible stabilisation with insulin. The blood sugar should be monitored during and after operation. ■ There is no scientific evidence in the literature to support the premise that well-controlled, or even moderately well-controlled, non-ketotic diabetic patients (controlled by diet) are prone to infection when undergoing uncomplicated dentoalveolar surgery. In these patients, routine administration of prophylactic antibiotics should be considered only in situations where prophylactic antimicrobials would be used for a non-diabetic patient.

Table 3.45 **Management of diabetics requiring general anaesthesia**

	Non-insulin-dependent diabetics*	Non-insulin-dependent diabetics	Insulin-dependent diabetics
Procedure	Minor operations, e.g. few extractions	Major operations, e.g. maxillofacial surgery	Any operation
Preop	Stop biguanides. If on chlorpropamide, change to tolbutamide 1 week preop	Stabilise on at least b.d. insulin for 2–3 days preop One day preop use only short-acting insulin (Actrapid soluble or neutral)	
Periop	Omit oral hypoglycaemic Estimate blood glucose level	Do not give sulphonylurea or subcutaneous insulin on day of operation Estimate blood glucose level Set up intravenous infusion of 10% glucose 500 mL containing Actrapid or Leo neutral insulin 10 units plus KCl 1 g at 8.00 a.m. Infuse over 4 h Estimate blood glucose and potassium levels 2-hourly Adjust insulin and potassium to keep glucose at 5–10 mmol/L and the patient normokalaemic	
Postop	Estimate blood glucose 4 h postop	Continue infusion 4-hourly Estimate blood glucose 4-hourly Estimate potassium 8-hourly	
On resuming normal diet	Start sulphonylurea or other usual regimen	Stop infusion Start Actrapid or Leo neutral insulin and over the next 2 days Start sulphonylurea Start normal insulin regimen	

*If well controlled, otherwise treat as insulin-dependent.

Diabetics controlled by diet and oral hypoglycaemics A similar regimen is used for both well- and poorly-controlled patients in this category as for those described for diabetics controlled by diet only.

Diabetics on insulin ■ In a well-controlled patient, providing that normal diet has, and can, be taken, it is feasible to carry out: ● minor surgical procedures, such as simple single extractions under local anaesthesia, as long as the procedure is carried out within 2 hours of breakfast and the morning insulin injection, with no change in the insulin regimen ● more protracted procedures such as multiple extractions must only be carried out in hospital ● prophylactic antimicrobials may be considered ● minor operations under general anaesthesia, by operating early in the morning and withholding both food and insulin from the previous midnight, until after the procedure ● major operations under general anaesthesia. The patient is put on an insulin sliding scale from the morning of the day of operation until a normal feeding regimen is possible. ■ In a poorly-controlled diabetic, all surgical treatment should be carried out in hospital.

Pain and anxiety control **Local anaesthesia** Local anaesthesia can usually be safely used. The dose of epinephrine used in dental local anaesthetic solution is unlikely to increase blood glucose levels significantly. **Conscious sedation** Conscious sedation can usually be safely used. Benzodiazepines have been recommended. **General anaesthesia** General anaesthesia for the diabetic is a matter for the specialist anaesthetist since it may be complicated especially by: ■ hypoglycaemia ■ chronic renal failure ■ ischaemic heart disease ■ severe autonomic neuropathy (carries a risk of cardiorespiratory arrest if a general anaesthetic is given). An example of a protocol employed for undertaking GA in diabetic patients is outlined in Table 3.45.

Table 3.46 **Key considerations for dental management in diabetes mellitus (see text)**

	Management modifications*	Comments/possible complications
Risk assessment	2	Hypoglycaemia; angina; hypotension; cardiac arrest
Appropriate dental care	2/4	Type and severity of the diabetes; type of anaesthetic; extent of surgery; the diabetician should advise on the regimen
Pain and anxiety control		
– Local anaesthesia	0	
– Conscious sedation	0	
– General anaesthesia	3/4	See Table 3.45
Patient access and positioning		
– Access to dental office	0	
– Timing of treatment	1	Early to mid-morning after breakfast and antidiabetic treatment
– Patient positioning	1	Postural hypotension
Treatment modification		
– Oral surgery	2	
– Implantology	2	
– Conservative/Endodontics	1	
– Fixed prosthetics	1	
– Removable prosthetics	1	Denture-induced stomatitis
– Non-surgical periodontology	2	
– Surgical periodontology	2	
Hazardous and contraindicated drugs	2	Avoid aspirin, steroids and tetracyclines

*0 = No special considerations. 1 = Caution advised. 2 = Specialised medical advice recommended in some cases. 3 = Specialised medical advice mandatory. 4 = Only to be performed in hospital environment. 5 = Should be avoided.

Patient access and positioning **Timing of treatment** ■ If normal eating will be resumed at lunchtime, appointments should be early to mid-morning after a normal breakfast and normal antidiabetic treatment. An early morning appointment will also minimise the risk of stress-induced hypoglycaemia. ■ If normal eating will not be resumed at lunchtime, appointments should be early to mid-morning after a normal breakfast and half the normal antidiabetic treatment, in consultation with the patient's physician. **Patient positioning** Autonomic neuropathy in diabetes can cause orthostatic hypotension; therefore the supine patient should be slowly raised upright in the dental chair.

Treatment modification **Implantology** Implant success rates are slightly reduced at 86–96%; there is no evidence that diabetes is a contraindication to implants, but medical advice should be taken first. The use of chlorhexidine and antibiotic prophylaxis has been recommended. **Removable prosthetics** Dentures must not be worn at night. Removable prostheses with large acrylic surfaces should be carefully cleaned and possibly replaced to prevent denture-related stomatitis. **Periodontology** There is some evidence that severe periodontitis may upset glycaemic control and that the plasma glycosylated haemoglobin decreases after periodontal treatment.

Drug use ■ Drugs should be sugar-free ■ Doxycycline and other tetracyclines may enhance insulin hypoglycaemia ■ Amoxicillin is the antibiotic of choice ■ Drugs that can disturb diabetic control (aspirin and steroids) must be avoided; aspirin increases the effect of oral hypoglycaemic agents ■ Acetaminophen alone or combined with codeine is the analgesic of choice.

Further reading ● Fiske J 2004 Diabetes mellitus and oral care. Dent Update 31:190–198 ● Manfredi M, McCullough M J, Vescovi P, Al-Kaarawi Z M, Porter S R 2004 Update on diabetes mellitus and related oral diseases. Oral Dis 10:187–200 ● Vernillo A T 2001 Diabetes mellitus: Relevance to dental treatment. Oral Surg Oral Med Oral Pathol Oral Radiol Endod 91:263–270.

DOWN SYNDROME

Definition Down syndrome is the most frequent genetic cause of mild to moderate learning disability. It is a chromosomal disorder caused by an error in cell division that results in the presence of an additional third chromosome 21' or 'trisomy 21'.

General aspects

■ This was named after John Langdon Down, the physician who identified the syndrome in 1866 ■ Down syndrome (DS) appears in one out of 800 live births, in all races and economic groups.

Aetiopathogenesis The aetiology of the syndrome remains unclear, however, in 88% of individuals with DS, the extra copy of chromosome 21 is derived from the mother. DS is usually due to a random event during formation of the ovum or sperm. ■ Three genetic variations can cause DS: ● In 92%, DS is caused by an extra chromosome 21 in all cells (trisomy 21) ● In 2–4%, DS is due to mosaic trisomy 21, when the extra chromosome 21 is present only in some cells. The range of physical problems varies, depending on the proportion of cells carrying the additional chromosome 21. ● In 3–4%, material from one chromosome 21 is translocated onto another chromosome (translocation trisomy 21), either before or at conception. In such situations, cells have two normal chromosomes 21, but also have additional chromosome 21 material on the translocated chromosome. ■ The probability that another child with DS will be born in a subsequent pregnancy is about 1%, regardless of maternal age. The likelihood that a reproductive cell will contain an extra copy of chromosome 21 increases dramatically as a woman ages. Only about 9% of total pregnancies occur in women 35 years or older each year, but about 25% of babies with DS are born to women in this age group.

Clinical presentation The characteristic features of DS are: ■ learning disability (100%) ■ mongoloid face (85%) ■ short stature (85%) ■ brachycephaly (80%) ■ muscular hypotonia (80%) ■ increased joint flexibility (80%) ■ pelvic dysplasia (70%) ■ clinodactyly (short fifth finger; 45%) ■ simian (single) palmar creases (45%) ■ Brushfield's spots in the iris (40%).

DS affects many if not most organs and may result in multiple disabilities including: ■ Neuropsychiatric disease: ● learning disability ● dementia, or memory loss and impaired judgment similar to that occurring in Alzheimer's disease patients, may develop ■ Endocrine: people with Down syndrome are especially vulnerable to thyroid disease ■ Sensory deficits: ● hearing loss – the external ear and the bones of the middle and inner ear may develop differently in DS and thus up to 90% have hearing loss of greater than 15–20 decibels in at least one ear ● visual defects: cataracts occur in approximately 3% of children with DS, but can be surgically removed; nystagmus and strabismus are not unusual ■ Seizure disorders: these affect 5–13% of individuals with DS, a 10-fold greater incidence than in the general population ■ Cardiac problems: approximately 50% of people with DS have cardiac disorders associated with early onset of pulmonary hypertension. Congenital heart disease is common: the main types are atrial septal defect, mitral valve prolapse or, less often, atrioventricular canal and ventricular septal defect. ■ Spinal problems: ● atlantoaxial instability can cause spinal cord compression if the neck is not handled considerately ● susceptibility to transient myelodysplasia, or defective development of the spinal cord ■ Malignant disease: ● people with DS are 10–15 times more likely than others to develop leukaemia ● predisposition to develop retinoblastoma ■ Immune defects: there are multiple immunological defects (IgA and T lymphocyte function defects) so that infections of the skin, gastrointestinal and respiratory tracts are common, especially in institutionalised patients who are also liable to be hepatitis B carriers (persistence of HBsAg in about 40% of individuals). Chronic respiratory infections in DS may include recurrent middle ear, tonsil, nasal and sinus infections and tuberculosis. ■ Premature aging.

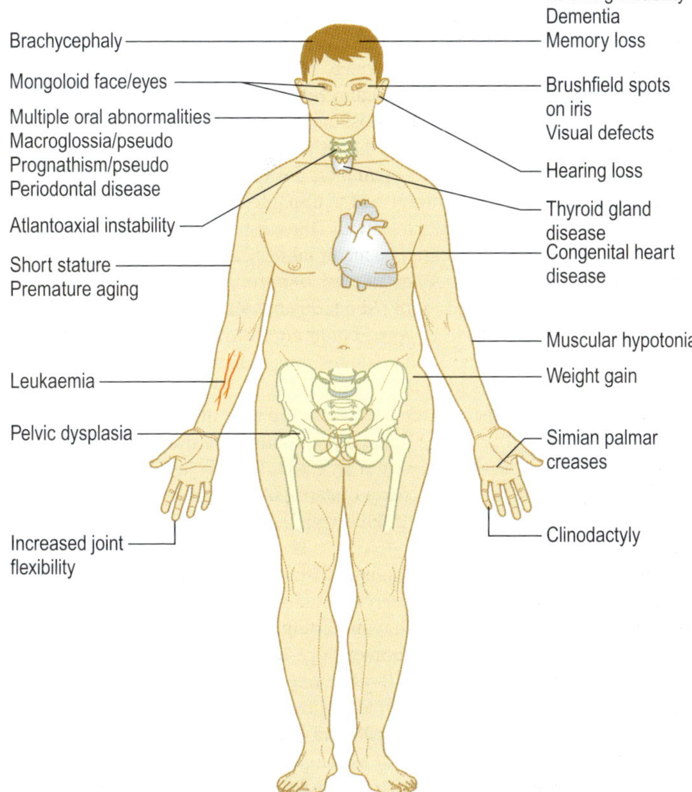

Figure 3.13 **Clinical presentation of Down syndrome**

Diagnosis ■ Many specialists recommend that women who become pregnant at age 35 or older undergo prenatal testing for DS ■ Prenatal screening for DS is available and includes, after counselling: • simple, non-invasive blood screening for maternal serum alpha fetoprotein (MSAFP; reduced in DS), chorionic gonadotropin (hCG; raised in DS) and unconjugated oestriol (uE3; reduced in DS) • amniocentesis • chorionic villus sampling • percutaneous umbilical blood sampling – to confirm the diagnosis, a chromosomal karyotype is carried out to determine if extra material from chromosome 21 is present.

Prognosis Although the life expectancy for people with DS has increased substantially to age 50 and beyond ■ about one-third of infants with DS die in the first few years of life from cardiac disease ■ a 12-fold higher mortality rate from infectious diseases exists, particularly from pneumonia ■ haematological malignancies may also influence the prognosis, and reduce life expectancy.

Oral findings

There are many oral abnormalities including: ■ An open-mouth posture with a protrusive tongue – the tongue may be absolutely or relatively large and is often fissured ■ The lips tend to be thick, dry and fissured with a poor anterior oral seal ■ The maxillae and malars (zygomatic bone) are small and the mandible is protrusive ■ Class III malocclusion is common, but 46% are class I ■ Anterior open bite, posterior crossbite and other types of malocclusion are common ■ Although the palate often appears to be high, with horizontal palatal shelves (the omega palate), a short palate is more characteristic ■ There is also an increased incidence of bifid uvula, cleft lip and cleft palate ■ As in all other aspects of their development, people with DS have delayed tooth formation and delayed/disordered eruption. The first dentition may begin to appear only after 9 months and may take 5 years to complete, if ever. The deciduous molars may erupt before the deciduous incisors and deciduous lateral incisors are absent in about 15%. The eruption of the permanent teeth is often also irregular. ■ Missing teeth are common, although, as in the general population, the third molars and lateral incisors are most often absent ■ Up to 30% have morphological abnormalities in both dentitions, particularly teeth with short, small crowns and roots. The occlusal surfaces of the deciduous molars may be hypoplastic and both dentitions may be hypocalcified. ■ The most significant dental disorder is severe early onset periodontal disease. Lower anterior teeth are usually severely affected and lost early. Acute necrotising ulcerative gingivitis is also seen. Individuals with DS have a raised prevalence of periodontal disease compared with otherwise normal, age-matched control groups and other patients with learning disability. The exaggerated immune-inflammatory response of the tissues cannot be explained by poor oral hygiene alone and might be the result of an impaired cell-mediated and humoral immunity and a deficient phagocytic system. As far as the progression and severity of destruction, this is consistent with an aggressive periodontitis disease pattern. ■ In contrast, caries incidence is usually low in both dentitions, possibly related to the high salivary bicarbonate and pH.

Dental management

Risk assessment Risk of dental management includes consideration of: ■ bacterial endocarditis prophylaxis ■ infection control ■ aggressive elimination of any dental infection.

Appropriate dental care ■ All people with Down syndrome have learning disability to some degree, but many are amiable and cooperative most of the time and are generally more easily managed than many other types of patients with learning disability. Rarely, some non-cooperative DS patients have to be treated under GA. ■ Most patients can be instructed in regular oral hygiene habits ■ Caregivers and parents play a key role in oral health education.

Pain and anxiety control **Local anaesthesia** Many can be treated under local anaesthesia. **Conscious sedation** Sedation can be a very

Table 3.47 **Key considerations in dental management in Down syndrome (see text)**

	Management modifications*	Comments/possible complications
Risk assessment	2	Bacterial endocarditis; infection
Appropriate dental care	2	Antibiotic prophylaxis; infection control; oral hygiene education
Pain and anxiety control		
– Local anaesthesia	0	
– Conscious sedation	1	Respiratory function/ infection
– General anaesthesia	3–5	Cardiac defects; respiratory disease; difficult intubation; chest infections; anaemia; atlantoaxial subluxation; hepatitis B
Patient access and positioning		
– Access to dental office	0	
– Timing of treatment	0	
– Patient positioning	1	Avoid neck hyperextension
Treatment modification		
– Oral surgery	1	
– Implantology	1/5	Periodontal disease; neglected oral hygiene
– Conservative/Endodontics	1/5	Severe periodontitis
– Fixed prosthetics	1/5	Severe periodontitis
– Removable prosthetics	1	
– Non-surgical periodontology	1	Periodontitis may progress despite therapy
– Surgical periodontology	1/5	
Hazardous and contraindicated drugs	1	Some patients receive platelet aggregation inhibitors

*0 = No special considerations. 1 = Caution advised. 2 = Specialised medical advice recommended in some cases. 3 = Specialised medical advice mandatory. 4 = Only to be performed in hospital environment. 5 = Should be avoided.

useful adjunct, although careful assessment must be made of respiratory function/infection. **General anaesthesia** General anaesthesia must be administered by a specialist anaesthetist, in view of other management difficulties which may include: ■ cardiac defects predisposing to infective endocarditis ■ respiratory disease ■ difficulty in intubation because of the hypoplastic midface; congenital anomalies of the respiratory tract and increased susceptibility to chest infections ■ anaemia ■ atlantoaxial subluxation (care needed when extending neck) ■ hepatitis B carriage.

Patient access and positioning **Patient positioning** Avoid neck hyperextension.

Treatment modification **Preventive dentistry** A well-planned preventive dental health programme should be successful in the prevention of dental diseases, and may include: ■ dental check-up once every 3 months ■ regular professional tooth cleaning (increased dental calculus accumulation) ■ diet counselling ■ oral hygiene and motivation. **Implantology** Prognosis of dental implants is influenced by oral hygiene and periodontal status. **Fixed prostheses** Fixed prostheses may be indicated in cases with favourable oral hygiene, morphology and periodontal health of the remaining natural teeth. **Periodontology** Due to the severity and early onset of periodontal disease, periodontal treatment is a priority, although, in some patients, periodontitis progresses despite therapy. Regular chlorhexidine mouthwashes are recommended. **Orthodontics** The orthodontic prognosis is often poor because of learning disability, parafunctional habits and severe periodontal disease. However, an early palatal widening with removable appliances may be useful in selected patients. **Paediatric dentistry** Removable orofacial stimulation plates (e.g. Castillo-Morales) have been recommended in young children to improve orofacial muscular tone and tongue position.

Drug use Some patients are under treatment with platelet aggregation inhibitors (for cardiac defects).

Further reading
● Chung E M, Sung E C, Sakurai K L 2004 Dental management of the Down and Eisenmenger syndrome patient. J Contemp Dent Pract 5:70–80 ● Fiske J, Shafik H H 2001 Down's syndrome and oral care. Dent Update 28:148–156 ● Kieser J, Townsend G, Quick A 2003 The Down syndrome patient in dental practice, part I: Pathogenesis and general and dental features. NZ Dent J 99:5–9 ● Scully C, Van Bruggen W, Dios P D, Porter S R, Davison M 2002 Down syndrome; lip lesions and *Candida albicans*. Br J Dermatol 147:37–40.

DRUG ALLERGIES

Definition Drug allergy is an adverse drug reaction mediated by an immunological mechanism.

General aspects

■ Almost any drug may produce unwanted or unexpected adverse reactions, but many adverse reactions are probably not, at present, recognised as drug-related ■ Most drug reactions occur in adult females and those individuals who are frequently exposed to multiple medications ■ A skin rash is the most common type of drug reaction ■ Most allergic antibiotic drug reactions occur to beta-lactam (e.g. penicillin) antibiotics ■ Reactions to radio contrast media (RCM) and aspirin or non-steroidal anti-inflammatory agents are frequent causes of allergic-like (and non-immunological) reactions.

Aetiopathogenesis Virtually all drugs can produce an allergic reaction, but some are considered 'high potential risk drugs' (e.g. penicillin or cephalosporins) and others 'low potential risk drugs' (e.g. erythromycin or lidocaine). In drug allergy, the allergen is often a complex made up from the drug (hapten) and a host protein (transporter).

Some risk factors that may increase the likelihood of developing a drug allergy include: ■ Composition of drug (e.g. presence of additives) ■ Grade of exposure (risk increases with repeated exposure) ■ Route of administration (risk of a reaction increases with parenteral administration) ■ Patient's susceptibility (conditioned by genetics, age, previous episodes of drug allergy and systemic immune disorders). Allergic drug reactions are more common in adults than children. Although atopy is not a risk factor, being atopic predisposes to a more severe reaction. ■ Immunosuppression – may inhibit suppressor T cells regulating IgE antibody synthesis and so enhance the sensitising potential of some drugs. HIV disease has become a major risk factor for adverse drug reactions – over half of patients with AIDS develop adverse reactions when treated with trimethoprim-sulfamethoxazole. The incidence of reactions to ampicillin is inversely proportional to CD4+ cell counts. Several other drugs have a higher than expected tendency to produce adverse reactions in HIV-infected patients. Most are mild-to-moderate skin eruptions, but the risk of anaphylaxis and even toxic epidermal necrolysis may also be enhanced in HIV infection. ■ Sjögren's syndrome – an association between primary Sjögren's and allergy has been suggested, with those individuals who are anti-Ro positive more at risk.

Classification Drug allergy reactions are classified as types I to IV. ■ Type I or anaphylactic: the allergen reacts with mast cell IgE ■ Type II or cytotoxic: the allergen reacts with IgG or IgM of erythrocytes or platelets ■ Type III or immune complex mediated: the allergen-IgE reaction produces microprecipitates on the blood vessel walls which induce lysosome enzyme liberation from neutrophils ■ Type IV or cell-mediated or delayed hypersensitivity: the allergen reacts with sensitised T lymphocytes.

Clinical presentation The clinical presentation varies with the type of drug allergy. ■ Type I anaphylactic reactions typically present as an acute reaction which produces vasodilatation and smooth muscle contraction, provoking complications involving cardiovascular (cardiac arrhythmias), respiratory (bronchospasm), skin (urticaria, angioedema and pruritus) and gastrointestinal (abdominal pain, vomit and diarrhoea) systems. Penicillin may cause this type of reaction. ■ Type II reactions present typically as haematological disorders, including haemolytic anaemia, leucopenia and thrombocytopenia ■ Type III reactions may present as: ● erythema nodosum – often related to penicillin and sulphonamides ● drug-induced fever – sometimes with arthralgia, eosinophilia or rash ● allergic exanthema or urticarial rash ● disseminated vasculitis – procainamide and methicillin have been implicated ■ Type IV reactions usually present as contact reactions, e.g. cheilitis due to lip cosmetics ■ Other reactions ● erythema multiforme ● photosensitivity – described with tetracyclines and sulphonamides.

Diagnosis ■ Skin tests for allergens (prick and patch testing) ■ Laboratory tests for IgE levels (paper radio-immunosorbent test [PRIST] and radio-allergosorbent test [RAST]).

Treatment ■ Drug withdrawal ■ Emergency treatment of anaphylactic reactions and angioneurotic oedema: ● call for medical assistance ● place patient in supine position ● ensure airway clear ● give oxygen by mask 10 L/min ● give epinephrine 1:1000, 0.5 mL intramuscularly into lateral thigh (some patients may carry an Epipen auto-injector) ● give 10 mg chlorpheniramine intramuscularly ● give 200 mg hydrocortisone intramuscularly ● additionally, in bronchospasm, give salbutamol 400 μg via volumetric flask repeated every 5 minutes ■ Antihistamines such as chlorpheniramine (4–10 mg) or diphenhydramine (50 mg) or hydroxyzine (25–100 mg) are prescribed in patients with a rash ■ Severe urticaria may be treated with prednisone or prednisolone (60 mg per day).

Prognosis ■ A severe anaphylactic reaction can lead to death within minutes (in about 10% of patients) ■ Urticaria and other lesser complications usually resolve with drug withdrawal and adequate treatment.

Oral findings

Oral findings related to allergic reactions may include: ■ angioneurotic oedema involving the lips ■ erythema multiforme ■ lichenoid reactions ■ orofacial granulomatosis. Mucosal erythema and ulceration are usually not related to drugs but rather to type IV reactions associated with latex or dental materials (impression materials, amalgam, composites, eugenol, acrylic monomer, gold or nickel).

Dental management

Risk assessment ■ Reaction types I and IV are the most common in dentistry ■ Patients with allergy to one drug, and probably those patients with Sjögren's syndrome or HIV disease, may be particularly liable to drug allergies.

Appropriate dental care ■ Always take a full medical history and ask specifically about adverse drug reactions, since this may influence the choice of drugs used ■ Any suggestion of previous drug reaction or allergy, and particularly any adverse reaction during anaesthesia, must be taken seriously (allergist consultation).

Pain and anxiety control Local anaesthesia ■ Anaphylactoid reactions have been registered in relation to parabens (a preservative formerly used in local anaesthetics) and sulphites (incorporated to prevent oxidation). Prilocaine with felypressin is a good alternative, as it does not contain sulphites and is preservative-free. ■ Allergic reactions have only rarely been definitively demonstrated with amides (methylparabens-free and without vasoconstrictor) such as lidocaine, mepivacaine or prilocaine ■ In a dental emergency, or in patients with allergy to several local anesthetics, 1% diphenhydramine (with 1:100 000 epinephrine) may be used as a local anaesthetic.

Table 3.48 **Key considerations in dental management in drug allergies (see text)**

	Management modifications*	Comments/possible complications
Risk assessment	2	Reaction types I or IV
Appropriate dental care	2	Medical history; allergist consultation
Pain and anxiety control		
– Local anaesthesia	2	Amides without epinephrine are recommended
– Conscious sedation	2	
– General anaesthesia	3/4	
Patient access and positioning		
– Access to dental office	0	
– Timing of treatment	0	
– Patient positioning	0	
Treatment modification		
– Oral surgery	1	
– Implantology	1	
– Conservative/Endodontics	1	
– Fixed prosthetics	1	
– Removable prosthetics	1	
– Non-surgical periodontology	1	
– Surgical periodontology	1	
Imaging	2	Avoid radiological contrast medium
Hazardous and contraindicated drugs	2	Avoid aspirins (other NSAIDs) and penicillin; some patients are on corticosteroids and/or antihistamines

*0 = No special considerations. 1 = Caution advised. 2 = Specialised medical advice recommended in some cases. 3 = Specialised medical advice mandatory. 4 = Only to be performed in hospital environment. 5 = Should be avoided.

Conscious sedation Caution is advisable when undertaking CS, not only in terms of possible allergies with the concurrent use of LA, but also in view of reaction to sedative agents. **General anaesthesia** Local anaesthetics are used extensively to facilitate GA, and dental LA to minimise postoperative discomfort. Caution and medical advice are required.

Drug use ■ For patients allergic to penicillin, alternative antibiotics such as clindamycin are recommended (cephalosporins give cross-reactions in about 10% of penicillin-allergic patients) ■ Aspirin and other salicylates produce allergic reactions in 2 per 1000 patients, especially in people with asthma; cross-sensitivity with other NSAIDs has been described ■ Patients can be allergic to iodine, such as in some radiological contrast media and some antiseptics ■ Many patients with allergic problems are on corticosteroids and/or antihistamines.

Further reading ● Abdollahi M, Radfar M 2003 A review of drug-induced oral reactions. J Contemp Dent Pract 4:10–31 ● Chiu C Y, Lin T Y, Hsia S H, Lai S H, Wong K S 2004 Systemic anaphylaxis following local lidocaine administration during a dental procedure. Pediatr Emerg Care 20:178–180 ● Duque S, Fernandez L 2004 Delayed-type hypersensitivity to amide local anesthetics. Allergol Immunopathol (Madr) 32:233–234 ● Scully C, Bagan J V 2004 Adverse drug reactions in the orofacial region. Crit Rev Oral Biol Med 2004;15:221–239.

EATING DISORDERS

Definition Eating disorders involve serious disturbances in eating behaviour, such as extreme and unhealthy reduction of food intake or severe overeating, as well as feelings of distress or extreme concern about body shape or weight.

General aspects

Aetiopathogenesis Eating disorders usually develop during adolescence or early adulthood and most often in females. Genetic, cultural, and psychiatric factors have been implicated. It has been hypothesised these disorders result from inappropriate emotional input from the limbic system to the hypothalamus. Serotonin may also play a role, linking leptin and neuropeptide Y inhibition.

Classification Eating disorders include: ■ *Anorexia nervosa* (self-imposed starvation) – anorexia is failure to eat, in the absence of any physical cause, to the extent that >15% of body weight is lost; it may become life-threatening ■ *Bulimia nervosa* (binge eating and dieting) – bulimia is binge eating, which may be associated with self-induced vomiting and purgative abuse ■ Overlap anorexia and bulimia syndromes have been described and some authors consider bulimia as a variant of anorexia nervosa ■ Eating disorders frequently co-exist along with other psychiatric problems such as depression, substance abuse, and anxiety disorders.

Clinical presentation **Anorexia** Features of anorexia nervosa include: ■ Intense fear of gaining weight or becoming fat, even though underweight. Body image may be distorted, so the emaciated patient considers herself normal or even fat. There is resistance to maintaining body weight at or above a minimally normal weight for age and height. People with anorexia may repeatedly check their body weight. ■ Disturbance in body image – the way in which one's body weight or shape is experienced, undue influence of body weight or shape on self-evaluation, or denial of the seriousness of the current low body weight ■ Obsession in the process of eating and development of unusual habits, such as avoiding food and meals, picking out a few foods and eating these in small quantities, or carefully weighing and portioning food ■ Engaging in techniques to control weight, such as intense and compulsive exercise, or purging by means of vomiting, or abuse of laxatives, enemas, appetite suppressants, diuretics and even thyroid hormones ■ Medical complications include (Fig. 3.14): ● anaemia ● endocrine

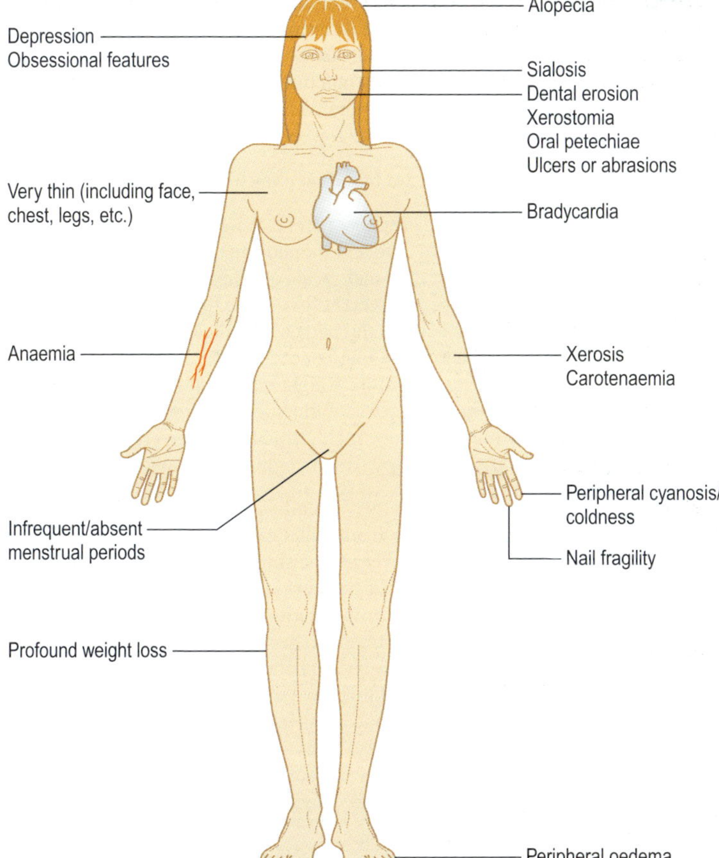

Figure 3.14 **Medical complications of anorexia nervosa**

disturbances • peripheral oedema and electrolyte depletion (especially hypokalaemia) • infrequent or absent menstrual periods (in females who have reached puberty) are common; girls with anorexia often experience a delayed menarche • peripheral cyanosis and coldness with bradycardia are common • depression is common but lacks the classic features of depression in adults • obsessional features • alopecia, hypertrichosis, xerosis, carotenaemia and nail fragility are not uncommon in advanced cases.

Bulimia Unlike people with anorexia, these patients usually weigh within the normal range for their age and height, but like individuals with anorexia, may fear gaining weight, desire to lose weight, and feel intensely dissatisfied with their bodies. Features of bulimia nervosa include: ■ eating an excessive amount of food within a discrete period of time ■ a sense of lack of control over eating during the episode, plus recurrent inappropriate compensatory behaviour in order to prevent weight gain, such as self-induced vomiting or misuse of laxatives, diuretics, enemas, or other medications (purging), fasting, or excessive exercise ■ performing the behaviours in secret, feeling disgusted and ashamed when bingeing, yet relieved once purged ■ binge eating and inappropriate compensatory behaviours are both practised, on average, at least twice a week for 3 months.

Diagnosis Diagnostic criteria are based on clinical features.

Treatment ■ Patients with eating disorders require a comprehensive treatment plan involving medical care and monitoring, psychosocial interventions, nutritional counselling and, when appropriate, medication ■ The acute management of severe weight loss is usually provided in hospital, where feeding plans address the person's medical and nutritional needs; in some cases, intravenous feeding is needed ■ Selective serotonin reuptake inhibitors (SSRIs) are helpful for weight maintenance and for resolving mood and anxiety symptoms in anorexia; antidepressant drugs are also often effective in treating bulimia ■ Once malnutrition has been corrected and weight gain has begun, psychotherapy (often cognitive–behavioural or interpersonal psychotherapy) may be of benefit.

Prognosis **Anorexia** The course and outcome in people with anorexia nervosa is variable. Some fully recover after a single episode (50% achieve normal weight); some have a fluctuating pattern of weight gain and relapse. However, others experience a chronically deteriorating illness over many years. The mortality rate is about 12 times higher than the population with normal weight – cardiac arrest, electrolyte imbalance, or suicide are the main causes. **Bulimia** Patients with bulimia have a poor prognosis, because of severe psychiatric disturbances. Complications include aspiration, oesophageal or gastric rupture, hypokalaemia, cardiac arrhythmias, pancreatitis and cardiomyopathy. About 40% of patients remain bulimic after treatment and recurrences are frequent. Bulimic patients have a high suicide rate.

Oral findings

■ Erosion of teeth (perimyolysis) may result from repeated vomiting and may cause hypersensitivity. The erosion is usually most severe on lingual, palatal and occlusal surfaces. Full-coverage plastic splints may be needed to protect the teeth. ■ Parotid enlargement (sialosis) and angular stomatitis may develop, as in other forms of starvation. The parotid swellings tend to subside if the patient returns to a normal diet. ■ Oral petechiae, ulcers or abrasions, particularly in the soft palate, may be caused by fingers or other objects used to induce vomiting ■ Xerostomia is common ■ Poor oral hygiene, dental caries and periodontal disease are often seen in bulimic patients.

Dental management

Risk assessment Patients may have poor compliance and display signs of associated behavioural problems.

Table 3.49 **Key considerations in dental management in eating disorders (see text)**

	Management modifications*	Comments/possible complications
Risk assessment	2	Vomiting; behaviour problems; poor compliance
Appropriate dental care	2	Eating disorder patient recognition; start elective care when the vomiting cycle has finished
Pain and anxiety control		
– Local anaesthesia	0	
– Conscious sedation	1	Anaemia; hypokalaemia; arrhythmias
– General anaesthesia	3/4	Anaemia; hypokalaemia; arrhythmias
Patient access and positioning		
– Access to dental office	0	
– Timing of treatment	0	
– Patient positioning	0	
Treatment modification		
– Preventive dentistry	1	Bicarbonate rinsing; daily sodium fluoride gel
– Oral surgery	0	
– Implantology	1/5	Neglected oral hygiene; poor compliance
– Conservative/Endodontics	1	Monitor amalgams closely
– Fixed prosthetics	1	Select resistant materials
– Removable prosthetics	0	
– Non-surgical periodontology	0	
– Surgical periodontology	0	
Hazardous and contraindicated drugs	1	Avoid paracetamol/ acetaminophen

*0 = No special considerations. 1 = Caution advised. 2 = Specialised medical advice recommended in some cases. 3 = Specialised medical advice mandatory. 4 = Only to be performed in hospital environment. 5 = Should be avoided.

Appropriate health care ■ The general dental practitioner may be the first to become aware of the eating disorder ■ Individuals with anorexia may use pain from dental erosion as a reason not to eat ■ The individual may request cosmetic dentistry (including tooth whitening techniques) to improve the appearance of an already acceptable dentition ■ Restorative procedures in bulimics can start when the vomiting cycle has finished; planning complex dental treatment is best done when the patients have recovered from their illness ■ The possibility of losing the individual from the dental practice is something for which the dental practitioner must be prepared.

Pain and anxiety control **Local anaesthesia** LA may be used with the usual routine precautions. **Conscious sedation** Caution is advised if there are significant medical complications.
General anaesthesia Anaemia and the possibility of hypokalaemia and consequent arrhythmias must be remembered if a general anaesthetic is considered necessary for dental treatment.

Treatment modification **Preventive dentistry** Rinsing with bicarbonate after each vomiting episode (rather than brushing the teeth), may reduce the dental damage. Topical daily sodium fluoride gel applications or a 0.05% sodium fluoride mouthwash may help to reduce tooth sensitivity.
Fixed prosthetics and conservation Erosion will cause margination of amalgams, such that they appear raised from the tooth. Resin-bonded ceramic veneers/crowns have been used to restore severe tooth erosion.
Endodontics Endodontics and cast restorations are recommended where little clinical crown remains.

Drug use There is some evidence that repeated doses of paracetamol/acetaminophen may be hepatotoxic in anorexia nervosa, and thus doses should be kept to the minimum.

Further reading
● Burgess J 2004 Bulimia and the role of the dentist. Hawaii Dent J 35:7–8 ● Faine M P 2003 Recognition and management of eating disorders in the dental office. Dent Clin North Am 47:395–410 ● Little J W 2002 Eating disorders: dental implications. Oral Surg Oral Med Oral Pathol Oral Radiol Endod 93:138–143. Milosevic A 1999 Eating disorders: a dentists' perspective. Eur Eating Dis Rev 7:103–110

ELDERLY PATIENTS

Definition A growing proportion of the population in many countries is over the age of 65 (a chronological criterion of elderly), accounting for some 15% of the population in Western Europe. The sex differences in life expectancy are resulting in a rise in the proportion of elderly females, many of whom are single.

General aspects

■ Up to 75% of those over 65 years of age have one or more chronic diseases. Many have difficulty in accessing health care. Some 3% are bed-ridden, 8% walk with difficulty and 11% are house-bound. ■ Nevertheless, elderly patients are often reluctant to demand attention, especially if they are apathetic or fear consequent hospitalisation and further loss of independence.

Clinical presentation ■ Many physical disorders affect the elderly, particularly a greater incidence and severity of arthritis and cardiovascular disease ■ Ataxia, fainting and falls are common and may be due to transient cerebral ischaemic attacks, Parkinsonism, postural hypotension, cardiac arrhythmias or epilepsy ■ Mental and emotional disorders are also important and are often also caused by underlying physical disease, especially if the symptoms are of recent onset. An acute confusional state may result from disorders as widely different as minor cerebrovascular accidents, respiratory or urinary tract infections, or left ventricular failure. A chronic confusional state may result from such conditions as diabetes mellitus, Alzheimer's disease, hypothyroidism, carcinomatosis, anaemia, uraemia or drug use. Intellectual deterioration, impaired mood and depression (sometimes related to hypothyroidism or drug-induced) are other common findings. ■ Defects of hearing or sight are common and there may be declining senses of smell and taste ■ Atypical symptomatology, polypharmacy and abnormal reactivity towards many drugs further complicate the situation ■ Many disorders in the elderly cause non-specific effects such as general malaise, social incompetence, a tendency to fall and mild amnesia. Disease may present in a less florid and dramatic way in elderly people. Even severe infections, for example, may cause little or no fever.

Classification Based on the capacity to carry out activities of ordinary life (to dress, to eat, to bathe, etc), which is assessed with specific tests (e.g. Activities of Daily Living Scale (ADLS), Katz), the elderly are classified as *functionally independent* or *dependent*. This has implications in relation to access to dental services and appropriate oral and other health care.

Treatment/complications ■ Drug reactions and interactions are common and account for about 10% of admissions to geriatric units ■ Inappropriate treatment, poor supervision, excessive dosage, drug interactions and polypharmacy, or impaired drug metabolism, may all contribute to adverse drug reactions; compliance with drug treatment can be very poor, not least because of forgetfulness or apathy ■ Drugs may precipitate or aggravate the physical disorders. For example, drugs with antimuscarinic activity, such as atropine or antidepressants, may precipitate glaucoma, may cause dry mouth or, if there is prostatic enlargement, cause urinary retention. Phenothiazines may worsen or precipitate Parkinsonism, or may cause hypotension, hypothermia, apathy, excessive sedation or confusion. Drowsiness, excessive sedation or confusional states may also be caused by the benzodiazepines, by barbiturates or by tricyclic antidepressants, while depression and postural hypotension not uncommonly follow the use of hypotensive agents.

Oral findings

■ Many elderly people are edentulous but, of those with remaining teeth, at least 75% have periodontal disease ■ Coronal dental caries is usually, however, less acute but root caries is more common ■ Impaired salivation may contribute to a high prevalence of root caries and oral candidosis, which especially affect hospitalised patients; xerostomia is even more likely if there is medication with neuroleptics or antidepressants ■ Nutrition may be defective due to poverty, apathy, mental disease or dental defects; malnutrition may in turn lead to poor tissue healing and predispose to ill health ■ Oral malignant disease is mainly a problem of the elderly and is a reason for regular oral examination of these patients ■ Some studies have demonstrated mucosal lesions in up to 40% of elderly patients but most of these are fibrous lumps or ulcers, with a minority of potentially malignant lesions such as keratoses ■ Atypical facial pain (often related to depressive illness), migraine, trigeminal neuralgia, zoster and oral dysaesthesias are more common as age advances.

Dental management

Risk assessment ■ The possibility of physical or mental disorders that may complicate management should always be considered and drug treatment should be carefully controlled, with the possibility of poor compliance and of adverse reactions always in mind ■ Arrhythmias are common in ambulatory elderly people – but they are typically benign.

Appropriate health care ■ The major goals are preventive and conservative treatment, and the elimination/avoidance of oral infections ■ Many elderly people are edentulous with little alveolar bone to support dentures, a dry mouth and a frail, atrophic mucosa. Inability to cope with dentures, or a sore mouth for any reason, readily demoralises the elderly patient, and may tip the balance between health and disease. However, by no means all patients complain of oral symptoms or denture-related difficulties. The dentist has an important role in supporting morale and contributing to adequate nutrition. ■ Independent individuals usually have no serious medical problems and may be treated in the general dental practice ■ Elderly dependent persons may need domiciliary dental care with portable dental equipment. When significant medical problems are present, the patient may be best seen in a hospital environment. However, this raises the issues of adequate transportation, and availability of escorts.

Preventive dentistry ■ Adapted and electric toothbrushes are useful ■ Chlorhexidine is recommended for daily use; spray, gel and varnish are especially indicated for dependent patients ■ Fluoride varnish is useful to prevent root caries ■ Salivary stimulants and substitutes are recommended in persons with dry mouths.

Patient education (and help groups) ■ Food can become tasteless and unappetising for geriatric patients as the result of declining taste and smell perception. Geriatric patients should be encouraged to add seasonings to their food instead of relying on excessive consumption of salt and sugar to give their food flavour. ■ Adequate nutrition, tongue cleaning and smoking cessation are recommended.

Pain and anxiety control **Local anaesthesia** It is better to use LA where possible, since the risks of general anaesthesia are greater than in the young patient, not least because of associated medical problems. LA used in recommended dosages has no effect on cardiac arrhythmias in the ambulatory elderly patient. **Conscious sedation** Elderly patients are often anxious about treatment and should therefore be sympathetically reassured and, if necessary, sedation provided. Benzodiazepines are preferable to opioids for sedation. Intravenous sedation in the dental chair is best avoided if there is any evidence of cerebrovascular disease, as a hypotensive episode may cause cerebral ischaemia. **General anaesthesia** Benzodiazepines are preferable to opioids for the induction of GA, which may be continued with nitrous oxide-oxygen supplemented with halothane or an equivalent. After long operations and GA, elderly patients are prone to deep vein thrombosis and pulmonary embolism, and to pulmonary complications, such as atelectasis.

Patient access and positioning **Access to dental surgery** Despite much evidence of need, many elderly people actually receive little or no dental attention. Access to dental care can be a major difficulty for people who are frail or have limited mobility, and is compounded by problems obtaining adequate transport or escorts. It can take a long time for a patient in a wheelchair, or using a Zimmer frame, to get into the surgery, and on to the dental chair. Domiciliary care may be more appropriate and also avoids the physical and psychological problems of a hospital or clinic visit. Handling of elderly patients may demand immense patience. **Patient positioning** Treatment is often best carried out with the patient sitting upright, as few like reclining for treatment, and some may become breathless and/or panic.

Treatment modification **Surgery** Hypercementosis, brittle dentine, low bone elasticity and impaired tissue healing may complicate surgical procedures. Older people, especially women, bruise readily if tissues are not carefully handled. **Implantology** Dental implants may be very useful to support prostheses in elderly patients. Age alone does not influence the results of implant placement or the prevalence of complications. However, careful assessment is required, with particular attention regarding associated medical problems that may make surgery problematic. **Endodontics** Endodontic therapy may be more difficult in view of secondary dentine deposition. **Fixed prosthetics and conservation** It is important to conserve sound teeth, even if they are simply endodontically treated roots, as these can serve, at least for a few years, as overdenture abutments or retainers for prostheses. Of note: ■ Attrition and brittleness of the teeth may complicate treatment, and it may be necessary to provide cuspal coverage in complex or large restorations ■ Glass-ionomer cements may be indicated in patients with a high caries risk ■ Amalgam with a spherical particle alloy is recommended since a lower condensation force is needed ■ Partial crowns may be indicated in cases of gingival recession ■ Interlock may help in cases of long fixed prostheses ■ In general, second molars should not be replaced on a fixed prosthesis. A missing first molar should be replaced by a premolar. **Removable prosthetics** It may be unwise to alter radically the shape or occlusion of dentures where they have been worn for years. A copy technique for replacement prostheses is advisable. It is wise to label the dentures with the name of the patient, particularly for those living in sheltered or other residential accommodation or those with dementia, since otherwise dentures can easily be mislaid or mixed up between patients.

Drug use ■ Elderly patients frequently have difficulties in understanding their medication and in remembering to keep to a regimen ■ Polypharmacy must be minimised, not only because of the danger of drug interactions but also because of the practical difficulties that the patient may have in taking the correct doses at the correct times ■ If it appears possible that there is

Table 3.50 **Key considerations for dental management in the elderly (see text)**

	Management modifications*	Comments/possible complications
Risk assessment	2	Poor compliance; adverse reactions; arrhythmias
Appropriate dental care	2	Systemic diseases condition dental treatment; dependent persons may need domiciliary dental care
Pain and anxiety control		
– Local anaesthesia	0	
– Conscious sedation	1	Oral benzodiazepines
– General anaesthesia	3/4	Avoid opioids, vascular and pulmonary complications
Patient access and positioning		
– Access to dental office	1	Evaluate need for domiciliary care
– Timing of treatment	0	
– Patient positioning	1	Upright position
Treatment modification		
– Preventive dentistry	1	Adapted and electric toothbrushes; chlorhexidine; fluoride varnish; salivary stimulants
– Oral surgery	1	Hypercementosis; low bone elasticity; impaired tissue healing
– Implantology	1	
– Conservative/Endodontics	1	Attrition; brittle dentine
– Fixed prosthetics	1	Material selection
– Removable prosthetics	1	Do not alter shape and occlusion; label appliance
– Non-surgical periodontology	1	Poor compliance
– Surgical periodontology	1	Impaired wound healing
Hazardous and contraindicated drugs	2	Avoid polypharmacy; possibly dosage reduction

*0 = No special considerations. 1 = Caution advised. 2 = Specialised medical advice recommended in some cases. 3 = Specialised medical advice mandatory. 4 = Only to be performed in hospital environment. 5 = Should be avoided.

hepatic or renal disease likely to impair drug metabolism or excretion, drug dosage must be reduced appropriately.

Further reading ● Allen P F, Whitworth J M 2004 Endodontic considerations in the elderly. Gerodontology 21:185–194 ● Chiappelli F, Bauer J, Spackman S et al 2002 Dental needs of the elderly in the 21st century. Gen Dent 50:358–363 ● Diz Dios P, Rodríguez Ponce A 2003 Endodoncia en pacientes de edad avanzada. In: Rodríguez Ponce

A (ed) Endodoncia. Consideraciones Actuales. Amolda, Madrid ● Henriksen B M, Ambjornsen E, Laake K, Axell T E 2004 Oral hygiene and oral symptoms among the elderly in long-term care. Spec Care Dentist 24:254–259 ● Scully C, Porter S R, Hodgson T 2000 Mouth conditions in the elderly; part 1. The Practitioner 244:938–953 ● Scully C, Hodgson T, Porter S R 2000 Mouth conditions in the elderly; part 2. The Practitioner 244:1050–1055 ● Shay K 2004 The evolving impact of aging America on dental practice. J Contemp Dent Pract 5:101–110 ● Tomás Carmona I, Limeres Posse J, Diz Dios P, Mella Pérez C 2003 Bacterial endocarditis of oral etiology in an elderly population. Arch Gerontol Geriatr 36:49–55.

END OF LIFE CARE

Definition The guiding principle in end of life care is that the quality of life is as important as, or more important than, its duration.

General aspects

Every effort should be made to make the individual as comfortable as possible in every way. Communication with patient, partners, family and friends is crucial since many different persons are involved in the care. All should be aware of: ■ the prognosis ■ how much the patient understands about his/her disease ■ their psychological reactions to their disease ■ the adverse effects of treatment.

Psychological care In any incurable disease, hope is all-important and management must include particular attention to psychological aspects. Careful assessment is required. Patients may or may not know, or may not want to know, that they have malignant or other terminal or incurable disease. Even if they are aware of it, they may not appreciate, or be willing to accept, the prognosis. Dignity is extremely important, and this can be lost in terminal disease. Patients are thus subject to considerable distress and up to a third have anxiety or depression, which may even lead to suicide. Counselling is especially important but should include family members and partners.

Feeding Feeding can be a problem, especially if there is dysphagia, when nasogastric intubation may be needed. Percutaneous endoscopic gastrostomy (PEG) is a better long-term solution as it avoids the fear of choking and aspiration pneumonia.

Pain control Pain control is of paramount importance. Potent analgesics, such as narcotics, sedatives or antidepressants, may be needed and are certainly warranted in terminal disease. The World Health Organization (WHO) three-step analgesic ladder is a guideline for cancer pain management that has been shown to be effective in relieving pain for approximately 90% of patients with cancer and over 75% of cancer patients who are terminally ill. The five essential concepts in the WHO approach to drug therapy of cancer pain are: ■ by the mouth ■ by the clock ■ by the ladder ■ for the individual ■ with attention to detail. Adjuvant drugs to enhance analgesic efficacy, treat concurrent symptoms that exacerbate pain, and provide independent analgesic activity for specific types of pain may be used at any step: ■ *Step 1*, for mild to moderate pain, involves the use of paracetamol/ acetaminophen, aspirin, or another NSAID ■ *Step 2*, when pain persists or increases, advises that an opioid such as codeine or hydrocodone should be added (not substituted) to the analgesic regimen. When higher doses of opioid are necessary, the third step is used. ■ *Step 3*, for pain that is still persistent or moderate to severe, involves giving opioid and non-opioid analgesics separately, in order to avoid exceeding maximally recommended doses of paracetamol/ acetaminophen or NSAIDs. Drugs such as codeine or hydrocodone are used initially but may need to be replaced with more potent opioids (usually morphine, hydromorphone, oxycodone, methadone, fentanyl, or levorphanol) (Table 3.51). Morphine and diamorphine are the drugs of choice for severe pain but hydromorphone and oxycodone are of comparable efficacy and tolerability. Phentazocine may be valuable in patients intolerant of, or allergic to, morphine. Pethidine has too short an action and the metabolite norpethidine can accumulate in renal failure and then cause convulsions. Buprenorphine is a partial agonist and should be avoided. Dextromoramide is only very short-acting but can be useful to 'cover' painful procedures. Carbamazepine or tricyclic antidepressants may relieve pain due to the tumour infiltrating nerves. Transdermal fentanyl skin patches are increasingly used since they have an effect comparable with morphine and a duration of action of around 3 days.

■ Medications for persistent cancer-related pain should be administered on an around-the-clock basis, with additional 'as-needed' doses, because regularly scheduled dosing maintains a constant level of drug in the body and helps to prevent a recurrence of pain.

■ Patient-controlled analgesia (PCA), can be accomplished by mouth, inhalation, subcutaneously, or epidurally, but is usually delivered via continuous systemic infusion, which allows patients to control the amount of analgesia they receive. Intravenous and subcutaneous PCA is contraindicated for sedated and confused patients.

Oral findings

See Bedbound patients.

Dental management

See Bedbound patients. The type of oral health care must be planned in relation to the interest that the patient has in their oral state. Just because patients are dying does not mean that they should be allowed to suffer from pain or that their appearance or comfort be neglected. Indeed, the provision of oral hygiene, attention to halitosis, and dental care, for example the construction of a new denture, may all help the patient's morale.

Further reading ● Anonymous 2005 Opioid analgesics for cancer pain in primary care. Drugs Therap Bull 43:9–12 ● Chiodo G T, Tolle S W, Madden T 1998 The dentist's role in end-of-life care. Gen Dent 46:560–565 ● Griffiths J, Lewis D 2002 Guidelines

Table 3.51 **Drugs for severe pain treatment**

	Buccal	Intravenous	Per rectum	Subcutaneous	Sublingual	Transdermal
Buprenorphine	+	+			+	+
Fentanyl	+					+
Hydromorphone		+	+	+		
Morphine		+	+	+	+	
Oxycodone			+			

Table 3.52 **Key considerations for dental management in end of life care (see text)**

	Management modifications*	Comments/possible complications
Risk assessment	3/4	Related to the systemic condition; aspiration pneumonia
Appropriate dental care	3–5	Individualised oral health care plan
Pain and anxiety control		
– Local anaesthesia	2	
– Conscious sedation	3–5	
– General anaesthesia	3–5	
Patient access and positioning		
– Access to dental office	2/4	Possibly domiciliary care
– Timing of treatment	1	
– Patient positioning	1	
Treatment modification		
– Oral surgery	3/4	Only simple procedures at home
– Implantology	5	
– Conservative/Endodontics	5	
– Fixed prosthetics	5	
– Removable prosthetics	1/5	Individualised evaluation
– Non-surgical periodontology	3–5	Individualised evaluation
– Surgical periodontology	5	
Hazardous and contraindicated drugs	2	Antibiotic selection; some patients receive anticoagulants or corticosteroids

*0 = No special considerations. 1 = Caution advised. 2 = Specialised medical advice recommended in some cases. 3 = Specialised medical advice mandatory. 4 = Only to be performed in hospital environment. 5 = Should be avoided.

for the oral care of patients who are dependent, dysphagic or critically ill. J Disability Oral Health 3:30–33 ● Hecker D M, Wiens J P, Cowper T R et al 2002 Can we assess quality of life in patients with head and neck cancer? A preliminary report from the American Academy of Maxillofacial Prosthetics. J Prosthet Dent 88:344–351 ● World Health Organization 1996 Cancer pain relief, with a guide to opioid availability, 2nd edn. WHO, Geneva, 1996.

ENDOCARDITIS

Definition Infective endocarditis (IE) is a rare, but dangerous, infection of the endocardial surface of the heart. It predominantly affects one or more heart valves, especially where there is turbulent blood flow because of valve damage. The earlier term 'subacute bacterial endocarditis' is now rarely used.

General aspects

Aetiopathogenesis **Pathophysiology** Platelets and fibrin deposits accumulate at endothelial sites where there is turbulent blood flow (non-bacterial thrombotic endocarditis) to produce sterile 'vegetations'. If there is a subsequent bacteraemia, these sterile 'vegetations' can readily be infected. Infective endocarditis predominantly affects natural heart valves (native valve endocarditis), sometimes those damaged by disease such as rheumatic carditis, or congenitally defective valves. Cardiac valves already damaged by infective endocarditis, or prosthetic cardiac valves, are particularly susceptible (prosthetic valve endocarditis). An uncommon but particularly dangerous type of infective endocarditis may occur in intravenous drug users. Highly virulent bacteria such as staphylococci, or occasionally fungi, can be introduced into the bloodstream with the addict's needle and can cause particularly severe endocarditis, usually on the right side of an apparently previously healthy heart. The causative organisms are: ■ Viridans streptococci (oral) 50–60% ■ Enterococci (faecal strep) 10% ■ Staphylococci (skin) 20–30% ■ Others 10% ■ Gram-negative bacteria (including the HACEK group – *Haemophilus* species (*H. parainfluenzae*, *H. aphrophilus*, and *H. paraphrophilus*), *Actinobacillus actinomycetemcomitans*, *Cardiobacterium hominis*, *Eikenella corrodens*, and *Kingella* species) ■ Fungi ■ *Coxiella burnetti* (Q fever) ■ Culture negative.

Association with dentistry ■ Dental procedures can initiate a bacteraemia, which could lead to endocarditis. Oral bacteraemias occur mainly after dental procedures associated with bleeding, such as a tooth extraction or periodontal scaling. They are generally transient and usually last for less than 15 minutes, but occasionally last for up to 1 hour.

■ The most common types of bacteraemia in patients with infective endocarditis involve: ● *S. mutans* and *S. sanguis*, both of which are *Streptococcus viridans*, found in dental plaque. They account for nearly 40% of the many different causative organisms of infective endocarditis. They have complex attachment mechanisms that may enable them to adhere to the endocardium. ● Gram-negative bacilli, mainly the HACEK group that are difficult to culture, are occasionally implicated.

■ The widespread but simplistic idea that bacteraemia is virtually synonymous with infective endocarditis is a common misapprehension: if that were so, it would be necessary to give antibiotic cover even for brushing the teeth. In simple terms, therefore, bacteria from the teeth and elsewhere can enter the bloodstream on many occasions, but only rarely infect the heart. In statistical terms, the chance of dental extractions causing infective endocarditis, even in a patient with valvular disease, may be as low as 1 in 3000.

■ Few healthy ambulant patients acquire infective endocarditis as a result of dental treatment, as shown by: ● large surveys that have shown that dental treatment precedes only 5–10% of cases ● the steady decline in the frequency of a history of dentally related cases since before the penicillin era ● the fact that some of the patients are edentulous ● the increasing variety of non-dental causes of bacteraemia.

■ It is clear that bacteria are released into the blood from the mouth (and other sites) on innumerable occasions, unrelated to operative intervention, but usually cause no harm. The variables that determine whether microorganisms will infect the heart are unclear, but the number released into the bloodstream is probably a deciding factor.

Clinical presentation In the previously healthy patient who acquires endocarditis due to Viridans streptococci, the clinical picture is likely to be that, 3 or 4 weeks after a medical–surgical manipulation procedure, there is insidious onset of low fever and mild malaise. Pallor (anaemia) or light (café-au-lait) pigmentation of the skin, joint pains and hepatosplenomegaly are typical. However the symptoms of endocarditis are highly variable/vague and include: ■ fever and chills ■ anorexia, weight loss, malaise ■ headache, myalgias, night sweats ■ shortness of breath, cough, or joint pains ■ chest pain (particularly in intravenous drug users) ■ secondary effects due to embolic phenomena – up to 20% of cases present with focal neurological complaints/stroke syndromes. **Common signs** ■ Fever (90%); possibly low-grade and intermittent ■ Heart murmurs (85%) ■ One/more classic signs (50%) ■ Petechiae – common but non-specific finding ■ Splinter haemorrhages – dark red linear lesions on the nailbeds ■ Osler nodes – tender subcutaneous nodules on the distal pads of the digits ■ Janeway lesions – non-tender maculae on the palms and soles ■ Roth spots – retinal haemorrhages with small, clear centres ■ Signs of embolic phenomena: haematuria, cerebrovascular occlusion ■ Signs of congestive heart failure ■ Signs of immune complex formation from the antigens' resultant antibodies which can lead to vasculitis, arthritis and renal damage.

Diagnosis ■ Changing murmurs ■ ECG ■ Echocardiography (Doppler and transoesophageal) ■ Blood culture positive (15% of cases are blood culture-negative).

Treatment ■ The patient should be admitted to hospital ■ Early treatment is needed to minimise cardiac damage; the usual treatment is penicillin with gentamicin by injection for 2 weeks or more if Viridans streptococci are the cause, but the bacteriological findings determine the choice of antibiotics ■ In severe cases, such as prosthetic valve or candidal endocarditis, early removal of the infected valves and insertion of a sterile replacement can be highly effective.

Prognosis Without treatment, infective endocarditis may be fatal in about 30% of individuals. Young patients, penicillin-sensitive isolates and early treatment are considered good prognostic factors.

Endocarditis prophylaxis

From the purely dental standpoint, it is obligatory to try to prevent the onset of infective endocarditis in view of the high morbidity and mortality, and this depends on: ■ identification of patients at risk ■ planned preventive dental care ■ deciding which treatments require antimicrobial cover

■ giving the appropriate antibiotic(s) at the appropriate time ■ It is important to note that there is significant variation in the protocols applied within parts of Europe and the USA.

Identification of patients at risk ■ In the UK, identification of patients at risk of infective endocarditis following dental procedures has changed significantly. The recommendations of the British Society for Antimicrobial Chemotherapy (BSAC) 1992 and those of the British Cardiac Society/Royal College of Physicians (BCS-RCP) 2004, place individuals in risk categories and require antibiotic prophylaxis to be given to a large group of patients with various cardiac defects and/or surgery. ■ However, BSAC revised this advice in April 2006 in view of the lack of evidence of the benefit for prophylactic antibiotics to prevent endocarditis associated with dental procedures. BSAC 2006 recommends that antibiotic prophylaxis for dental treatment should be restricted to those patients in whom the risk of developing endocarditis is the highest, namely those who have or have had ● a history of previous endocarditis ● cardiac valve replacement surgery ● a surgically constructed systemic or pulmonary shunt or conduit (Table 3.53). ■ An attempt should be made to elicit a relevant history, and patients should therefore be asked if they have or have had: ● a previous episode of infective endocarditis ● heart surgery (and its nature).

Planned preventive care ■ Good oral hygiene is probably the most important factor in reducing the risk of endocarditis in susceptible individuals.

Table 3.53 **Infective endocarditis prophylaxis and dental procedures**

Cardiac risk factors for antibiotic prophylaxis	Dental procedures requiring antibiotic prophylaxis	Antibiotic regimens for endocarditis prophylaxis
Previous infective endocarditis	All dental procedures involving dento-gingival manipulation	Amoxicillin 3g orally one hour before the dental procedure: ≥ 5 < 10 years of age 1.5g < 5 years of age 750mg
Cardiac valve replacement surgery i.e. mechanical or biological prosthetic valves		**If allergic to penicillin:** Clindamycin 600mg orally one hour before the dental procedure: ≥ 5 < 10 years of age 300mg < 5 years of age 150mg
Surgically constructed systemic or pulmonary shunt or conduit		**Patients allergic to penicillin or unable to swallow capsules:** Azithromycin 500mg orally one hour before the dental procedure: ≥ 5 < 10 years of age 300mg < 5 years of age 200mg

Based on the recommendations of the British Society for Antimicrobial Chemotherapy (BSAC April 2006; www.bsac.org.uk/_db/_documents/ENDOCARDITIS.doc; J Antimicrobial Chemo, 2006. doi:10.1093/jac/dk1121).

Patients at risk for endocarditis should receive intensive preventive oral health care, to try and minimise the need for dental intervention ■ There is no reliable evidence to suggest that electric toothbrushes pose a risk ■ The aim is to keep periodontal infection at its lowest possible level, to obviate the need for extractions or, if extractions are unavoidable, to lessen the severity of the bacteraemia by keeping the gingiva healthy ■ However, it must be appreciated that scaling also requires antibiotic cover ■ Unfortunately, this aspect of care is frequently neglected; a very high proportion of patients attending cardiology clinics have periodontal disease.

Deciding which treatments require antibiotic cover ■ There has been much debate regarding which dental procedures require antibiotic cover ■ In a survey of nearly 5000 cases of infective endocarditis attributable to dental treatment, it was found to have followed dental extractions in 95% of cases ■ There is only one published study really supporting antibiotic prophylaxis, that of a series of patients with cardiac valve prostheses – only about half of whom received antimicrobial prophylaxis before subsequent surgical or dental procedures. There were no cases of endocarditis in those receiving prophylaxis, but a few cases developed in the group receiving no antimicrobial. ■ A study in the USA suggests that the mortality from penicillin anaphylaxis far exceeds that of infective endocarditis ■ BSAC 1992 recommended that antibiotic cover was given for all procedures associated with bleeding, most notably dental extractions and scaling ■ The BCS-RCP recommendations in 2004 suggest antibiotic prophylaxis should be given for all bacteraemic dental procedures, and they have produced detailed guidance on this issue (Box 3.8) ■ BSAC 2006 have simplified their advice by recommending that for the high risk patients they

Box 3.8 Dental and oral procedures requiring antimicrobial prophylaxis in persons at risk from endocarditis*

- Periodontal probing
- Scaling or polishing of teeth (any method)
- Root planing and any other subgingival procedure (e.g. placement of retraction cords or antibiotic fibres)
- Surgical procedures such as tooth extraction, exposure, reimplantation of avulsed tooth, periodontal and implant surgery and any involving mucoperiosteal flaps (biopsy, incision and drainage of abscess and suture removal do *not* require antibiotic cover)
- Rubber dam, matrix band and wedge placement
- Root canal instrumentation beyond the apex
- Orthodontic tooth separation
- Sialography
- Intraligamentary local anaesthesia

*Based on the recommendations of the British Cardiac Society and Royal College of Physicians (Dental Aspects of Endocarditis Prophylaxis, 2004; http://www.bcs.com/library)

Table 3.54 **Choices of prophylactic antibiotic regimens against infective endocarditis for treatment under local anaesthesia**

Recommending authority*		Regimen**
BSAC***	1992	(a) Amoxicillin: 3g 1h before treatment
		(b) Clindamycin: 600mg 1h before treatment
EUROPEAN CONSENSUS***	1995	(a) Amoxicillin: 3g 1h before treatment
		(b) Clindamycin: 300–600mg 1h before treatment
AHA***	1997	(a) Amoxicillin: 2g 1h before treatment
		(b) Clindamycin: 600mg 1h before treatment
BCS-RCP	2004	(a) Amoxicillin: 3g 1h before treatment
		(b) Clindamycin: 600mg 1h before treatment
BSAC	2006	(a) Amoxicillin: 3g 1h before treatment
		(b) Clindamycin: 600mg 1h before treatment

*AHA = American Heart Association. BSAC = British Society for Antimicrobial Chemotherapy. BCS-RCP = British Cardiac Society and the Royal College of Physicians.
**(a) = penicillin non-allergic. (b) = penicillin allergic.
***Does not include highest risk patients.

have identified, antibiotic prophylaxis should be given for dental procedures involving dento-gingival manipulation or endodontics (Table 3.53).

Giving the appropriate antibiotic at the right time The most widely applied protocols are those of the American Heart Association (AHA) and the British Society for Antimicrobial Chemotherapy (BSAC) (available in the British National Formulary) (Tables 3.53 and 3.54). A further regimen has been proposed by the British Cardiac Society (BCS) and the Royal College of Physicians (RCP) (Table 3.54). Details may be found at: www.rcseng.ac.uk/dental/fds/clinical_guidelines/ie_recs.pdf. The most recent recommendations from BSAC 2006 allow antibiotic cover to be given orally for the 3 high risk groups identified (Table 3.53), although they recognise that in some situations it may be logistically easier to administer antibiotic via the intravenous route (www.bsac.org.uk/_db/_documents/ENDOCARDITIS.doc; J Antimicrobial Chemo, 2006. doi:10.1093/jac/dk1121).

Additional measures ■ Application of an antiseptic such as 10% povidone-iodine or 0.5% chlorhexidine gel to the gingival crevice or chlorhexidine 0.2% mouth rinses for 1 minute before the dental procedure may reduce the severity of any resulting bacteraemia and may usefully supplement antibiotic prophylaxis in those at risk ■ Good dental health should reduce the frequency and severity of any bacteraemias and also reduce the need for extractions ■ It is essential that, even when antibiotic cover has been given, patients at risk should be instructed to report any unexplained illness. Infective endocarditis is often exceedingly insidious in origin and can develop two or more months after the operation that might have precipitated it. Late diagnosis considerably increases both the mortality and morbidity among survivors. ■ For patients requiring sequential dental procedures, these should ideally be performed at intervals of at least 14 days to allow healing of oral mucosal surfaces and limit the emergence of antibiotic-resistant microorganisms. If further dental procedures cannot be delayed, amoxicillin and clindamycin should be alternated. In this scenario, if the patient has a penicillin allergy expert advice should be sought. ■ Patients at risk should carry a warning card to be shown to their dentist at each visit to indicate the danger of infective endocarditis and the need for antibiotic prophylaxis.

In summary: ■ infective endocarditis only rarely follows dental procedures ■ it has not been proven that antimicrobial prophylaxis effectively prevents endocarditis ■ there is always a risk of adverse reactions to the drug ■ the risk:benefit ratio of antimicrobial prophylaxis for endocarditis remains questionable.

Nevertheless, it remains mandatory to give such prophylaxis to patients at risk, and administration should be supervised in view of the possible risk of anaphylaxis. It must be accepted that, although neither the need nor the efficacy of antibiotic prophylaxis can be established in any given case, antibiotics must be given to patients with a recognised predisposing cardiac disorder before extractions, scaling and surgery involving the periodontal tissues. In addition, it is essential to warn patients (whether or not antimicrobial prophylaxis has been given) to report back if even a minor febrile illness develops after dental treatment.

It must be remembered that patients at risk from infective endocarditis may also have a heart lesion that makes them a poor risk for general anaesthesia, and some are on anticoagulant treatment or on other drugs.

Further reading ● Carmona I T, Dios P D, Scully C 2002 An update on the controversies in bacterial endocarditis of oral origin. Oral Surg Oral Med Oral Pathol Oral Radiol Endod 93:660–670 ● Holmstrup P, Poulsen A H, Andersen L, Skuldbol T, Fiehn N E 2003 Oral infections and systemic diseases. Dent Clin North Am 47:575–598 ● Oliver R, Roberts G J, Hooper L 2004 Penicillins for the prophylaxis of bacterial endocarditis in dentistry. Cochrane Database Syst Rev (2):CD003813 ● Seymour R A, Whitworth J M 2002 Antibiotic prophylaxis for endocarditis, prosthetic joints, and surgery. Dent Clin North Am 46:635–651 ● Tomás Carmona I, Diz Dios P, Seoane Lestón J, Limeres Posse J 2001 Pautas de profilaxis antibiótica de la endocarditis bacteriana en pacientes sometidos a tratamiento odontológico. Rev Clin Esp 201:21–24 ● Tomás Carmona I, Diz Dios P, Limeres Posse J, González Quintela A, Martínez Vázquez C, Castro Iglesias A 2002 An update on infective endocarditis of dental origin. J Dent 30:37–40 ● www.bsac.org.uk/_db/_documents/ENDOCARDITIS.doc ● J Antimicrobial Chemo, 2006. doi: 10.1093/jac/dk1121

EPILEPSY

Definition Epilepsy is not a disease entity but a chronic manifestation of brain damage that results in abnormal electrical brain activity and electrical discharges. It is common, with at least 3% of the UK population having two or more epileptic seizures during their life. It may manifest as: ■ changes in consciousness ■ altered or lost muscle control ■ convulsions, predominantly violent muscular contractions.

General aspects

Epileptic seizures result in interruptions or abnormalities in brain function, which may affect the level of consciousness, movement, sensation, and/or result in autonomic or psychic phenomena. They are usually self-limiting. Seizures may be provoked but usually appear to be spontaneous. Convulsions are physical signs of seizure activity described as forceful involuntary contractions of voluntary muscles. Convulsions may be preceded by hallucinations, changes in mood or behaviour (aura), disorientation, slurring of speech and blinking.

Aetiopathogenesis Some neuropathological factors may underlie epilepsy, including: ■ increased neuronal excitability ■ decreased inhibition of the motor cortex ■ metabolic disorders of cerebral neurones. The initiation, continuation and suppression of seizures are mediated by neurotransmitters such as glutamate, which is excitatory, and gamma-aminobutyric acid (GABA), which is inhibitory. **Causes of epilepsy** ■ Idiopathic epilepsy ■ Symptomatic or secondary epilepsy: ● Febrile convulsions ● Intracranial causes: space-occupying lesions, trauma, vascular defects, infections, cerebral palsy, rubella syndrome, phakomatoses (neurofibromatosis, epiloia), AIDS meningitis ● Systemic causes: hypoxia, hypoglycaemia, inborn errors of metabolism, drug withdrawal (anticonvulsants, barbiturates, alcohol, opioids, benzodiazepines).

Classification The diagnosis and classification of seizures and epilepsy syndrome follow the guidelines suggested by the International League against Epilepsy. Epilepsy may be classified in three main groups (Table 3.55): ■ generalised seizures ■ partial seizures ■ others, which are distributed in several subtypes. Seizures may occasionally result in learning disability, e.g. **West syndrome or infantile spasm** Associated with a characteristic appearance of hypsarrhythmia (a chaotic mixture of high amplitude EEG slow waves with variable spike and sharp waves) and spasms, with most children having severe learning disabilities when they grow up. **Gastaut syndrome** Presents with intractable seizures, learning disability and a characteristic EEG appearance; may follow on from West syndrome. Many of the children affected have learning disabilities in the long term.

Clinical presentation

Grand mal (tonic-clonic) epilepsy Grand mal epilepsy usually begins in the pre-school child, or occasionally at puberty. It manifests with a warning

Table 3.55 **Epilepsy – different types and features**

Type	Sub-type	Main features
Generalised seizures	Tonic-clonic (Grand mal)	Loss of consciousness Tonic phase Clonic phase Tongue biting Incontinence Seizure lasts < 5 minutes
	Absences (Petit mal)	Brief period of unresponsiveness Episode lasts < 30 seconds
Partial seizures	Simple (Jacksonian epilepsy)	Motor, sensory, autonomic or psychic features
	Complex (Temporal lobe epilepsy)	Impaired consciousness Automatic repetitive acts
Others	Myoclonic	
	Atonic	

(aura), followed by loss of consciousness, tonic and clonic convulsions, and finally a variably prolonged recovery. ■ The aura may consist of a mood change, irritability, brief hallucination or headache, or even the sensation of a strong smell (e.g. burning rubber) ■ The attack then begins suddenly with total body tonic spasm and loss of consciousness. The sufferer falls to the ground and is in danger of injury. Initially the face becomes pale and the pupils dilate, the head and spine are thrown into extension (opisthotonous) and glottic and respiratory muscle spasm may cause an initial brief cry and cyanosis. There may also be incontinence and biting of the tongue or lips. The tonic phase passes, after less than a minute, into the clonic phase. ■ In the clonic phase there are repetitive jerking movements of trunk, limbs, tongue and lips. Salivation is profuse with bruxism, sometimes tongue-biting and, occasionally, vomiting. There may be urinary or faecal incontinence, and autonomic phenomena such as tachycardia, hypertension and flushing. ■ Clonus is followed by a state of flaccid semi-coma for a further 10–15 minutes, and then recovery. Confusion and headaches are common afterwards and the patient may sleep for up to 12 hours or more before full recovery. The attack may occasionally be followed by a transient residual paralysis (Todd's palsy) or by automatic or aggressive behaviour. This full sequence is, however, not always completed.

■ Most seizures end without mishap but complications of major convulsions can be trauma, respiratory embarrassment or brain damage, or they may pass into status epilepticus.

■ Status epilepticus is defined as a seizure lasting for more than 30 minutes, or repeated seizures over the same period without intervening periods of consciousness. This is a particularly dangerous form of epilepsy in which there is a danger from inhalation of vomit and saliva, or brain damage due to cerebral hypoxia; death may result.

Petit mal seizures Petit mal seizures occur most often during childhood. It interferes little with activities of daily living but many patients who have petit mal also have grand mal attacks. Petit mal epilepsy is characterised by: ■ minimal or no movements (usually, except for 'eye blinking') – may appear like a blank stare ■ brief sudden loss of awareness or conscious activity – lasts only seconds ■ recurs many times ■ decreased learning (child often thought to be daydreaming). **Simple partial (focal) seizures** Simple partial (focal) seizures can be motor, sensory or behavioural and typically remain confined to one area. They may present as: ■ Muscle contractions of a specific body part. Localised motor seizures (focal motor epilepsy) may take the form of clonic movements of a limb or group of muscles, usually in the face, arm or leg. The clonus may spread (march) to adjacent muscles on the same side of the body (Jacksonian epilepsy). ■ Abnormal sensations ■ May also be nausea, sweating, skin flushing, and dilated pupils ■ May be other focal (localised) symptoms.

Complex partial seizures Complex partial seizures, or temporal lobe epilepsy (psychomotor epilepsy) are characterised by: ■ automatism (automatic performance of complex behaviours) such as lip smacking and chewing movements, or facial grimacing ■ abnormal sensations ■ may be nausea, sweating, skin flushing, and dilated pupils ■ may be other focal symptoms ■ recalled or inappropriate emotions ■ changes in personality or alertness ■ may or may not be disorientation, confusion and amnesia or loss of consciousness ■ olfactory (smell) or gustatory (taste) hallucinations or impairments.

Diagnosis The diagnosis of epilepsy is essentially clinical, based largely on an accurate description of events from carers. CT and EEG (electroencephalogram) are also helpful.

Treatment Anticonvulsants are the treatment of choice, especially gamma-aminobutyric acid (GABA) potentiators and neuronal inhibitors (Table 3.56). Carbamazepine and sodium valproate are the most widely used anticonvulsants but newer drugs are being used more frequently either in monotherapy (lamotrigine) or as an adjunct (vigabatrin, gabapentin, topiramate, tiagabine). Phenytoin and phenobarbitone are no longer drugs of first choice. In severe cases, protective headgear may be worn to limit injury to the CNS during seizures (Fig. 3.15). Surgical treatment may also be considered, such as temporal lobe lobotomy for intractable temporal lobe epilepsy. People with epilepsy face some legal restrictions, notably in the areas of driving and employment. They are prohibited from entering specific occupations, such as becoming an aircraft pilot, ambulance driver or soldier.

Prognosis Prognosis in epilepsy is influenced by the underlying disease, extent of brain damage, and severity and frequency of seizures. Status epilepticus may result in aspiration of material into the lungs, and cerebral hypoxia, and has a mortality rate of 5–20%.

Table 3.56 **Anticonvulsant treatment of epilepsy**

Drug type	Drug
GABA potentiators	Barbiturates
	Benzodiazepines
	Gabapentin
	Primidone
	Tiagabine
	Valproate
	Vigabatrin
Neuronal inhibitors	Carbamazepine
	Fosphenytoin
	Lamotrigine
	Phenytoin
	Topiramate

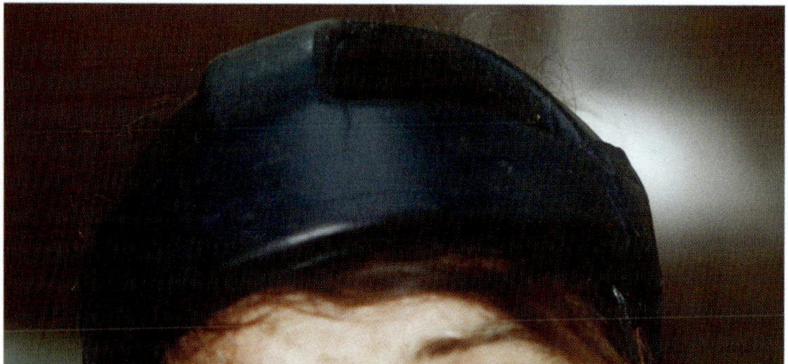

Figure 3.15 **Protective headgear worn by a patient with severe epilepsy**

Oral findings

■ Convulsions may have craniofacial sequelae, from trauma that frequently results from a grand mal attack when the patient falls unconscious, or from the muscle spasm. Such injuries can include: • periorbital subcutaneous haematomas in the absence or presence of facial fractures • injuries to the face from falling (lacerations, haematomas, fractures of the facial skeleton) • fractures, devitalisation, subluxation or loss of teeth (a chest radiograph may be required) • subluxation of the TMJ • lacerations of lips, tongue or buccal mucosa. ■ Undesirable effects of treatment include: • phenytoin-induced gingival swelling and/or ulcers secondary to folic acid deficiency anaemia • palatal petechiae, as a consequence of platelet aggregation inhibition due to valproic acid • ulcers due to agranulocytosis from carbamazepine depression of the bone marrow.

Dental management

Risk assessment ■ Do not misinterpret seizure for lack of cooperation/antisocial behaviour ■ Epileptics can have good and bad phases and it is sensible for dental treatment to be carried out in a good phase, when attacks are infrequent ■ Various factors can precipitate attacks including: ● withdrawal of anticonvulsant medication ● epileptogenic drugs ● fatigue ● starvation ● stress ● infection ● menstruation ● flickering lights (television, strobe lights) ■ Those who have infrequent seizures, or who are dependent upon others (such as those with a learning impairment), may fail to take regular medication and thus be poorly controlled.

Appropriate health care ■ Advise the patient that it is sensible to cancel the appointment if they feel that their seizures are poorly controlled on the day, or if they are tired/fatigued ■ When carrying out dental treatment in a known epileptic, a strong mouth prop attached to a chain may be kept in position and the oral cavity kept as free as possible of debris; as much apparatus as possible should be kept away from the area around the patient ■ Patients with poorly controlled epilepsy are classed as ASA III, and are best treated in a hospital-based clinic where medical support is available ■ Temporal lobe (psychomotor) epilepsy in particular is associated with paranoid and schizophrenic features. Antisocial and psychopathic behaviour may then make dental management difficult.

Appropriate management of a patient undergoing tonic-clonic seizure includes: ■ Summon help ■ Stop treatment ■ Lay the patient flat in the chair; do not try to move the patient while they are actively fitting ■ Protect the patient from injury: ● do *not* attempt to force a spoon or tongue depressor or other hard object between the teeth because you can cause more damage than that you are trying to prevent ● clear the area of equipment, furniture or other objects that may cause injury during the seizure ● do *not* attempt to restrain or hold the person down during the seizure ■ If the patient is having difficulty breathing or becoming cyanosed, maintain the airway by gently extending the neck ■ CPR or mouth-to-mouth breathing cannot be performed during the seizure and is rarely needed after seizures ■ In an uncomplicated seizure no other treatment is necessary ■ However, if the fit continues for longer than normal, or >10 minutes, midazolam 10mg should be given intramuscularly ■ If the fit does not resolve within the next 5 minutes, an ambulance should be called, as status epilepticus may develop and is a medical emergency ■ While waiting, the airway should be protected where possible, with suction to remove excess saliva, and high flow oxygen 10–15L/min administered.

Pain and anxiety control **Local anaesthesia** Large doses of lidocaine given intravenously may occasionally cause convulsions and, therefore, an over-enthusiastic casualty officer may blame a dental LA for causing a fit. There is no evidence that this can happen; indeed, intravenous lidocaine has been advocated for the *control* of status epilepticus. It is best to avoid electronic dental analgesia, as this could induce a fit. **Conscious sedation** Conscious sedation in epilepsy should be safe and stress reduction should reduce the chance of a fit. Benzodiazepines such as midazolam are anti-epileptogenic. However, seizures have occasionally been recorded in epileptics undergoing intravenous sedation with midazolam. Flumazenil is potentially epileptogenic. Nitrous oxide can increase the CNS depression in patients on anticonvulsants, and cause nausea and vomiting in patients under phenytoin. **General anaesthesia** Some GA agents may enhance the toxic effects of anticonvulsants.

Patient access and positioning Patients may be more likely to have seizures at certain times of the day (e.g. early morning). It is important to assess this for each individual, so that appointments can be scheduled when fits are less likely to occur.

Treatment modification **Preventive dentistry** Frequent plaque removal may reduce gingival swelling related to the use of phenytoin. Chlorhexidine mouthwash/gel/spray may be of additional benefit. **Fixed prosthetics and conservation** Fixed prostheses with increased metal structure (better than porcelain) are recommended. **Removable prosthetics** There is a risk of oral injury and airway obstruction if removable prostheses fracture during a seizure. As a consequence, prostheses may be contraindicated in severe epilepsy and any prosthesis for an epileptic should be constructed of radio-opaque materials. **Periodontal surgery** Surgical excision is the usual approach to phenytoin-related gingival swelling.

Drug use Drugs that can be epileptogenic, interfere with anticonvulsants or whose own activity can be altered by anticonvulsant therapy include some analgesics and antimicrobials commonly prescribed in dentistry (Box 3.9).

Box 3.9 Drug problems in epilepsy

Drugs that can be epileptogenic and therefore are contraindicated
• alcohol • chlorpromazine • enflurane • flumazenil • fluoxetine • ketamine • lidocaine (large doses) • metronidazole • propofol • quinolones • tramadol • tricyclic antidepressants

Drugs used in dentistry that can increase anticonvulsant activity, leading to overdose
• aspirin and other NSAIDs – can interfere with phenytoin, can increase the bleeding tendency induced by valproate • azole antifungals – can interfere with phenytoin • erythromycin – can interfere with carbamazepine, can increase the bleeding tendency induced by valproate • metronidazole – can interfere with phenytoin • propoxyphene – can interfere with carbamazepine

Drugs used in dentistry whose activity can be altered by anticonvulsants
• acetaminophen/paracetamol – hepatotoxicity may be increased by anticonvulsants • doxycycline – metabolism may be increased by carbamazepine

Table 3.57 **Key considerations for dental management in epilepsy (see text)**

	Management modifications*	Comments/possible complications
Risk assessment	2	Risk of epileptic attack
Appropriate dental care	2/4	Better in 'good phases'; avoid precipitating factors; behaviour control; use a mouth prop; management of status epilepticus
Pain and anxiety control		
– Local anaesthesia	1	Limit lidocaine dose; avoid electronic dental analgesia
– Conscious sedation	3/4	Avoid midazolam and nitrous oxide
– General anaesthesia	3/4	May enhance the toxic effects of anticonvulsants
Patient access and positioning		
– Access to dental office	0	
– Timing of treatment	1	Determine when seizures usually occur
– Patient positioning	0	
Treatment modification		
– Preventive dentistry	1	Frequent plaque removal and chlorhexidine are recommended
– Oral surgery	1/4	
– Implantology	1/4/5	
– Conservative/Endodontics	1/4/5	
– Fixed prosthetics	1/4	Increase metal structure
– Removable prosthetics	1/4/5	Risk of fracture; acrylic better than porcelain
– Non-surgical periodontology	1/4	
– Surgical periodontology	1/4	
Hazardous and contraindicated drugs	2	Avoid aspirin, acetaminophen and metronidazole (see Box 3.9)

*0 = No special considerations. 1 = Caution advised. 2 = Specialised medical advice recommended in some cases. 3 = Specialised medical advice mandatory. 4 = Only to be performed in hospital environment. 5 = Should be avoided.

Further reading • Karolyhazy K, Kovacs E, Kivovics P, Fejerdy P, Aranyi Z 2003 Dental status and oral health of patients with epilepsy: an epidemiologic study. Epilepsia 44:1103–1108 • Stoopler E T, Sollecito T P, Greenberg M S 2003 Seizure disorders: update of medical and dental considerations. Gen Dent 51:361–366.

GLUCOSE-6-PHOSPHATE DEHYDROGENASE (G6PD) DEFICIENCY

Definition ■ Glucose-6-phosphate dehydrogenase (G6PD) deficiency is the most common human enzyme deficiency ■ G6PD normally functions in catalysing the oxidation of glucose-6-phosphate to 6-phosphogluconate, while concomitantly reducing nicotinamide adenine dinucleotide phosphate ($NADP^+$ to NADPH), the first step in the pentose phosphate pathway which produces the 5-carbon sugar ribose, an essential component of both DNA and RNA ■ G6PD is also responsible for maintaining adequate levels of reduced nicotinamide adenine dinucleotide phosphate (NADPH), needed to keep glutathione in its reduced form to act as a scavenger for dangerous oxidative metabolites.

General aspects

Aetiopathogenesis G6PD deficiency is a sex-linked disorder, fully expressed in the heterozygote male and homozygote female. G6PD deficiency occurs especially in people from Africa, the Mediterranean, and the Middle and Far East. When red cells are exposed to oxidising agents, e.g. various drugs, broad beans (*Vicia fava*) or naphthalene, there is oxidation damage to haemoglobin and red blood cell membranes causing methaemoglobinaemia and haemolysis.

Clinical presentation ■ Mostly asymptomatic ■ Drugs and intercurrent infections may precipitate a haemolytic episode with myalgia, malaise, weakness, anaemia and jaundice ■ Drugs that can be dangerous are shown in Box 3.10 but include: ● analgesics: aspirin and acetaminophen/paracetamol in large doses ● antibiotics: sulphonamides, ciprofloxacin, sulphones, nitrofurantoin, chloramphenicol ● antimalarials: primaquine, quinacrine, quinine.

Classification There are more than 300 G6PD variants. Three grades of severity have been described: ■ mild – > 10% residual G6PD activity ■ moderate – < 10% residual G6PD activity ■ severe – no residual G6PD activity.

Diagnosis The diagnosis is suspected from screening tests, such as the methaemoglobin dye reduction test, and confirmed by G6PD assay.

Treatment ■ Fluid balance and alkalinisation are strongly recommended ■ Blood transfusions and splenectomy are occasionally needed.

Prognosis Haemolysis is usually self-limiting but, in severe cases, it may produce metabolic acidosis and renal damage.

Oral findings

No specific oral findings have been described, other than occasional oral pallor.

Box 3.10 Drugs that may precipitate haemolysis in G6PD deficiency

Analgesics/Antipyretics
• acetanilid • acetaminophen • acetophenetidin (phenacetin) • amidopyrine (aminopyrine) • antipyrine • aspirin • phenacetin • probenicid • pyramidone

Antimalarials
• chloroquine • hydroxychloroquine • mepacrine (quinacrine) • pamaquine • pentaquine • primaquine • quinine • quinocide

Cardiovascular drugs
• procainamide • quinidine

Sulphonamides/sulphones
• dapsone • sulphacetamide • sulphamethoxypyrimidine • sulphanilamide • sulphapyridine • sulphasalazine • sulphisoxazole

Miscellaneous
• alpha-methyldopa • ascorbic acid • dimercaprol (BAL) • hydralazine • mestranol • methylene blue • nalidixic acid • niridazole • phenylhydrazine • pyridium • toluidine blue • trinitrotoluene • urate oxidase • vitamin K (water soluble)

Cytotoxic/antibacterial
• chloramphenicol • furazolidone • furmethonol • nalidixic acid • neoarsphenamine • nitrofurantoin • nitrofurazone • para-aminosalicylic acid

Dental management

Appropriate health care *Risk assessment* It is vital to avoid oxidant drugs that can precipitate haemolysis, particularly the sulphonamides (including co-trimoxazole). However, there is little evidence to suggest that short-term therapeutic administration of analgesics will pose a threat of haemolytic reaction in dental patients.

Patient education (and help groups) Patients should be informed about drugs and foods that can trigger a haemolytic episode.

Pain and anxiety control **Local anaesthesia** Prilocaine may, in large doses, induce methaemoglobinaemia, and is therefore best avoided. **Conscious sedation** Conscious sedation is usually safely given as relative analgesia. **General anaesthesia** Metabolic acidosis causes haemolysis and must be avoided during GA.

Drug use ■ Aspirin and acetaminophen/paracetamol may precipitate haemolysis when used in high dosage and so codeine is better used for analgesia ■ Topical toluidine blue for oral cancer screening has not been recorded as causing haemolysis, but it is best to avoid it.

Further reading • Alexander R E, Vosskuhler R J 1991 Analgesic concerns in glucose-6-phosphate dehydrogenase-deficient dental patients: myth or reality? Mil Med 156:681–684 • Kostopoulou M, Papagiannoulis-Alexandrides L, Kouvelas N 1984

Table 3.58 **Key considerations in dental management in G6PD deficiency (see text)**

	Management modifications*	Comments/possible complications
Risk assessment	1	Avoid oxidant drugs
Appropriate dental care	2	Avoid oxidant drugs
Pain and anxiety control		
– Local anaesthesia	1	Avoid prilocaine
– Conscious sedation	1	
– General anaesthesia	3/4	
Patient access and positioning		
– Access to dental office	0	
– Timing of treatment	0	
– Patient positioning	0	
Treatment modification		
– Oral surgery	0	
– Implantology	0	
– Conservative/Endodontics	0	
– Fixed prosthetics	0	
– Removable prosthetics	0	
– Non-surgical periodontology	0	
– Surgical periodontology	0	
Hazardous and contraindicated drugs	2	Avoid aspirin, acetaminophen, sulphonamides and topical toluidine blue

*0 = No special considerations. 1 = Caution advised. 2 = Specialised medical advice recommended in some cases. 3 = Specialised medical advice mandatory. 4 = Only to be performed in hospital environment. 5 = Should be avoided.

Patients with glucose 6-phosphate dehydrogenase (G-6-PD) deficiency and their dental treatment. Odontostomatol Proodos 38:149–154 ● Taylor M H, Peterson D S 1982 Erythrocyte glucose-6-phosphate dehydrogenase deficiency: precautions for dental treatment. J Pedod 6:330–336.

GOUT

Definition Gout is a painful joint disease caused by impaired uric acid excretion leading to high blood uric acid levels (hyperuricaemia), deposition of crystals of sodium monourate, and subsequent lysosomal enzyme release from neutrophil leucocytes as they attempt phagocytosis of the crystals.

General aspects

Aetiopathogenesis ■ Hyperuricaemia results from accelerated purine metabolism, disturbed renal clearance, or increased intake ■ Attacks are precipitated by: ● trauma ● starvation ● infection ● diuretics (thiazide).

Clinical presentation ■ Acute gout or gouty arthritis present with severe pain, redness and swelling, often in a single joint ■ It is seen usually in males over 50 years and involves mainly the first metatarsophalangeal (big toe) joint; the ankle, knee, wrist, and elbow may also be involved ■ In chronic tophaceous gout there are nodules on the cartilage of the elbow joint and the ear due to deposits of urate crystal ■ When crystals deposit in the kidney, this may result in renal calculi and obstructive renal disease.

Classification ■ Primary gout has a genetic basis and is associated with hypertriglyceridaemia, hypertension, atherosclerosis and diabetes ■ Secondary gout is related to severe systemic diseases such as lymphoma, leukaemia and sickle cell anaemia.

Diagnosis ■ Serum uric acid – typically raised ■ Synovial fluid – urate crystals ■ Radiology – juxta-articular radiolucencies.

Treatment ■ NSAID (indometacin not aspirin) or colchicine ■ Probenecid has been used in chronic gout ■ To prevent new episodes, use uricosuric agents such as allopurinol ■ Avoid purine-rich food, alcohol and diuretics.

Table 3.59 **Key considerations for dental management in gout (see text)**

	Management modifications*	Comments/possible complications
Risk assessment	2	Underlying disease
Appropriate dental care	1	Avoid elective oral care during acute attacks
Pain and anxiety control		
– Local anaesthesia	0/2	Underlying disease
– Conscious sedation	0/2	
– General anaesthesia	0/2	
Patient access and positioning		
– Access to dental office	0/1	
– Timing of treatment	0	
– Patient positioning	1	
Treatment modification		
– Oral surgery	0	
– Implantology	0	
– Conservative/Endodontics	0	
– Fixed prosthetics	0	
– Removable prosthetics	0	
– Non-surgical periodontology	0	
– Surgical periodontology	0	
Hazardous and contraindicated drugs	1	Avoid aspirin and ampicillin

*0 = No special considerations. 1 = Caution advised. 2 = Specialised medical advice recommended in some cases. 3 = Specialised medical advice mandatory. 4 = Only to be performed in hospital environment. 5 = Should be avoided.

Oral findings

■ Drugs used for the treatment of gout, particularly allopurinol, can occasionally cause oral ulceration ■ Gout affects the temporomandibular joint only rarely; sudden pain on mouth opening is the main symptom ■ Gingivitis has been observed in relation to probenecid intake ■ Lesch–Nyhan syndrome is a rare inborn error of metabolism in which hyperuricaemia is associated with learning disability, choreoathetosis and compulsive self-mutilation. In Lesch–Nyhan syndrome the lips are chewed and self-inflicted injuries, especially to the face and head (despite the pain it obviously causes), are typical.

Dental management

Risk assessment Underlying diseases, such as hypertension, ischaemic heart disease, cerebrovascular disease, diabetes mellitus and renal disease, may affect dental management.

Appropriate health care During acute attacks, only emergency dental treatment should be provided.

Pain and anxiety control There are no specific contraindications to LA, CS or GA, although the underlying disease process must be considered.

Patient access and positioning Gout may be associated with painful, tender joints. This may impact on access to the dental clinic, such that transport may have to be arranged. Furthermore, the patient's position in the dental chair should be carefully adjusted to minimise discomfort from involved joints.

Drug use ■ Aspirin is contraindicated as it interferes with uricosuric agents ■ The incidence of rashes with ampicillin, but not other penicillin allergies, is increased in patients on allopurinol ■ Probenecid increases penicillin plasma levels.

Further reading ● Marbach J J 1979 Arthritis of the temporomandibular joints. Am Fam Phys 19:131–139.

GRAFT VERSUS HOST DISEASE (GVHD)

Definition Graft versus host disease (GVHD) is a severe complication following allogeneic haematopoietic stem cell transplantation (HSCT) ■ Acute GVHD is a syndrome of dermatitis, hepatitis and enteritis developing within 100 days ■ Chronic GVHD describes a more diverse syndrome developing after day 100.

General aspects

Aetiopathogenesis In HSCT recipients whose immune system has been damaged by iatrogenic immunosuppression (chemotherapy with or without total-body irradiation [TBI]), lymphocytes transferred to the host attempt to destroy the host's tissues. Chronic GVHD is viewed as an extension of acute GVHD, but also may occur *de novo* in patients who never showed clinical evidence of acute GVHD, or it may emerge following a quiescent interval after acute GVHD resolution. The most important risk factor for chronic GVHD is prior history of acute GVHD.

Clinical presentation **Acute GVHD** ■ Acute GVHD may manifest initially with a pruritic or painful rash ■ *Liver involvement:* asymptomatic elevation of bilirubin, alanine aminotransferase (ALT), aspartate aminotransferase (AST), and alkaline phosphatase, similar to cholestatic jaundice ■ *Gastrointestinal involvement:* affects the distal small bowel and colon, resulting in diarrhoea, intestinal bleeding, cramping abdominal pain, and ileus (intestinal immobility) ■ *Other findings:* increased risk of infectious and non-infectious pneumonia and sterile effusions, haemorrhagic cystitis with infective agents, thrombocytopenia, and anaemia, and a haemolytic–uraemic syndrome (thrombotic microangiopathy) ■ It may be graded (grades I–IV) in terms of severity. **Chronic GVHD** ■ Chronic GVHD (Fig. 3.16) has manifestations similar to those of systemic progressive sclerosis, systemic lupus erythematosus, lichen planus, Sjögren's syndrome, eosinophilic fasciitis, rheumatoid arthritis, and primary biliary cirrhosis ■ Chronic GVHD can lead to lichenoid skin lesions or sclerodermatous thickening of the skin, sometimes causing contractures and limitation of joint mobility ■ *Ocular manifestations:* symptoms of burning, irritation, photophobia, and pain from lack of tear secretion ■ *Oral and gastrointestinal manifestations:* dryness, dysphagia, sensitivity to acidic or spicy foods, and increasing pain ■ *Pulmonary manifestations:* obstructive lung disease with symptoms of wheezing, dyspnoea, and a chronic cough that usually is non-responsive to bronchodilator therapy ■ *Neuromuscular manifestations:* weakness, neuropathic pain, and muscle cramps ■ Autoimmune phenomena are sometimes observed and include myasthenia gravis or polymyositis.

Treatment ■ Most patients undergoing allogeneic stem cell transplantation are on prophylaxis for GVHD with ciclosporin or tacrolimus in combination with methotrexate and/or prednisone/prednisolone ■ Acute GVHD is treated with methotrexate IV for as long as 14 days ■ Chronic GVHD is treated with oral prednisone alone or in combination with ciclosporin.

Prognosis ■ Overall the grade of acute GVHD predicts outcome, with the highest rates of mortality in those with grade IV, or severe, GVHD ■ Chronic GVHD is a major cause of morbidity and mortality in long-term survivors of allogeneic HSCT. Chronic GVHD mortality rates are increased in patients with extensive disease, progressive-type onset, thrombocytopenia, and HLA-non-identical marrow donors. The overall survival rate is about 40%, but patients with a progressive onset of chronic GVHD have only a 10% survival rate.

Oral findings

Oral GVHD may be associated with: ■ hyposalivation ■ increased caries risk ■ altered taste ■ candidosis ■ herpes infections ■ lichenoid

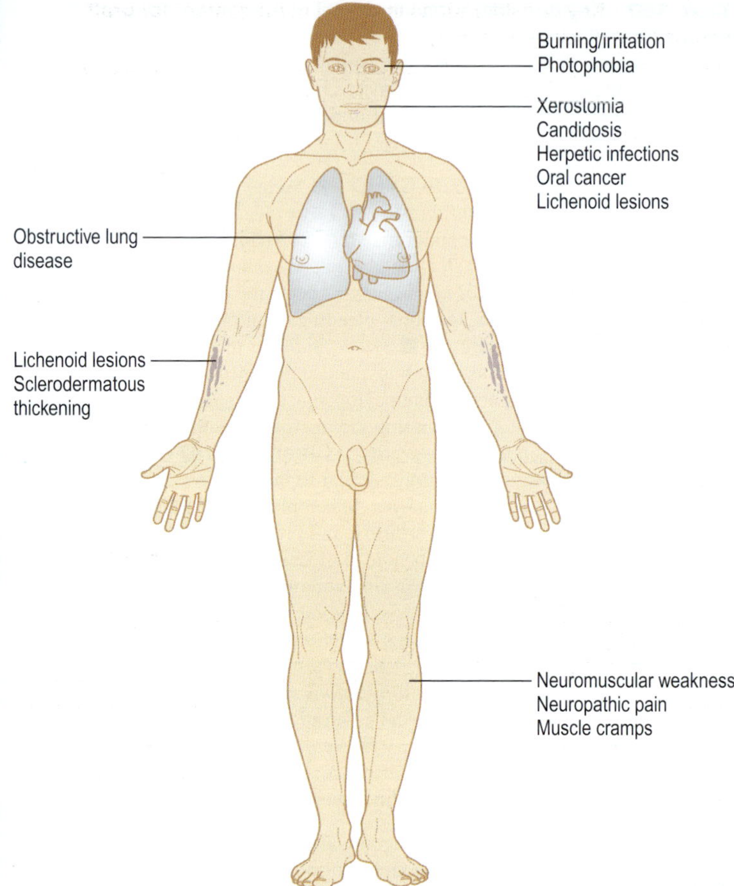

Figure 3.16 **Features of chronic graft versus host disease**

lesions ■ progressive systemic sclerosis-like changes ■ oral pain ■ oral cancer (squamous cell carcinoma).

Oral lesions due to GVHD treatment include: ■ methotrexate-induced mucositis ■ ciclosporin-induced gingival swelling.

Dental management

Risk assessment ■ There is an increased risk of oral infections due to immunosuppression ■ Liver involvement and thrombocytopenia may cause a bleeding tendency.

Table 3.60 **Key considerations in dental management for graft versus host disease (see text)**

	Management modifications*	Comments/possible complications
Risk assessment	3	Infection; bleeding tendency
Appropriate dental care	3/4	Only emergency oral care during acute phase; individualised assessment
Pain and anxiety control		
– Local anaesthesia	1	
– Conscious sedation	2	
– General anaesthesia	3/4	
Patient access and positioning		
– Access to dental office	0	
– Timing of treatment	0	
– Patient positioning	1	Upright position if pulmonary involvement
Treatment modification		
– Oral surgery	3/4	Dryness; GVHD prognosis
– Implantology	3–5	
– Conservative/Endodontics	3	GVHD prognosis
– Fixed prosthetics	3/5	GVHD prognosis
– Removable prosthetics	3/5	Mucosal involvement
– Non-surgical periodontology	3–5	GVHD prognosis
– Surgical periodontology	3–5	GVHD prognosis
Hazardous and contraindicated drugs	2	Some patients receive methotrexate, ciclosporin or corticosteroids

*0 = No special considerations. 1 = Caution advised. 2 = Specialised medical advice recommended in some cases. 3 = Specialised medical advice mandatory. 4 = Only to be performed in hospital environment. 5 = Should be avoided.

Appropriate health care ■ Only emergency dental care (antibiotics and analgesics) should be performed during acute GVHD ■ An individualised evaluation should be performed if complex dental treatment is considered, since GVHD morbidity and mortality rates are high. Surgery is best performed in a hospital environment.

Pain and anxiety control **Local anaesthesia** Caution is advised when planning treatment with the use of LA as oral lesions may be present, and patient tolerance poor. **Conscious sedation** Specialist medical advice is recommended prior to undertaking CS, particularly as pulmonary function may be compromised. **General anaesthesia** GA is a high-risk procedure, not only due to the complications of GVHD, but also the primary disease. It should only be undertaken after a thorough assessment by the anaesthetist and consultation with the patient's physician.

Patient access and positioning The patient should be treated upright in the dental chair if GVHD is associated with pulmonary involvement.

Drug use Some patients are on corticosteroids in addition to immunosuppressants.

Further reading ● Elad S, Or R, Garfunkel A A, Shapira M Y 2003 Budesonide: a novel treatment for oral chronic graft versus host disease. Oral Surg Oral Med Oral Pathol Oral Radiol Endod 95:308–311 ● Majorana A, Schubert M M, Porta F, Ugazio A G, Sapelli P L 2000 Oral complications of pediatric hematopoietic cell transplantation: diagnosis and management. Support Care Cancer 8:353–365 ● Melkos A B, Massenkeil G, Arnold R, Reichart P A 2003 Dental treatment prior to stem cell transplantation and its influence on the post-transplantation outcome. Clin Oral Invest 7:113–115 ● Uderzo C, Fraschini D, Balduzzi A et al 1997 Long-term effects of bone marrow transplantation on dental status in children with leukaemia. Bone Marrow Transplant 20:865–869.

HAEMOPHILIA A

Definition ■ Haemophilia A is a congenital X-linked disorder resulting from a deficiency in blood clotting factor VIII, a key component of the coagulation cascade ■ Haemophilia A therefore affects males ■ Sons of carriers have a 50:50 chance of developing haemophilia while daughters of carriers have a 50:50 chance of being carriers – all daughters of an affected male are carriers but sons are normal ■ Carriers rarely have a clinically manifest bleeding tendency ■ Haemophilia A, with a prevalence of about 5 per 100 000 of the population, is about 10 times as common as haemophilia B (see Christmas disease) except in some Asian populations, where frequencies are almost equal. A family history can be obtained in only about 65% of cases.

General aspects

Aetiopathogenesis Some 150 different point mutations have been characterised in the factor VIII gene in haemophilia A. Most of these are inherited, although spontaneous mutations may occur.

Clinical presentation ■ The characteristic feature of haemophilia is excessive bleeding particularly after trauma, and sometimes spontaneously ■ Haemorrhage in haemophiliacs appears to stop immediately after the injury (as a result of normal vascular and platelet response) but, after an hour or more, intractable oozing or rapid blood loss starts and persists ■ Haemorrhage is dangerous either because of loss of blood or, if haemorrhage is internal, because of damage to joints, muscles and nerves, or vital organs ■ Haemarthroses can cause joint damage and cripple the patient ■ Abdominal haemorrhage may simulate an acute abdomen ■ Bleeding into the cranium, or compression of the larynx and pharynx following haematoma formation in the neck, can be fatal ■ Dental extractions or deep lacerations are followed by persistent oozing for days or weeks and, in the past, have been fatal. The haemorrhage cannot be controlled by pressure and, although clots may form in the mouth, they fail to stop the bleeding.

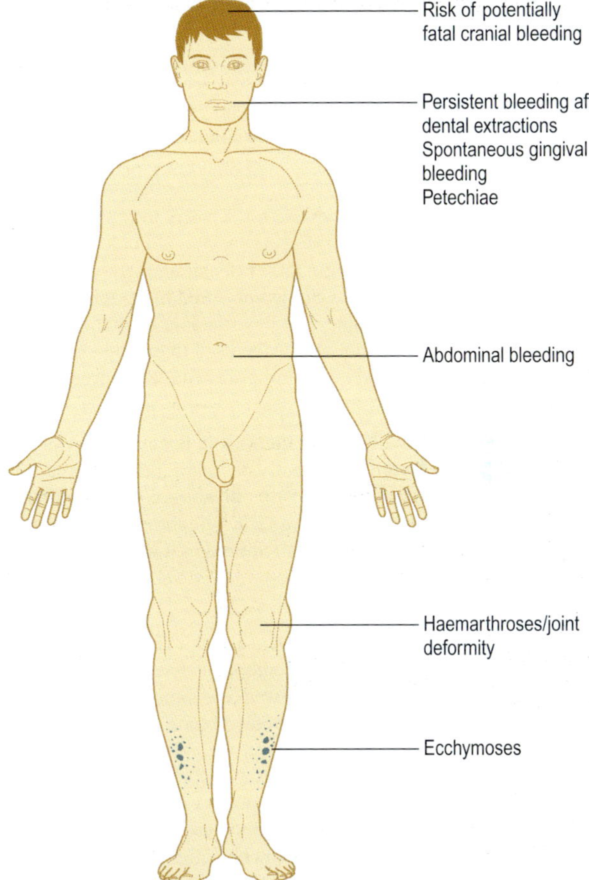

Figure 3.17 **Clinical presentation of haemophilia A**

Classification ■ Normal plasma contains 1 unit of Factor VIII per mL, a level defined as 100% ■ There are severe, moderate or mild forms of haemophilia – the severity of the disease being variable but correlating well with the Factor VIII level in the plasma (Table 3.61) ■ Factor VIII activity of less than 1% (FVIIIC <1 IU/dL) (severe haemophilia) results in spontaneous bleeding, which typically becomes apparent in childhood with bleeding into muscles or joints (haemarthroses), easy bruising and prolonged bleeding from wounds following injuries ■ Factor VIII activity of 1–5% (FVIIIC level 1–5 IU/dL) is moderate haemophilia ■ Factor VIII level above 5% (FVIIIC >5 IU/dL), is mild disease but comparatively minor trauma

Table 3.61 **Severity, Factor VIII activity, and haemorrhage type in haemophilia**

Classification	Factor activity, %	Cause of haemorrhage
Mild	>5	Major trauma or surgery
Moderate	1–5	Mild-to-moderate trauma
Severe	<1	Spontaneous, haemarthroses

can lead to persistent bleeding. Bleeding after dental extractions is sometimes the first or only sign of mild disease. Some very mild haemophiliacs may not bleed excessively even after a simple dental extraction, so that the absence of post-extraction haemorrhage cannot always be used to exclude haemophilia. Most will, however, bleed excessively after more traumatic surgery, such as tonsillectomy.

Diagnosis The diagnostic laboratory findings in haemophilia can be summarised as follows: ■ prolonged activated partial thromboplastin time (APTT) ■ normal prothrombin time (PT) ■ normal bleeding time ■ low Factor VIIIC but normal VIIIR:Ag (von Willebrand factor) and R:RCo (ristocetin co-factor); Factor VIII assay is required as even the APTT may be normal in mild haemophilia.

Treatment

■ Replacement of the missing clotting factor is achieved with porcine Factor VIII or genetically engineered (recombinant) Factor VIII.

■ In the past, fresh plasma, frozen plasma, cryoprecipitate or fractionated human factor concentrates obtained from pooled blood sources were used, but these had, and may still occasionally have, the potential to carry blood-borne pathogens such as hepatitis viruses, HIV and various herpes viruses.

■ Regular prophylactic replacement of Factor VIII is used when possible but necessitates daily injections as the half-life is around 12 hours. This has implications as regards to cost and patient inconvenience. Furthermore, its use may be complicated by antibody formation. As a result, many patients receive replacement Factor VIII less frequently, with additional doses being provided perioperatively when procedures associated with bleeding are undertaken (e.g. surgery, periodontal treatment). Some patients are able to self-administer their factor replacement, considerably improving their quality of life and convenience.

■ Gene therapy of haemophilia is still very much in its infancy.

■ Desmopressin (deamino-8-D arginine vasopressin: DDAVP) is a synthetic analogue of vasopressin that induces the release of Factor VIIIC, von Willebrand factor (vWF) and tissue plasminogen activator (tPA) from storage sites in endothelium. Desmopressin cover just before surgery, and repeated 12-hourly if necessary for up to 4 days, is useful to cover minor surgery in some very mild haemophiliacs. It is given as an intranasal spray of 1.5 mg desmopressin per mL with each 0.1 mL pump spray delivering a 100–150 μg dose, or as a slow intravenous infusion over 20 minutes of 0.3–0.5 μg/kg. Multiple infusions of desmopressin have been associated with a reduced response (tachyphylaxis). This suggests that maximal responses are achieved short-term. Additional doses may be minimally effective and may even increase the bleeding time.

■ Tranexamic acid (which is not FDA approved for use on the US market, where epsilon amino caproic acid is an alternative), is a synthetic derivative of the amino acid lysine, which exerts an antifibrinolytic effect through the reversible blockade of lysine binding sites on plasminogen molecules. Tranexamic acid significantly reduces blood loss after surgery in patients with haemophilia and can be used topically or systemically. Systemically, it is given in a dose of 1 g (30 mg/kg) orally, 4 times daily starting at least 1 hour preoperatively for surgical procedures, or as infusion 10 mg/kg in 20 mL normal saline over 20 minutes, then 1 gm tds orally for 5 days (child dose is 20 mg/kg). However, nausea is a common adverse effect and antifibrinolytics must not be used systemically where residual clots are present, because clots may form in the urinary tract or intracranially. These problems have led to the development of topical preparations, typically 5% solutions w/v, often used as a mouthwash 10 mL qds for 1–2 weeks after dental extractions and/or applied to gauze swabs placed over the bleeding socket.

Haemophiliacs with inhibitors ■ The haematologists must always be consulted ■ Factor VIII inhibitor levels should be checked preoperatively ■ In general, patients with low titre inhibitors can have dental treatment in the same way as those who have no antibodies ■ In those with high titre inhibitors, surgery needs special care. Traumatic procedures must be avoided unless absolutely essential. Human Factor VIII Inhibitor Bypassing Fractions (FEIBA) can often be effective; these are usually either non-activated prothrombin complex concentrates (PCC) or activated prothrombin complex concentrates (APCC) which act by activating Factor X directly, bypassing the intrinsic pathway of blood clotting. The danger with these products is of uncontrolled coagulation with thromboses. Currently, the choice is usually either prothrombin-complex concentrates (e.g. FEIBA), or recombinant factor VIIa. In some cases, desmopressin is an effective alternative, and antifibrinolytics may help.

Prognosis The severity of bleeding in haemophilia is dependent on the level of Factor VIII coagulant (VIIIC) activity, and degree of trauma. Spontaneous bleeding in severe haemophilia is frequent and may be life-threatening.

Oral findings

Petechiae, ecchymoses, spontaneous gingival bleeding and prolonged bleeding after surgical procedures are common findings

Dental management

Risk assessment Difficulties in the management of haemophiliacs may include: ■ dental neglect necessitating frequent dental extractions ■ trauma, surgery and subsequent haemorrhage ■ Factor VIII inhibitors ■ hazards of anaesthesia, especially nasal intubation, and intramuscular injections ■ risks of hepatitis, and liver disease ■ HIV infection (in older haemophiliacs; blood and blood products are now screened to exclude known infectious agents) ■ risk of vCJD increased if blood transfusions received ■ aggravation of bleeding by drugs ■ anxiety ■ drug dependence as a result of chronic pain.

Appropriate health care ■ To ensure safe and comprehensive oral care is provided, close cooperation between the dental practitioner and the patient's haematologist is essential ■ In all but severe haemophiliacs, non-surgical dental treatment can usually be carried out with minimal problems, with the occasional use of antifibrinolytic cover (usually tranexamic acid) if required ■ In all but the most mild haemophiliacs, Factor VIII replacement is required before regional LA (see below) and surgery ■ In severe or moderate haemophilia, Factor VIII must be replaced to a level adequate to ensure haemostasis if bleeding starts or is expected ■ In mild haemophilia, there is increasing reliance on use of desmopressin and antifibrinolytics such as tranexamic acid.

Preventive dentistry ■ Oral health education of patient or parents is critical ■ It should be started as early as possible in the young child, when the teeth begin to erupt ■ This will minimise dental operative intervention that can cause severe, or occasionally fatal, complications ■ The use of fluorides, fissure sealants, dietary advice on the need for sugar restriction and regular dental inspections from an early age are crucial to the preservation of teeth ■ Prevention of periodontal disease is also imperative ■ Comprehensive dental assessment is needed at the age of about 12–13, to decide how best to forestall difficulties resulting from overcrowding, or misplaced third molars or other teeth.

Pain and anxiety control **Local anaesthesia** ■ Local anaesthesia regional blocks (inferior dental or posterior superior alveolar), lingual infiltrations, or injections in the floor of the mouth must not be used in the absence of Factor VIII replacement since they can cause haemorrhage which can compromise the airway and be life-threatening ■ Alternative methods of LA should be explored (e.g. intraligamentary, intraosseous, papillary or electronic dental anaesthesia) ■ If regional LA is required, Factor VIII replacement therapy should be given to ensure that the Factor level is maintained above 30% ■ Infiltration LA may be used without Factor replacement; however, as even submucosal LA infiltrations may occasionally cause widespread haematoma formation, lingual infiltration should be avoided to minimise the risk to the airway. **Conscious sedation** Nitrous oxide relative analgesia and oral sedation are preferable, as intravenous sedation may be complicated by haematoma formation. **General anaesthesia** A thorough preoperative assessment by the anaesthetist, in close consultant with the haematologist and dental practitioner, is required. Issues such as appropriate factor replacement, availability of blood products at the time of operation, joint deformity and hence access and positioning issues, need to be addressed. Nasal intubation should be avoided if possible.

Treatment modification **Dentoalveolar surgery** ■ Dentoalveolar surgery should be carefully planned and ideally all necessary surgery (and other dental treatment) should be performed at one operation. A Factor VIII level of between 50 and 75% is required for dental extractions or dentoalveolar surgery. ■ A detailed radiological survey should be taken to identify any other teeth with unsuspected lesions that may also require extractions, to prevent future problems ■ Local measures are important to minimise the risk of postoperative bleeding, namely: ● Surgery should be carried out with minimal trauma to both bone and soft tissues ● Careful mouth toilet postoperatively is essential ● Suturing is desirable to stabilise gum flaps and to prevent postoperative disturbance of wounds by eating. A non-traumatic needle must be used, and the number of sutures minimised. Vicryl sutures are preferred as they usually remain *in situ* for over 4 days. Non-resorbable sutures such as black silk, if used, should be removed at 4–7 days. ● Although suturing carries with it the risk, if there is postoperative bleeding, of causing blood to track down towards the mediastinum with danger to the airway, this complication is usually an indication of inadequate preoperative replacement therapy, or more rarely the presence of Factor VIII inhibitors ● In the case of difficult extractions, when mucoperiosteal flaps must be raised, the lingual tissues in the lower molar regions should preferably be left undisturbed since trauma may open up planes into which haemorrhage can track and endanger the airway. The buccal approach to lower third molars is therefore safer. ● Minimal bone should be removed and the teeth should be sectioned for removal where possible ● Topical haemostatic agents introduced into the base of the sockets may be of use. Agents used include collagen, cyanoacrylate, fibrin glues, and oxidised cellulose soaked in tranexamic acid (Table 3.62). Fibrin sealant, which consists mainly of fibrinogen and thrombin, provides rapid haemostasis as well as tissue sealing and adhesion (commercial, viral-inactivated products are available in Europe, Canada, and Japan). Liquid fibrin sealant (LFS) has been used but fibrin glue is unavailable in USA, because of the risk of viral infections, and concern regarding CJD; recombinant fibrin glues are becoming available. ● Tranexamic acid mouthwash (used either as a mouthwash, or as a swish/swallow technique) is a helpful adjunct ● Postoperatively, a diet of cold liquid and pureed/soft solids should be taken for up to 5–10 days ● Infection may also induce fibrinolysis by secondary haemorrhage, so antimicrobials, such as

Table 3.62 **Topical haemostatic agents**

Agent (®)	Main constituent	Source
Avitene	Collagen	Bovine origin
Beriplast	Fibrin	Various
Colla-Cote	Collagen	Bovine origin
Cyclokapron	Tranexamic acid	Synthetic
Gelfoam	Gelatin	Bovine origin
Helistat	Collagen	Bovine origin
Instat	Collagen	Bovine origin
Surgicel	Cellulose	Synthetic
Thrombinar	Thrombin	Bovine origin
Thrombogen	Thrombin	Bovine origin
Thrombostat	Thrombin	Bovine origin

oral penicillin V 250 mg or amoxicillin 500 mg 4 times daily given postoperatively for a full course of 7 days, may be considered ● Acrylic protective splints are now rarely used, in view of their liability to cause mucosal trauma and to promote sepsis, but they are sometimes useful in sites such as the palate ■ Care should be taken to watch for haematoma formation that may manifest itself by swelling, dysphagia or hoarseness. The patency of the airway must always be ensured. ■ Compounding factors, such as thrombocytopenia in HIV-infected haemophiliacs, should be considered.

Maxillofacial surgery ■ Factor VIII replacement is essential for all haemophiliacs ■ The dose of factor VIII given before operation depends both on the severity of haemophilia and the amount of trauma expected. A Factor VIII level of between (at least) 75% and (better) 100% is required for maxillofacial surgery. Factor VIII must be given 1 hour preoperatively and regularly at least twice daily postoperatively for major surgery. ■ Before maxillofacial surgery, the patient is assessed by haemostatic screening (APTT, PT, platelet count), Factor VIII assay, specific antibody test, fibrinogen estimation, hepatitis B, C and HIV tests, and liver function tests
■ Blood is also grouped and cross-matched for use in emergency
■ Bleeding is most likely on the day of operation or from 4 to 10 days

Table 3.63 **Guidelines for management of oral health care procedures in the haemophilias**

Procedure*		Haemophilia**		
		Mild	*Moderate*	*Severe*
LA	Intraligamentary	–	–	–
	Buccal infiltration	–	–	–
	Lingual infiltration	–	FR	FR
	Regional block	FR	FR	FR
Non-surgical care without regional LA	Prosthetics	–	–	–
	Conservation	–	–	–
	Root canal therapy	–	–	FR
	Orthodontics	–	–	–
Surgical care with or without LA	Scaling	± T	T	FR + T
Trauma	Soft tissue	–	FR	FR
	Bone	FR	FR	FR
Surgery	Soft tissue	FR + T	FR + T	FR + T
	Periodontal	FR + T	FR + T	FR + T
	Exodontia	FR + T	FR + T	FR + T
	Dentoalveolar	FR + T	FR + T	FR + T
	Implant	FR + T	FR + T	FR + T
	Major	FR + T	FR + T	FR + T

*If in doubt, consult haematologist.
**Minimal requirements, assuming no additional bleeding tendency (liver disease etc).
LA = local anaesthesia. FR = Factor replacement. T = Tranexamic acid 5% mouthwash used qds for 5 days post-procedure.

postoperatively. **Trauma to the head and neck** ■ Haemophiliacs with head and neck injuries are at risk from bleeding into the cranial cavity or into the fascial spaces of the neck – they must, therefore, be given Factor VIII to achieve a level of 100% prophylactically after head or facial trauma

Table 3.64 **Key considerations for dental management in haemophilia (see text)**

	Management modifications*	Comments/possible complications
Risk assessment	3	Haemorrhage; Hazards of anaesthesia; hepatitis, liver disease and HIV infection; anxiety
Appropriate dental care	3/4	Factor replacement; desmopressin; tranexamic acid
Pain and anxiety control		
– Local anaesthesia	2	Avoid regional blocks and lingual infiltrations
– Conscious sedation	2	Avoid IV sedation
– General anaesthesia	3/4	Assess joint involvement, mobility; avoid nasal intubation
Patient access and positioning		
– Access to dental office	1	Joint involvement
– Timing of treatment	1	1 hour after factor replacement
– Patient positioning	1	Joint involvement
Treatment modification		
– Oral surgery	3/4	Factor replacement; minimal trauma; topical haemostatic agents; avoid catgut
– Implantology	5	
– Conservative/Endodontics	2	Avoid local bleeding; intracanal LA with epinephrine
– Fixed prosthetics	2	Avoid local bleeding
– Removable prosthetics	1	
– Non-surgical periodontology	3/4	Factor replacement; topical haemostatic agents
– Surgical periodontology	3/4	See oral surgery
Imaging	1	Do not rest radiographs on the floor of the mouth
Hazardous and contraindicated drugs	2	Avoid aspirin, indometacin and other NSAIDs; avoid intramuscular injections

*0 = No special considerations. 1 = Caution advised. 2 = Specialised medical advice recommended in some cases. 3 = Specialised medical advice mandatory. 4 = Only to be performed in hospital environment. 5 = Should be avoided.

■ If there are only lacerations that need suturing, a minimum level of Factor VIII of 50% is required at the time, with further cover for 3 days. **Fixed prosthetics and conservation** ■ Soft tissue trauma must be avoided. Care must be taken not to let the matrix band cut the periodontal tissues and start gingival bleeding. A rubber dam is useful to protect the mucosa from trauma but the clamp must be carefully applied. Cotton wool rolls should be moistened to avoid adherence to the mucosa, which may result in mucosal bleeding when they are removed. High-speed vacuum aspirators and saliva ejectors must be used with caution in order to avoid production of haematomas. Trauma from the saliva ejector can be minimised by resting it on a gauze swab placed in the floor of the mouth. Tranexamic acid mouthwash may be of use to control local bleeding. ■ Subgingival restorations may be placed with the use of haemostatic solutions such as for gingival retraction (e.g. Racestyptine) or locally applied LA containing epinephrine, to control gingival bleeding. **Endodontics** ■ Endodontic treatment may obviate the need for extractions and can usually be carried out without special precautions other than care to avoid instrumenting through the tooth apex ■ Intracanal injection of LA solution containing epinephrine or topical application (with paper points) of epinephrine 1:1000 may be useful to minimise bleeding ■ However, in severe haemophilia, bleeding from the pulp and periapical tissues can be persistent and troublesome, and factor replacement may need to be considered. **Periodontology** ■ In all but severe haemophiliacs, scaling can usually be carried out under antifibrinolytic cover ■ Periodontal surgery necessitates LA and factor replacement; a Factor VIII level of between 50 and 75% is required. **Orthodontics** ■ There is no contraindication to the movement of teeth in haemophilia. However, care must be taken to ensure that there are no sharp edges to orthodontic appliances or fixtures, as these may traumatise the mucosa and cause bleeding.

Drug use ■ Intramuscular injections should be avoided unless replacement therapy is being given, as they can cause large haematomas. Oral alternatives are satisfactory in most instances. ■ The bleeding tendency can be aggravated by drugs such as aspirin or other non-steroidal anti-inflammatory drugs such as indometacin; safer choices appear to be paracetamol/acetaminophen and codeine-based analgesics.

Further reading ● Blanco J, Liñares A, Batalla P, Diz P 2004 Morbidity and economic complications following mucogingival surgery in a hemophiliac HIV-infected patient. J Periodontol 75:1413–1416 ● Brewer A K, Roebuck E M, Donachie M et al 2003 The dental management of adult patients with haemophilia and other congenital bleeding disorders. Haemophilia 9:673–677 ● Scully C, Watt-Smith P, Dios P D, Giangrande P L 2002 Complications in HIV-infected and non-HIV-infected haemophiliacs and other patients after oral surgery. Int J Oral Maxillofac Surg 31:634–640 ● Scully C, Dis Dios P, Giangrande P, Lee C 2002 Oral health care in haemophilia and other bleeding tendencies. World Federation on Hemophilia Treatment of Hemophilia Monograph Series, No. 27 ● Scully C, Diz Dios P, Shotts R 2004 Oral health care in patients with the most important medically compromising conditions; 2. congenital coagulation disorders. CPD Dentistry 5:8–11.

HEARING IMPAIRMENT

Definition Hearing impairment occurs when there is a problem with one or more parts of the ear, or the main sensory pathway ■ *Conductive hearing loss* results from problems in the external or middle ear. Sound levels seem lower. ■ *Sensorineural hearing loss* results from damage to the inner ear (cochlea), auditory nerve or the central connections. This type of hearing loss is permanent. The affected person has difficulty hearing clearly, understanding speech, and interpreting various sounds. ■ *Mixed hearing loss* occurs when a person has both conductive and sensorineural hearing problems.

General aspects

Aetiopathogenesis **Conductive hearing loss** May occur in association with: ■ craniofacial congenital disorders (e.g. first arch defects, cleft palate) ■ chronic infection ■ trauma ■ 'glue' ear in children. **Sensorineural hearing loss** May be consequence of: ■ genetic disorders interfering with the development of the inner ear and auditory nerve ■ injuries, such as a skull fracture ■ complications during pregnancy or birth, such as infections (e.g. rubella) or other illnesses; premature babies are at increased risk for hearing impairment ■ infections or illnesses: mumps, measles, chickenpox, repeated otitis media ■ brain tumours ■ drugs, such as some antibiotics (e.g. aminoglycosides, including gentamicin) and chemotherapy drugs ■ loud noise – a sudden loud noise (e.g. explosion) or exposure to high noise levels over time (e.g. pop music or road drills) can cause permanent damage to the cochlea.

Clinical presentation ■ About one in 10 people have hearing impairment but the degree of disability can vary widely from person to person ■ Prevalence is similar in males and females ■ One or both ears may be affected, and the impairment may be worse in one ear than in the other ■ Hearing loss can be sudden or progressive ■ Some people have partial hearing loss, meaning that the ear can detect some sounds; others have complete hearing loss, meaning that the ear cannot hear at all (they are considered deaf) ■ The timing of the hearing loss can also vary. Congenital hearing loss is present at birth or within the first few days of life. Acquired hearing loss occurs later in life, often appearing slowly over time. ■ The higher the frequency of the sound, the louder the sound has to be, in order for the hearing-impaired person to hear it.

Diagnosis Otorhinolaryngological and audiological examinations are typically required.

Treatment ■ Conductive hearing loss can often be corrected with medications or surgery ■ Sensorineural hearing loss may be treated with hearing aids or, in severe cases, a cochlear implant. Hearing aids are essentially wearable miniature amplifiers that give an amplification of approximately +40 decibels.

Prognosis ■ Conductive hearing loss can have a good prognosis ■ Sensorineural hearing loss typically has a prognosis that is less good, depending on the cause, and in some cases this condition is irreversible.

Dental management

Risk assessment ■ The main problem to overcome is communication. The patient with a hearing impairment may exhibit fear or hostility if they feel they do not hear/understand instructions, and may pretend to hear in order to avoid embarrassment. ■ There has been concern over possible auditory damage from dental rotary and ultrasonic instruments. However, the evidence for damage from air turbines is equivocal, and ultrasonic scalers are not considered to have a negative effect on the hearing of dental hygienists at 500, 1000, 2000, 4000, 6000 and 8000 Hz – though there may be hearing loss at 3000 Hz.

Appropriate dental care ■ Speech communications are easier for the hearing-impaired person if (Fig. 3.18): ● there is bright lighting ● the speaker is facing them directly and not wearing a face mask ● the speaker is not moving their head around ● the speaker talks slowly, preferably one phrase at a time ● the speaker is at the optimal distance from the person (between 1 and 2 metres) ● there is as little background noise as possible, i.e. turn off the high-volume evacuator, saliva ejector, radio or piped-in music. ■ Hearing devices can be adversely affected by the high-pitched tone of the handpiece or ultrasonic scaler, which may make the device useless and cause

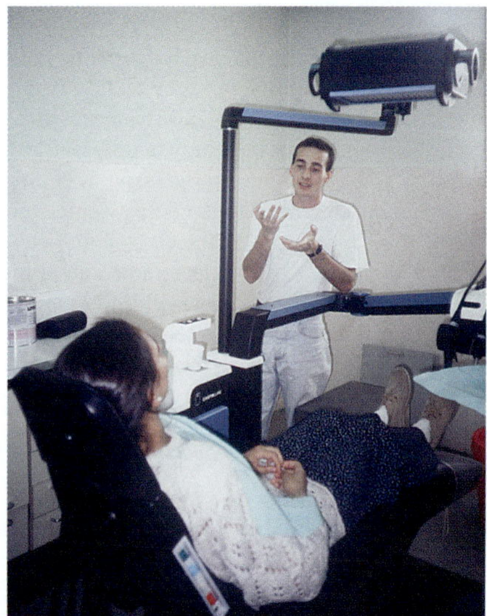

Figure 3.18 **Communication with a dental patient who has a hearing impairment**

the patient to be less cooperative ■ Communication can be helped by cued speech – which uses hand symbols for each sound, and is used in conjunction with lip reading ■ Use mirrors, models, drawings and written information to augment communication ■ A sign language interpreter can be very valuable ■ Sometimes it is easier to use a notepad or a keyboard to communicate ■ Other aids include E-mail, Blackberry, Voice-To-Text Phone Service or Text-To-Voice Phone Service, or Text Telephone (TDD/TTY) a special telephone called a Telecommunications Device for the Deaf (TDD) or a TeleTypewriter (TTY), Internet Relay Service, Voice Carry Over (VCO) and Captioned Telephones ■ The patients may prefer to have their hearing device turned off before clinical procedures begin – especially if dental rotary or ultrasonic instruments are going to be used.

Pain and anxiety control **Local anaesthesia** Local anaesthesia may be used with routine precautions **Conscious sedation** It may be difficult to monitor the patient's state of consciousness through verbal communication and caution is advisable. **General anaesthesia** Care must be taken to

Table 3.65 **Key considerations for dental management in hearing impairment (see text)**

	Management modifications*	Comments/possible complications
Risk assessment	1	Communication
Appropriate dental care	1	Speech communication guidelines; hearing aids
Pain and anxiety control		
– Local anaesthesia	0	
– Conscious sedation	1	
– General anaesthesia	1	
Patient access and positioning		
– Access to dental office	0	
– Timing of treatment	0	
– Patient positioning	1	Light position; distance dentist–patient
Treatment modification		
– Oral surgery	1	
– Implantology	1	
– Conservative/Endodontics	1	
– Fixed prosthetics	1	
– Removable prosthetics	1	
– Non-surgical periodontology	1	
– Surgical periodontology	1	
Hazardous and contraindicated drugs	1	Avoid any ototoxic drugs

*0 = No special considerations. 1 = Caution advised. 2 = Specialised medical advice recommended in some cases. 3 = Specialised medical advice mandatory. 4 = Only to be performed in hospital environment. 5 = Should be avoided.

ensure that methods of communication are in place so that the patient may be assessed and monitored safely, both prior to GA and on recovery.

Further reading ● Diz Dios P, García García A, Fernández Feijoo J et al 1994 Prótesis auricular implantosoportada. Acta Otorrinolaring Esp 45:45–48 ● Hyson J M Jr 2002 The air turbine and hearing loss: are dentists at risk? J Am Dent Assoc 133:1639–1642 ● Oredugba F A 2004 Oral health care knowledge and practices of a group of deaf adolescents in Lagos, Nigeria. J Public Health Dent. 64:118–120 ● Peeters J, Naert I, Carette E, Manders E, Jacobs R 2004 A potential link between oral status and hearing impairment: preliminary observations. J Oral Rehabil 31:306–310 ● Skrinjaric I, Jukic J, Skrinjaric K, Glavina D, Legovic M, Ulovec Z 2003 Dental and minor physical anomalies in children with developmental disorders – a discriminant analysis. Coll Antropol 27:769–778 ● Trenter S C, Walmsley A D 2003 Ultrasonic dental scaler: associated hazards. J Clin Periodontol 30:95–101 ● Wilson J D, Darby M L, Tolle S L, Sever J C Jr 2002 Effects of occupational ultrasonic noise exposure on hearing of dental hygienists: a pilot study. J Dent Hyg 76:262–269.

HEART TRANSPLANTATION

Definition Cardiac transplantation is the treatment for end-stage cardiac disease (idiopathic cardiomyopathy, coronary artery disease, or valvular disease) that cannot be corrected by other medical or surgical means. The heart usually comes from a brain-dead human organ donor, although porcine heart transplantation may become a more viable option in the future and address the issue of limited donor availability.

General aspects

Clinical presentation Clinical manifestations due to immunosuppressive therapy may be seen after transplantation.

Diagnosis Selection of donor recipients is performed based on: ECG, echocardiogram and radionuclide scintillation studies. The success of the transplantation is evaluated by means of: endomyocardial biopsies, ECG and coronary angiography.

Treatment All transplant recipients require life-long immunosuppression to prevent a T-cell, alloimmune rejection response. The agents used usually include ciclosporin, mycophenolate or azathioprine, corticosteroids and antithymocyte globulin, or tacrolimus.

Prognosis ■ The one-year survival is variable (20–80%), although postoperative mortality and morbidity are falling ■ Coronary artery stenosis develops in about 30% of transplant patients within a few years.

Oral findings

Consequences of immunosuppressive drug treatment may include:
■ bacterial infections (also caries and periodontitis) ■ candidosis

■ mucormycosis ■ sinusitis ■ herpes virus infections ■ Kaposi's sarcoma ■ gingival swelling ■ transient perioral hyperaesthesia ■ oral hairy leukoplakia.

Dental management

Risk assessment ■ The patient will be immunosuppressed ■ If the patient is also on corticosteroids, additional doses may need to be given to facilitate stressful/surgical procedures ■ Due to the absence of cardiac innervation, angina is rare and patients may experience 'silent' myocardial infarction or sudden death ■ It has been argued that heart transplant patients cannot show a vasovagal reaction because the donor heart is transplanted completely deprived of any vagal or sympathetic innervation; however, one report has documented three episodes of vasovagal syncope in three heart transplant patients undergoing periodontal surgery ■ Patients may be anticoagulated or taking aspirin and dipyridamole to reduce platelet adhesion and thus have a prolonged bleeding time ■ A proportion of heart transplants require placement of pacemakers to optimise function.

Appropriate health care ■ Before heart transplantation most patients are considered ASA IV or V and therefore are best treated dentally in a hospital environment ■ A meticulous pre-surgery oral assessment is required and dental treatment undertaken with particular attention to establishing optimal oral hygiene and eradicating sources of potential infection ■ Dental treatment should be completed before surgery, including extraction of teeth with poor prognosis and adjustment of any dental prostheses ■ For 6 months after surgery, elective dental care is best deferred; if surgical treatment is needed during that period, antibiotic prophylaxis is probably warranted, although there is no conclusive evidence of this indication ■ The coagulation profile should be determined in advance of any operative dental treatment.

Preventive dentistry Sepsis is the main cause of death in heart transplant patients. Furthermore, there is some evidence that periodontal disease is a risk factor for cardiovascular disease and has been detected in higher frequency in patients requiring heart transplantation. Hence a meticulous oral hygiene programme is mandatory.

Pain and anxiety control **Local anaesthesia** There is increased sensitivity to catecholamines such as epinephrine, which should thus be avoided. **Conscious sedation** Benzodiazepines are the anxiolytics of choice, although relative analgesia may also be used safely. **General anaesthesia** GA should only be undertaken after advice from the patient's cardiac specialist, and a thorough assessment appointment with the anaesthetist. Ideally it should be undertaken within the specialised unit where the transplant was provided.

Drug use ■ Some patients are taking anticoagulants or aspirin ■ Some patients are on corticosteroids.

Further reading
● Meechan J G, Parry G, Rattray D T, Thomason J M 2002 Effects of dental local anaesthetics in cardiac transplant recipients. Br Dent J 192:161–163

Table 3.66 **Key considerations for dental management in heart transplantation (see text)**

	Management modifications*	Comments/possible complications
Risk assessment	2	Immunosuppression; steroid cover; anticoagulants/aspirin; silent angina, no vasovagal reactions; pacemakers; bleeding; infections
Appropriate dental care	2/4	Preferable before transplantation; delay 6 months after surgery; antibiotic prophylaxis for the first 6 months; coagulation profile
Pain and anxiety control		
– Local anaesthesia	1	Avoid epinephrine
– Conscious sedation	1	
– General anaesthesia	3/4	
Patient access and positioning		
– Access to dental office	0	
– Timing of treatment	1	Avoid elective treatment in the first 6 months
– Patient positioning	0	
Treatment modification		
– Oral surgery	2	
– Implantology	2	
– Conservative/Endodontics	1	
– Fixed prosthetics	1	
– Removable prosthetics	1	
– Non-surgical periodontology	2	
– Surgical periodontology	2	
Hazardous and contraindicated drugs	2	Some patients are taking anticoagulants, aspirin or corticosteroids

*0 = No special considerations. 1 = Caution advised. 2 = Specialised medical advice recommended in some cases. 3 = Specialised medical advice mandatory. 4 = Only to be performed in hospital environment. 5 = Should be avoided.

● Montebugnoli L, Prati C 2002 Circulatory dynamics during dental extractions in normal, cardiac and transplant patients. J Am Dent Assoc 133:468–472 ● Research, Science and Therapy Committee, American Academy of Periodontology 2002 Periodontal management of patients with cardiovascular diseases. J Periodontol 73:954–968 ● al-Sarheed M, Angeletou A, Ashley P F, Lucas V S, Whitehead B, Roberts G J 2000 An investigation of the oral status and reported oral care of children with heart and heart–lung transplants. Int J Paediatr Dent 10:298–305 ● Scully C, Diz Dios P, Shotts R 2004 Oral health care in patients with the most important medically compromising conditions; 4. patients with cardiovascular disease. CPD Dentistry 5:50–55.

HEPARINISATION

Definition ■ Heparin is a natural sulphated glycosaminoglycan, abundant in the mast cells that line the vasculature ■ It is released in response to injury, when it inhibits coagulation ■ Heparin was originally obtained from liver (hence the term heparin) but is now obtained from beef or porcine lung or gut, although recombinant oral heparin is being developed ■ It is heterogeneous with respect to molecular size, anticoagulant activity, and pharmacokinetic properties ■ The anticoagulant activity is heterogeneous because the anticoagulant profile and clearance of heparin are influenced by the chain length of the molecules, with the higher-molecular-weight species cleared from the circulation more rapidly than the lower-molecular-weight species. Hence, typically only one-third of heparin molecules administered to patients have anticoagulant function, with a half-life of 1–2 hours.

General aspects

Indications ■ Heparin is used as a parenteral anticoagulant administered subcutaneously or intravenously for: ● acute thromboembolic episodes and to prevent deep venous thrombosis and pulmonary emboli after major surgery (i.e. in-patient care) ● initial prophylactic prevention of thrombosis after a myocardial infarct ● low-dose heparin therapy (such as 'Minihep') to reduce risk of deep vein thrombosis ● in IV dialysis to prevent thrombosis in the pumps (e.g. renal dialysis) ■ Low molecular weight (LMW) may also be used for long-term outpatient prophylaxis for: ● pregnancy ● patients intolerant to/failed on warfarin ● lupus anticoagulant factor ■ Some heparins are also being used for other effects, such as immunosuppression.

Mechanism of action Heparin acts immediately on blood coagulation by ■ Inhibiting the thrombin–fibrinogen reaction; it does this by binding to and catalysing antithrombin III, which then inhibits the serine proteases of the coagulation cascade to inactivate thrombin ■ It also acts on activated factors IX–XII ■ It also decreases platelet aggregation by inhibiting thrombin-induced activation.

Classification Heparin is available as: ■ Standard or unfractionated heparin. This has an immediate effect on blood clotting which is usually lost within 6 hours of stopping heparin. ■ LMW heparins (certoparin, dalteparin, enoxaparin, tinzaparin). These interact predominantly with factor Xa, and are given once daily because they have a longer duration of action. They do not affect standard blood test results (APTT).

Laboratory findings ■ The prothrombin, activated partial thromboplastin (APTT) and thrombin times (TT) are prolonged in persons on heparin ■ Most patients are monitored with the APTT and are maintained at 1.5 to 2.5 times the control value (the therapeutic range) ■ Large doses of heparin can increase the INR (International Normalised Ratio) ■ Platelet counts should also be monitored if heparin is used for more than 5 days, since heparin can cause thrombocytopenia. Autoimmune thrombocytopenia can occur within 3–15 days, or sooner if there has been previous heparin exposure.

Dental management

Risk assessment Surgery is the main oral health care hazard to the patient, as they bleed excessively after trauma.

Appropriate health care ■ Warn the patient in advance of the procedure, of the increased risk of intra- and postoperative bleeding and intra/extraoral bruising ■ Any surgical intervention can cause problems, and thus the possibility of alternatives to surgery, e.g. endodontics (root canal therapy), should always be considered ■ Withdrawal of heparin is adequate to reverse anticoagulation where this is deemed necessary; however, the effects can be unpredictable, especially with LMW heparin ■ In an emergency, this can be reversed by intravenous protamine sulphate given in a dose of 1 mg per 100 IU heparin – but a medical opinion should be sought first. Protamine is less effective at reversing low molecular weight heparins. ■ Systemic conditions that may aggravate the bleeding tendency include a wide range of disorders, including coagulopathies, thrombocytopenias, vascular disorders such as Ehlers–Danlos syndrome, liver disease, renal disease, malignancy, and HIV infection.

Preventive dentistry Preventive care is especially important, in order to minimise the need for surgical intervention.

Pain and anxiety control **Local anaesthesia** Regional block LA injections may be a hazard since bleeding into the fascial spaces of the neck can threaten airway patency. If possible, use intraligamentary or intrapapillary injections instead. **Conscious sedation** Care must be taken if giving intravenous sedation, due to the increased risk of a haematoma. **General anaesthesia** Avoid nasal intubation.

Patient access and positioning ■ Any dental manipulation should be performed at least 6 hours after injection of standard or unfractionated heparin, however care must be taken as clinically profuse bleeding may still occur ■ Patients on daily LMW heparins may be instructed to take their dose after the completion of an invasive procedure, although advice from the haematologist must always be sought ■ In patients on renal dialysis, or having cardiopulmonary bypass or other extracorporeal circulation with heparinisation, surgery is best carried out on the following day as the effects of heparinisation have then ceased.

Treatment modification **Surgery** ■ For uncomplicated forceps extraction of 1–3 teeth there is usually no need to interfere with anticoagulant treatment involving heparin or low molecular weight heparins ■ Surgery should be carried out with minimal trauma to both bone and soft tissues ■ Local measures are important to protect the soft tissues and operation area and minimise the risk of postoperative bleeding (see Warfarinisation) ■ Prior to more advanced surgery in a heparin-treated patient, medical advice should be sought.

Table 3.67 **Key considerations for dental management in heparinisation (see text)**

	Management modifications*	Comments/possible complications
Risk assessment	2	Excessive bleeding
Appropriate dental care	2/3	Consider alternatives to surgery; in case of emergency use protamine
Pain and anxiety control		
– Local anaesthesia	1	Avoid regional block
– Conscious sedation	1	
– General anaesthesia	1	Avoid nasal intubation
Patient access and positioning		
– Access to dental office	0	
– Timing of treatment	1/2	Dental treatment should be performed at least 6 hours after injection; or the day after dialysis; or prior to the daily dose of a LMW heparin
– Patient positioning	0	
Treatment modification		
– Oral surgery	3	Local haemostatic measures
– Implantology	3/5	
– Conservative/Endodontics	1	
– Fixed prosthetics	1	
– Removable prosthetics	1	
– Non-surgical periodontology	3	
– Surgical periodontology	3	
Hazardous and contraindicated drugs	2	Avoid aspirin and other NSAIDs; avoid intramuscular injections

*0 = No special considerations. 1 = Caution advised. 2 = Specialised medical advice recommended in some cases. 3 = Specialised medical advice mandatory. 4 = Only to be performed in hospital environment. 5 = Should be avoided.

Drug use ■ Drugs causing an increased bleeding tendency (e.g. aspirin and other NSAIDs) should be avoided ■ Other interventions to avoid, if possible, include intramuscular injections.

Further reading ● Della Valle A, Sammartino G, Marenzi G et al 2003 Prevention of postoperative bleeding in anticoagulated patients undergoing oral surgery: use of platelet-rich plasma gel. J Oral Maxillofac Surg 61:1275–1278 ● Dunn A S, Turpie A G Perioperative management of patients receiving oral anticoagulants: a systematic review. Arch Intern Med 163:901–908 ● Scully C, Wolff A 2004 Oral surgery in patients on anticoagulant therapy. Oral Surg Oral Med Oral Pathol Oral Radiol Endod 94:57–64.

HEPATITIS

Definition 'Hepatitis' is the term for liver inflammation, and can result from a wide range of insults, from infections to drugs (e.g. halothane) and poisons. The most common recognised causes include viruses, autoimmune disorders and alcohol.

General aspects

A common feature is jaundice (yellowing of the skin and sclerae). In a patient with a past history of jaundice who requires dental treatment, it is wise to try to establish the probable diagnosis and whether there is any liver dysfunction (Box 3.11).

Viral hepatitis

Definition ■ Hepatitis viruses A, B, C, D, E, G, TTV (transfusion-transmitted virus) and SEN (named after the initials of the patient from whom it was isolated) have now been recognised, although the association of HGV, TTV and SEN with the development of hepatitis is less clear ■ The term 'viral hepatitis' usually refers to liver infection by hepatitis A (HAV), hepatitis B (HBV), or hepatitis C (HCV) viruses ■ Only HBV, HCV and HDV are of special significance in dentistry.

Aetiopathogenesis ■ The main types of hepatotrophic viruses and routes of transmission are detailed in Table 3.68.

Clinical presentation ■ All these viruses can cause acute, or short-term, viral hepatitis ■ HAV usually has no serious consequences ■ HBV, HCV and HDV (hepatitis D) have a small mortality in the early stages, and can also cause chronic hepatitis – in which the infection is prolonged, sometimes lifelong; HCV in particular can lead to cirrhosis and liver cancer ■ The major finding in viral hepatitis of any cause is jaundice, although anicteric hepatitis (i.e. no evident jaundice) may occur ■ Other common findings include malaise, fatigue, fever, arthralgia and urticaria.

Diagnosis Diagnosis is based on: ■ Clinical findings ■ Liver function tests (LFTs): ● serum bilirubin level – raised ● serum enzyme estimations, including aspartate transaminase (AST) and alanine transaminase (ALT) – raised in proportion to the severity of the illness ● serum alkaline

Box 3.11 Common causes of jaundice

- Just after birth – usually physiological and rarely of consequence
- During childhood – often caused by hepatitis A, usually of little consequence
- In the teenager or young adult – may be due to viral hepatitis
- In middle age or later – more likely to be obstructive, e.g. gallstones or pancreatic cancer

Table 3.68 **Comparative features of more common forms of viral hepatitis relevant to dentistry**

	A (infectious)	B (serum)	C (Non-A non-B-)	D (delta agent)	E	G
Prevalence in developed world	Common; 40% urban populations	Uncommon; about 5–10% of general populations	Uncommon; about 1–5% of general populations	In countries with low prevalence of chronic HBV infection, HDV prevalence is low among both HBV carriers (< 10%) and patients with chronic hepatitis (< 25%)	Rare, except in endemic areas in Far East	Uncommon; about 1–2% of general populations
Type of virus	Picornaviridae (RNA)	Hepadnaviridae (DNA)	Flaviviridae (RNA)	Delta virus (RNA)	RNA	Flaviviridae (RNA)
Incubation	2–6 weeks	2–6 months	2–22 weeks	3 weeks to 2 months	2–9 weeks	?
Main route of transmission	Faecal–oral	Parenteral	Parenteral	Parenteral	Faecal–oral	Parenteral
Vaccine available	+	+	–	–	–	–
Severity	Mild	May be severe	Moderate	Severe	May be severe	No consequences known
Complications	Rare Acute mortality 0.1%	Relatively few Chronic liver disease in 10–20% Hepatocarcinoma Polyarteritis nodosa Chronic glomerulonephritis Acute mortality 1–2%	Many Chronic liver disease in > 70% Hepatocarcinoma	Can cause fulminant hepatitis	Rare, except in pregnancy	–

phosphatase – raised if there is an obstructive element ■ Serological markers of viruses.

Treatment ■ Bed rest ■ High carbohydrate diet ■ Avoiding hepatotoxins, such as alcohol ■ Drugs including: ● lamivudine ● interferon.

Prognosis ■ Main complications and grade of severity are detailed in Table 3.68 ■ Coinfection with other blood-borne agents, such as other types of hepatitis virus, or HIV, is common, particularly in intravenous drug users ■ Some hepatitis viruses, notably HCV and HBV, may result in cirrhosis, may be associated with liver cancer (hepatoma or hepatocellular carcinoma) or can be responsible for aplastic anaemia.

Hepatitis B (serum hepatitis, homologous serum jaundice)

Background ■ Hepatitis B is caused by the hepatitis B virus (HBV) and is a serious disease since it can cause lifelong infection ■ Hepatitis B infection is endemic throughout the world, especially in institutions, in cities and in poor socioeconomic conditions ■ It is especially common in the developing world; Africa, South-East Asia and South America are the areas of highest endemicity. In parts of sub-Saharan Africa, Asia and the Pacific, nearly all children are infected. ■ The prevalence of carriers varies considerably, being low (about 0.2%) in Western Europe and North America, rising to 20% in southern and eastern Europe, up to 40% in some parts of West Africa, and even higher in Indo-China. Over 75% of some populations, such as Australian aborigines (hence the older term 'Australia antigen'), are carriers. ■ Approximately 1 in 1000 people in the UK are carriers of the hepatitis B virus. In certain inner city areas the prevalence may be as high as 1% – of these about 10% may be in the highly infective category, who are hepatitis B e antigen (HBeAg) positive. ■ Spread of hepatitis B is mainly parenteral via: ● intravenous drug abuse ● unscreened blood or blood product transfusions ● tattooing/ear-piercing ● sexual transmission (especially among promiscuous individuals who do not practise safe sex) ● perinatal transmission ● hepatitis B virus has been transmitted to patients and staff in health care facilities.

Aetiopathogenesis HBV is a DNA virus which belongs to the hepadnaviridae family. Electron microscopy shows three types of particle in serum from patients with hepatitis B: ■ the Dane particle probably represents intact hepatitis virus, and consists of an inner core containing DNA and core antigens (HBcAg), and an outer envelope of surface antigen (HBsAg) ■ the smaller spherical forms and the tubular forms represent excess HBsAg. The other antigen from hepatitis B is the e antigen (HBeAg), which represents the soluble form of HBcAg, and hence is detectable via blood tests.

Clinical presentation ■ The effects of HBV infection range from subclinical infections without jaundice (anicteric hepatitis), to fulminating hepatitis, acute hepatic failure and death ■ About 30% of persons with HBV infection have no signs or symptoms ■ Most patients with clinical hepatitis recover completely with no untoward effect, apart perhaps from some persistent malaise; viraemia precedes the clinical illness by weeks or months and lasts for some weeks thereafter, before clearing completely ■ The disease has an incubation period of 2–6 months ■ The prodromal period of 1–2 weeks is characterised by anorexia, malaise and nausea ■ As jaundice becomes clinically evident the stools become pale and the urine dark due to bilirubinuria. The liver is enlarged and tender, and pruritus may be troublesome. Muscle pains, arthralgia and rashes are more common in hepatitis B than hepatitis A, and there is often fever.

Diagnosis Diagnosis is made based on: ■ Clinical findings ■ Liver function tests ■ Serological markers; these are useful in the specific diagnosis of HBV infection, are of prognostic value and are outlined below and summarised in Table 3.69. **Antigens** ■ outer protein coat: **HBsAg** ■ inner protein coat: **HBcAg** ■ soluble **HbcAg** protein **HBeAg** (serum) ■ DNA polymerase. **Antibody response** ■ **Anti-HBc (IgM)** (2–5 months) ■ **Anti-HBc (IgG)** (3 months onwards) ■ **Anti-HBe** (5 months onwards) ■ **Anti-HBs** (7 months onwards).

Treatment ■ Patients with hepatitis B may benefit from: ● bed rest ● a high carbohydrate diet ● avoiding hepatotoxins such as alcohol ■ Chronic HBV infection can be treated with lamivudine or interferon. The former is usually better tolerated, but treatment for 1–3 years is usually needed and a mutant strain of the virus may emerge. Adefovir dipivoxil is also available but is very expensive and not widely used.

Prognosis ■ Hepatitis B has an acute mortality of < 2%, but in a very few outbreaks where there was also infection with hepatitis D virus, the death rate has been as high as 30% ■ Complications of hepatitis B include: mainly a carrier state, chronic infection, cirrhosis, carcinoma or death ■ A carrier state, in which HBV persists within the body for more than 6 months, develops in 5–10% of infected individuals. It is more frequent in anicteric infections or those contracted early in life. Although 5–10% of these carriers lose the hepatitis antigen each year, carriers may remain positive for up to 20 years and may not be suspected clinically. However, certain groups of patients – especially those who have received blood products, those infected with HDV and those who have immune defects – are predisposed to the carrier state. Most carriers are healthy but others, especially those with persistently abnormal liver function tests, develop chronic liver disease, which causes death in 15–25% of cases. ■ In the absence of complications, infection with hepatitis B virus confers immunity. Active immunity can therefore be acquired naturally.

Prevention Prevention of hepatitis B is best achieved by avoiding contact with HBV, and having the hepatitis B vaccine. ■ Steps to minimise contact with hepatitis include: ● use of condoms ● giving infants born to HBV-infected mothers HBIG (hepatitis B immune globulin) and vaccine within 12 hours after birth ● drug users should never share needles, syringes, water, or 'works', and should be vaccinated against hepatitis A and B ● personal care items that might have blood on them (razors, toothbrushes) should never be shared ● the risks from tattoo or body piercing should be considered ● health care workers should always follow standard precautions and safely handle needles and other sharps, and be vaccinated against hepatitis B ■ The hepatitis B vaccine confers 90% protection for

Table 3.69 **Serum markers of hepatitis B infection in relation to progress of disease**

	HbsAg	Anti-HBs	HBeAg*	Anti-HBe	HbcAg	Anti-HBc	DNA polymerase*
Late incubation	+	–	+	–	Liver only	–	++
Acute hepatitis	++	–	±	–	Liver only	++	+
Recovery (immunity)	–	++	–	+	–	+	–
Asymptomatic carrier state	++	–	–	±	–	++	±
Chronic active hepatitis	++	–	+	–	–	+	±

+ = serum level raised.
*Presence implies high infectivity.

years and possibly for life, and the need for serological testing and reinforcing doses has not been established. Many health care workers are, however, advised to receive reinforcing doses every 5 years according to local policy. ■ The current vaccine against HBV infection is a recombinant vaccine of HBsAg. Vaccination also protects, indirectly, against hepatitis D. It may not protect against newly reported (pre-core) variants of HBV. ■ Combined Hepatitis A and Hepatitis B vaccine is available for some travellers, users of injectable drugs, promiscuous individuals who do not practise safe sex, and persons with clotting factor disorders who receive therapeutic blood products.

Health care workers and HBV ■ Health care workers should always follow routine cross-infection control procedures, barrier precautions and procedures to safely handle needles and other sharps ■ All health care workers who perform exposure-prone procedures – including independent contractors such as GPs and dentists working outside the hospital setting, and all medical, dental, nursing and midwifery students – should be immunised against hepatitis B, unless immunity to hepatitis B as a result of natural infection or previous immunisation has been documented. Their response to the vaccine should subsequently be checked. ■ Staff whose work involves exposure-prone procedures and who fail to respond to the vaccine should be permitted to continue in their work, provided that they are not HBeAg positive. Newer vaccines are also being developed with the aim of improving response rates. ■ Health care workers who are HBeAg positive should not perform exposure-prone procedures in which injury to the worker could result in blood contaminating the patient's open tissues ■ Health care workers who are HBsAg positive but who are not HBeAg positive need not be barred from any area of work unless they have been associated with transmission of hepatitis B to patients whilst HBeAg negative ■ Health Authorities and Trusts should ensure that members of staff employed or taking up employment, or other health care workers contracted to provide a service which involves carrying out exposure-prone procedures, are immunised against the hepatitis B virus, that their antibody response is checked and that carriers of the virus who are HBeAg positive do not undertake such procedures ■ The response to vaccine should be checked 2–4 months after completion of the primary course. An anti-HBs level of 100 mIU/mL is considered to reflect an adequate response to the vaccine and to confer protective immunity. In the absence of natural immunity, levels of anti-HBs between 10 and 100 mIU/mL indicate a response to the vaccine but one that may not necessarily confer long-lasting immunity and which may require boosting. The specificity of levels of anti-HBs below 10 mIU/mL cannot be assured and such levels cannot be considered as evidence of a response to the vaccine. If there is a delay in checking the response, a booster dose should be given before anti-HBs titres are measured as levels of antibody gradually fall after immunisation.

Hepatitis C

Background ■ Hepatitis C virus (HCV) infection accounts worldwide for at least 90% of post-transfusion non-A non-B hepatitis and is responsible for much sporadic viral hepatitis, particularly in intravenous drug abusers, among whom its prevalence is rising. By contrast, transfusion-associated hepatitis C is declining and will presumably decline rapidly now that blood is routinely tested for it. ■ HCV now ranks second only to alcoholism as a cause of liver disease ■ HCV is responsible for many patients with chronic liver disease and may account for a significant number of those who were thought to have autoimmune hepatitis ■ Persons at special risk for hepatitis C include those who: ● have been notified they have received blood from a donor who later tested positive for hepatitis C ● have ever injected illegal drugs ● received a blood transfusion or solid organ transplant before about 1992 ● received a blood product for clotting disorders produced before about 1987 ● have ever been on long-term renal dialysis ● have evidence of liver disease (e.g. persistently abnormal ALT levels).

Aetiopathogenesis HCV is a RNA virus that belongs to flaviviridae family.

Clinical presentation ■ Hepatitis C has a similar incubation period to hepatitis B (usually less than 60 days, but may be as long as 150 days) ■ About 80–90% of patients infected with HCV have no signs or symptoms ■ Clinical hepatitis C is usually a less severe and shorter illness than hepatitis B ■ Patients infected with HCV are, in about 15% of cases, coinfected with hepatitis G virus (HGV). Coinfection with HBV is common.

Diagnosis ■ Serological tests (ELISAs) are available to detect HCV, but anti-HCV IgG is usually not detectable until 1–3 months after the acute infection and may take up to a year to appear ■ A more sensitive method, using the polymerase chain reaction (PCR) to detect viral sequences, has been developed, and suggests that most of those who are seropositive by immunoassay are viraemic and (despite the presence of antibody) are infective.

Treatment Currently, chronic hepatitis C may be treated with a combination of interferon alpha and ribavirin; about 40% of patients respond to this 'combination' therapy.

Prognosis ■ Some patients (25–80%) infected with HCV have abnormal liver function tests after one year ■ Many go on to chronic liver disease (75–85%) ■ Some develop liver cancer/die (< 3%).

Prevention ■ There is as yet no vaccine against hepatitis C ■ Hepatitis C prevention is therefore by: ● health care workers always following routine cross-infection control procedures, barrier precautions, and safely handling needles and other sharps ● drug addicts never sharing needles, syringes, or water for injection ● not sharing personal care items that might have blood on them (razors, toothbrushes) ● assessing the risks when considering getting a tattoo or body piercing ● not inhaling cocaine through contaminated straws ● using condoms: HCV can be spread by sex, but this is rare.

Hepatitis D

Definition ■ HDV infection may coincide with hepatitis B or superinfects patients with chronic hepatitis B; infection may produce a biphasic pattern with double rises in liver enzymes, and bilirubin ■ HDV spreads parenterally, mainly by shared hypodermic needles; risk groups are as for HBV ■ HDV is endemic especially in the Mediterranean littoral and among intravenous drug abusers, but is found worldwide. It is not endemic in Northern Europe or the USA, but some haemophiliacs and others have acquired the infection and the prevalence is rising.

Aetiopathogenesis Hepatitis D virus (HDV) or delta agent (δ agent) is an incomplete virus carried within the hepatitis B particle and will only replicate in the presence of HBsAg.

Clinical presentation ■ The incubation period of hepatitis D is unknown ■ 90% of infections are asymptomatic ■ HDV infection may not differ clinically from hepatitis B, although it is associated with more fulminant disease.

Diagnosis HDV antigen and antibody can now be assayed: delta antigen indicates recent infection; delta antibody indicates chronic hepatitis or recovery.

Treatment Drug treatment with alpha interferon is available.

Prognosis ■ HDV infection can cause fulminant disease with a high mortality rate ■ 70–80% of HBV carriers with HDV superinfection develop chronic liver diseases with cirrhosis, compared with 15–30% of patients with chronic HBV infection alone.

Prevention Vaccination against HBV protects indirectly against HDV.

Autoimmune hepatitis

Definition Autoimmune hepatitis is liver damage produced by antibodies against self antigens.

Aetiopathogenesis The aetiopathogenesis of autoimmunity is only partially known. Some possible mechanisms include: ■ self-antigens modified by infective agents or reacting with them ■ ectopic expression of class II major histocompatibility complex (MHC) molecules ■ release of antigens from their secluded sites ■ persistence of forbidden clones of lymphocytes.

Clinical presentation Features include: ■ acute hepatitis ■ fever, malaise, rash ■ polyarthritis ■ amenorrhoea ■ glomerulonephritis.

Classification Autoimmune disorders are either: ■ Type I: antinuclear and/or anti-smooth muscle antibodies (SMA) ■ Type II: anti-liver/kidney microsomes type 1 (LKM1) antibodies.

Diagnosis ■ Liver function tests – abnormal ■ Serum autoantibodies – positive ■ Liver biopsy.

Treatment Corticosteroids or azathioprine.

Oral findings

■ Discolouration of posterior palate and floor of the mouth along the lingual fraenum may be seen in icteric patients ■ In severe liver disease, petechiae and ecchymoses are common ■ HCV may be associated with sicca syndrome, non-Hodgkin's lymphoma, and with lichen planus in some populations.

Dental management

Risk assessment The main problems in management of all patients with viral hepatitis are bleeding tendencies and drug sensitivity (see Liver failure). Transmission of the viruses causing the hepatitis is also a major consideration: ■ Standard precautions against transmission of infection must always be employed. Many hepatitis viruses constitute a cross-infection risk in dentistry as they are transmitted parenterally. ■ Although HBV has been of greatest importance in dentistry, HCV has become a more serious problem due to the absence of a vaccine as yet.

Sources of infection by hepatitis B in the dental environment

■ Blood, plasma or serum can be infectious; indeed, as little as 0.0000001 mL of HBsAg-positive serum can transmit infection ■ The main danger is from needlestick injuries; some 25% of these (HBeAg-positive) may transmit infection ■ Saliva may contain HBV (presumably derived from serum via gingival exudate) and may be a source for non-parenteral transmission, but the risk appears to be low except where there is very close contact, as in families or children's nurseries, or sexual contact ■ HBV can be transmitted by human bites.

Risk of infection by HBV in dental personnel ■ There is clear evidence of unvaccinated dentists and other dental personnel contracting hepatitis, but several reports indicate that the risk is now low, since staff are immunised and standard infection control precautions are taken ■ There is a higher risk for oral surgeons and periodontologists, and for those working with high-risk patients, probably because of needlestick injuries.

Risk of transmission of HBV infection to patients ■ Dental procedures have in the past transmitted hepatitis B to patients ■ However, if standard precautions are taken, this is no longer a significant source of transmission: all clinical personnel must follow the standard precautions, and must wear protective clothing, gloves and mask ■ Most hepatitis viruses are destroyed by autoclaving, dry heat, or ethylene oxide gas, but not by cold or chemical sterilising solutions ■ Practitioners ill with hepatitis should stop dental practice until fully recovered. Testing for HBeAg may indicate those individuals likely to spread hepatitis B. HBeAg-positive dental surgeons and those who are HBeAg-negative but have greater than 1000 HBV viral particles per mL blood should discontinue practice involving exposure-prone procedures.

Needlestick injuries involving HBV to unvaccinated individuals

■ An injection of hepatitis B immune globulin within 24 hours of contact with HBV may help protect the individual from developing hepatitis ■ The injured person should also receive the first in a series of three shots of the hepatitis B vaccine.

HCV transmitted to patients and staff in health care facilities

■ HCV has been transmitted to dental patients ■ There has been a raised prevalence of HCV infection in some dental staff studied ■ HCV is present in blood and serum from infected persons ■ HCV is transmitted in about 10% of needlestick injuries ■ Hepatitis C virus has been found in saliva; there is no correlation between oral health status or HIV seropositivity, and the detection of HCV in saliva ■ HCV infection has followed a human bite. **Other hepatitis viruses** These are generally less problematic: ■ HDV has been transmitted to patients and staff in health care facilities and has been associated with serious sequelae ■ HGV is not known to be transmitted during dentistry ■ TTV and SEN viruses are not known to have been transmitted during dentistry.

Appropriate dental care

■ If there is clinical jaundice or if liver function tests are abnormal, operative intervention should be avoided unless imperative; the responsible physician should be consulted for the diagnosis

Table 3.70 **Key considerations for dental management in hepatitis (see text)**

	Management modifications*	Comments/possible complications
Risk assessment	2	Viral hepatitis transmission; bleeding tendency; drug sensitivity
Appropriate dental care	2	During acute hepatitis only emergency dental care; standard precautions; bleeding test (PT time)
Pain and anxiety control		
– Local anaesthesia	1	Avoid lidocaine
– Conscious sedation	1	Reduce benzodiazepine dosage
– General anaesthesia	3/4	Avoid halothane
Patient access and positioning		
– Access to dental office	0	Standard cross-infection control procedures
– Timing of treatment	0	
– Patient positioning	0	
Treatment modification		
– Oral surgery	2	Prolonged bleeding
– Implantology	2	Prolonged bleeding
– Conservative/Endodontics	1	Standard cross-infection control procedures
– Fixed prosthetics	1	
– Removable prosthetics	1	
– Non-surgical periodontology	2	Prolonged bleeding
– Surgical periodontology	2	Prolonged bleeding
Hazardous and contraindicated drugs	2	Avoid acetaminophen, erythromycin estolate and tetracycline; some patients are on corticosteroids or immunosuppressives

*0 = No special considerations. 1 = Caution advised. 2 = Specialised medical advice recommended in some cases. 3 = Specialised medical advice mandatory. 4 = Only to be performed in hospital environment. 5 = Should be avoided.

and for advice on management ■ Patients known to be incubating hepatitis, those with clinical hepatitis or patients in the convalescent stages of hepatitis should also have dental treatment deferred where possible until after recovery is complete ■ Any essential emergency dental care during incubation or acute hepatitis should be carried out in a hospital department ■ As patients with hepatitis may have a bleeding tendency, a prothrombin time test is mandatory; patients with normal prothrombin times and normal platelet counts can undergo dental intervention safely.

Pain and anxiety control **Local anaesthesia** The metabolism of lidocaine may be suppressed in patients with viral hepatitis, leading to high plasma levels and the risk of acute poisoning. Care should be taken to minimise the use of lidocaine for LA. **Conscious sedation** The benzodiazepine dosage should be reduced to reduce clearance via the liver if viral hepatitis is present. **General anaesthesia** The hepatologist should be consulted, particularly in view of the risk of bleeding and drug sensitivities. Halothane must be avoided.

Drug use ■ Some patients are on corticosteroid or immunosuppressive therapy ■ Due to impaired drug detoxification and excretion, the use of acetaminophen, erythromycin estolate and tetracycline should be minimised (see Liver failure).

Further reading

● Castro Ferreiro M, Diz Dios P, Hermida Prieto M 2004 Sporadic transmission of hepatitis C in dental practice. Med Clin (Barcelona) 123:271–275 ● Diz Dios P, Lodi G, Vázquez García E, Porter S R. 1997 El virus de la hepatitis C. Implicaciones en Odontología. Medicina Oral 2:209–218 ● Golla K, Epstein J B, Cabay R J 2004 Liver disease: current perspectives on medical and dental management. Oral Surg Oral Med Oral Pathol Oral Radiol Endod 98:516–521 ● Hermida Prieto M, Castro Ferreiro M, Barral Rodríguez S, Laredo Vázquez R, Castro Iglesias A, Diz Dios P 2002 Detection of HCV-RNA in saliva of patients with hepatitis C virus infection by using a highly sensitive test. J Virol Meth 101:29–35 ● Lodi G, Bez C, Porter S R, Scully C, Epstein J B 2002 Infectious hepatitis C, hepatitis G, and TT virus: review and implications for dentists. Spec Care Dentist 22:53–58 ● Palenik C J 2004 Hepatitis C virus and dental personnel. Dent Today 23:56–59.

HEROIN AND OTHER OPIOID ABUSE

Definition ■ Opioids such as morphine and heroin (diacetyl morphine), derived from the opium poppy, and synthetic compounds such as methadone, dipipanone, dihydrocodeine and pethidine, are widely used medically to provide potent analgesia, although heroin cannot be prescribed in the USA ■ Opioids can be used orally, sometimes smoked or sniffed, subcutaneously (skin popping), or intravenously – when maximum effect is obtained; opioids may also be used as snuff or as cigarettes ■ Heroin is a highly addictive opioid, processed from morphine, extracted from the seedpod of the Asian poppy, and differs from other opioids mainly in the difficulty in overcoming addiction; it can be sniffed, smoked from a tin-foil ('chasing the dragon') or injected.

General aspects

Pathogenesis ■ Opioids act by mimicking the natural brain peptides – enkephalins and endorphins ■ Opiates can activate the brain's reward system – the stimulation of opiate receptors results in feelings of reward and activates the pleasure circuit by causing greater amounts of dopamine to be released within the nucleus accumbens, which can lead to addiction.

Classification ■ Direct opium derivates: ● morphine (morphine sulphate, 'white stuff', 'M') ● codeine (methyl-morphine, 'school boy') ■ Morphine derivatives: ● heroin (diacetyl-morphine, 'horse', 'junk', 'smack', 'scag', 'stuff') ● dilaudid (dihydromorphinone) ■ semi-synthetics and synthetics: ● methadone (dolophine amidone, 'dolly') ● LAAM (levo-alpha-acetylmethadol) ● propoxyphene ● meperidine ● fentanyl.

Clinical presentation Opioid misuse leads to tolerance at an early stage, and dependence after some months. The most significant risks are from behavioural disturbances and psychoses. Other complications of opioid misuse include infections, neglect of general health and hygiene, and poor diet. Constipation, respiratory depression and orthostatic hypotension are common. Respiratory arrest may occur in overdose. Intravenous use of these drugs is further complicated by the risk of transmission of infections (HIV, hepatitis B), infective endocarditis, or septicaemia. ■ Findings that may indicate a drug addiction problem are as for amphetamine/LSD/MDMA abuse ■ Other common signs are: ● constricted pupils ● needle tracks or abscesses (wearing long sleeves when inappropriate) ● lymphadenopathy ■ Other drug-abuse associated diseases: ● psychosis ● osteomyelitis.
Heroin (Fig. 3.19) ■ The three basic signs of heroin use are: ● euphoria (intoxication) ● sedation ● analgesia (pain relief) ■ The short-term effects of heroin misuse appear soon after a single dose with a surge of euphoria ('rush') accompanied by a warm flushing of the skin, a dry mouth, and heavy extremities – probably due to histamine release ■ Following this initial euphoria, which can last up to 4 hours, the heroin user goes 'on the nod', an alternately wakeful and drowsy state; mental functioning becomes clouded due to the depression of the central nervous system ■ Long-term effects of intravenous use include collapsed veins, infective endocarditis, abscesses and cellulitis ■ Heroin is a respiratory depressant and its use predisposes also to pneumonia, lung abscesses and fibrosis ■ With regular heroin use, tolerance, physical dependence and addiction develop.

Severe adverse effects ■ The mortality among opioid addicts is 2–6% per annum; deaths are usually from overdose ■ Heroin misuse is associated with serious health conditions, including fatal overdose, spontaneous abortion, and infectious diseases, such as HIV/AIDS and hepatitis ■ 'Street' heroin contains only about 10% heroin; since additives do not readily dissolve they can result in infection or infarction in lungs, liver, kidneys or brain.

Withdrawal and treatment ■ Opioid withdrawal is unpleasant – though usually not dangerous ■ Early features include lacrimation, rhinorrhoea, sweating and persistent yawning ■ After about 12 hours

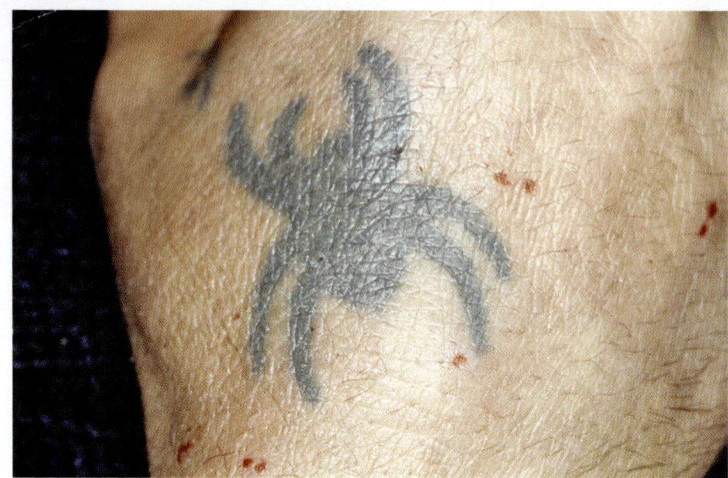

Figure 3.19 **The spider tattoo may be related to heroin drug use and/or sales**

the addict enters a phase of restless tossing sleep (yen) when there is pupil dilatation, tremor, gooseflesh (cold turkey), anorexia, nausea, vomiting, muscle spasms and pain, orgasms, diarrhoea and abdominal pains; pulse rate and blood pressure also rise ■ Once the main features have subsided, there may be weakness and insomnia for several weeks or months ■ Medical supervision and the use of opioid agonists such as oral methadone (now available in both a liquid and tablet form) and levo-alpha-acetylmethadol (LAAM), or antagonists such as naltrexone or lofexidine are needed in the management of opioid dependence.

Oral findings

■ There are no specific oral effects of opioid dependence but there is often oral neglect, advanced periodontal disease and caries ■ Advanced enamel loss and widespread black/brown carious lesions, which are not necessarily arrested, may be observed ■ Diet and sometimes medications predispose to caries; although methadone syrup is available now as a sugar-free preparation, some patients (and even pharmacists), may mix it with sweet drinks or sugar to disguise the bitter taste ■ Some agents such as lofexidine cause hyposalivation ■ Caries is often left untreated by the patient who, because of the opioid, may be undisturbed by the pain.

Dental management

Risk assessment ■ Recognition of individuals who may be abusing drugs is critical (Fig. 3.19). The opioid addict is said to be 'a depressed introvert with constricted pupils'. Hence highly suspicious features suggestive of opioid consumption include: • abnormal behaviour • persistently constricted pupils • outlining of veins. ■ Care should be taken with any patient who makes suspicious requests for medication (as detailed for amphetamine/ LSD/MDMA abuse) ■ Dental treatment can often be given to narcotic addicts without fear of complications, but possible difficulties include: • analgesia (see below) • feigning pain or stealing drugs or

Table 3.71 Key considerations for dental management in heroin or opioid abuse (see text)

	Management modifications*	Comments/possible complications
Risk assessment	2	Drug abusers recognition; abnormal behaviour; blood-borne infections; others (cardiac lesions, drug interactions, etc)
Appropriate dental care	2	Control behaviour; appropriate analgesia; universal cross-infection barriers; possibly bacterial endocarditis prophylaxis; select drugs
Pain and anxiety control		
– Local anaesthesia	2	Poor pain control
– Conscious sedation	3/4	Avoid opioids
– General anaesthesia	3/4	Avoid halothane, ketamine, suxamethonium, barbiturates and opioids; resistance to GA
Patient access and positioning		
– Access to dental office	0	
– Timing of treatment	1	Failed appointments
– Patient positioning	0	
Treatment modification		
– Oral surgery	1	
– Implantology	1/5	Neglected oral hygiene; periodontitis; xerostomia; heavy smokers
– Conservative/Endodontics	1	
– Fixed prosthetics	1/5	Neglected oral hygiene; heavy smokers
– Removable prosthetics	1	
– Non-surgical periodontology	1	
– Surgical periodontology	1/5	Neglected oral hygiene; heavy smokers
Hazardous and contraindicated drugs	1	Avoid opioids

*0 = No special considerations. 1 = Caution advised. 2 = Specialised medical advice recommended in some cases. 3 = Specialised medical advice mandatory. 4 = Only to be performed in hospital environment. 5 = Should be avoided.

prescription forms ● behavioural disturbances and withdrawal symptoms ● cardiac lesions ● maxillofacial injuries ● hepatitis or chronic liver disease ● infective endocarditis ● sexually transmitted diseases, including HIV infection ● venous thromboses making intravenous injection difficult ● tetanus ● bleeding tendency ● drug interactions ● drug intolerance.

Pain and anxiety control ■ Simulation of pain is a common manoeuvre to obtain narcotics – prescription pads may be stolen or drug cabinets raided ■ Dental drugs that may attract the addict include pethidine, codeine, pentazocine and dextropropoxyphene ■ In the established addict, non-narcotic analgesics may be ineffective in controlling dental pain, so that large doses of opioids may have to be given. Opioids should not be given or prescribed without first seeking expert advice – their only indication in dentistry is for severe postoperative pain. In most cases it is preferable to ask the medical practitioner to prescribe limited amounts and closely monitor the patient's usage and requirements. Pentazocine, being a narcotic antagonist, should not be used for such patients as it may precipitate a withdrawal syndrome. ■ Those under treatment for addiction have a period of several weeks during which they are particularly hypersensitive to pain and stress. In such patients, opioids must be avoided. Although the withdrawal syndrome subsides within about a week, the addict is, for a few weeks thereafter, intolerant of stress and pain. The respiratory response to carbon dioxide is reduced and general anaesthesia may then be hazardous. **Local anaesthesia/conscious sedation** Some addicts tolerate pain poorly and complain that local anaesthesia, even with the additional use of conscious sedation, is insufficient for operative procedures. General anaesthesia may therefore be preferred in these individuals, unless there are other medical contraindications. **General anaesthesia** If general anaesthesia is required, intravenous barbiturates should be avoided because they may induce convulsions, respiratory distress or coma. Opioids are also contraindicated.

Further reading ● Cornelius J R, Clark D B, Weyant R et al 2004 Dental abnormalities in children of fathers with substance use disorders. Addict Behav 29:979–982 ● van der Bijl P 2003 Substance abuse – concerns in dentistry: an overview. S Afr Dent J 58:382–385 ● Bullock K 1999 Dental care of patients with substance abuse. Dent Clin North Am 43: 513–526 ● Sandler N A 2001 Patients who abuse drugs. Oral Surg Oral Med Oral Pathol Oral Radiol Endod 91:12–14.

HIV/AIDS

Definition Infection with human immunodeficiency virus (HIV), a retrovirus, causes HIV disease and ultimately damages certain T lymphocytes, producing the acquired immune deficiency syndrome (AIDS).

General aspects

Aetiopathogenesis ■ There are two main types of human immunodeficiency virus – HIV-1 (most common) and HIV-2. Both infect cells expressing CD4 surface receptors, mainly the T-helper lymphocytes, and replicate within them, damaging them. ■ The geographic distributions of HIV-1 and HIV-2 differ markedly. HIV-1 is found in relative abundance throughout the world and is responsible for the global HIV pandemic, whereas the geographic distribution of HIV-2 is much more limited and it is found primarily in parts of Africa. ■ The World Health Organization (WHO) estimated the number of people living with HIV in 2005 to be around 40.3 million, and people newly infected with HIV in 2005 to be 4.9 million ■ At the end of 2004 an estimated 58 300 adults aged over 15 were living with HIV in the UK, 19 700 (34%) of whom were unaware of their infection. Since the epidemic began in the early 1980s about 16 728 deaths in HIV-infected individuals are known to have occurred in the UK. Currently the number of people living with diagnosed HIV is rising each year due to increased numbers of new diagnoses and decreasing deaths due to antiretroviral therapies. ■ HIV transmission is mainly sexual. Most new cases are via heterosexual intercourse rather than by men having sex with men, as was previously the case. Intravenous drug abuse, infected blood or blood products, or perinatal infection are other routes of infection.

Clinical presentation ■ In 1988 the Centers for Disease Control and Prevention, Atlanta, Georgia, USA classified the various presentations/stages of HIV infections into CDC stages 1–4b–d (Box 3.12). This classification was in 1993 replaced by a new one based on clinical findings and CD4 counts (p. 220) ■ HIV infection may be symptomless ■ HIV disease is symptomatic ■ The acute HIV syndrome may resemble glandular fever, and be characterised by fever, sweats, myalgias, lethargy, rash, sore throat, mouth ulcers, anorexia, nausea, vomiting, headache and diarrhoea but, as these features are non-specific, they may be misdiagnosed (Fig. 3.20) ■ AIDS is a lethal infection, defined as HIV infection plus one or more AIDS-defining illnesses (see below) and a CD4 T lymphocyte count $<200 \times 10^6$/L (or a CD4+ T-cell percentage of total lymphocyctes of <14%) ■ AIDS-defining illnesses are mainly infections, virally-related tumours or encephalopathy (Box 3.13) ■ The infections contracted by persons with HIV/AIDS to an extent depend upon their environmental exposure; thus TB is particularly common in people from Africa and in urban IV drug-users in the USA; leishmaniasis is common in persons from around the Mediterranean; mycoses such as penicillosis are seen mainly in northern Thailand ■ HIV-infected persons may also be at risk from viral hepatitis and other sexually transmitted diseases.

Box 3.12 1986 CDC classification of HIV/AIDS stages

- CDC* stage 1 – Primary seroconversion illness
- CDC stage 2 – Asymptomatic
- CDC stage 3 – Persistent generalised lymphadenopathy (PGL)
- CDC stage 4a – AIDS-related complex (ARC)
- CDC stage 4b–d – AIDS: opportunistic infections or tumours which are AIDS indicator illnesses

*CDC = Centers for Disease Control, Atlanta, Georgia, USA

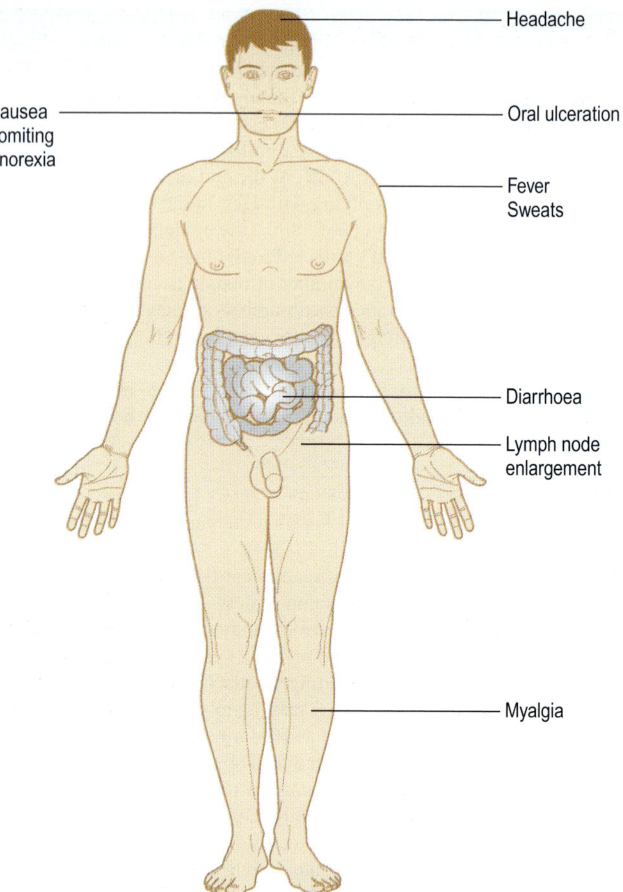

Figure 3.20 **Clinical features of acute HIV syndrome**

Classification Alongside the CDC staging of HIV infection in individuals, further classification may be made according to the clinical features present and the CD4 count. Based on clinical features patients are distributed in three categories: ■ A: asymptomatic, acute infection or persistent generalised lymphadenopathy ■ B: symptomatic, not A or C conditions ■ C: AIDS-defining illnesses. CD4 T-cell categories include: $> 500 \times 10^6$/L, $200–500 \times 10^6$/L, $< 200 \times 10^6$/L.

Diagnosis The diagnosis of HIV infection is suggested by clinical criteria and confirmed by laboratory specific tests. HIV infection must be confirmed carefully by testing for HIV (with appropriate counselling of patients) and all results must be kept confidential. Relatives cannot give consent for an HIV

Box 3.13 Some AIDS-defining illnesses

Fungi
- Candidosis: oesophageal • *Pneumocystis jiroveci* pneumonia
- Cryptococcosis • Histoplasmosis

Viruses
- Herpes simplex: chronic ulcers for more than a month
- Cytomegalovirus disease

Parasites
- Toxoplasmosis

Mycobacteria
- Tuberculosis: disseminated or extrapulmonary • Atypical mycobacterioses

Tumours
- Kaposi's sarcoma (HHV-8) • Lymphoma (EBV) • Cervical carcinoma (HPV)

Encephalopathy
- HIV-related

test. Investigations which are normally undertaken include: ■ whole blood count – lymphopenia ■ blood CD4 counts – low ■ blood CD4/CD8 ratio – reduced from a normal of about 2 to about 0.5 in AIDS ■ the 'AIDS test' – this is usually for serum HIV antibodies and involves ELISA and Western blot assays ■ techniques available to detect HIV nucleic acid can be used to clarify indeterminate Western blot results – for example, the polymerase chain reaction (PCR) is very sensitive and able to detect HIV in HIV-infected but seronegative persons ■ HIV can also be detected by viral culture or testing for the HIV reverse transcriptase enzyme (RT) but these are not simple tests and they lack the sensitivity and reproducibility needed for clinical work ■ the HIV viral load is also assayed.

It is important in diagnosis of HIV to: ■ apply at least two methodologically different assays for HIV infection ■ repeat the test 2–3 months later – no patient with signs of HIV infection should be discharged as uninfected solely on the basis of one negative HIV test result ■ treat the results of any of HIV tests and a diagnosis of HIV infection or AIDS with confidentiality.

Treatment **Management of HIV infection** There is as yet no effective treatment to eliminate HIV infection. Several drugs active against retroviruses (anti-retroviral drugs) are available though costly and often associated with resistance and/or adverse reactions. Some specific anti-retroviral agent combinations, the so-called highly active antiretroviral therapy (HAART), show an especially increased antiviral activity. Specific drug groups include nucleoside analogues, protease (proteinase) inhibitors and non-nucleoside reverse-transcriptase inhibitors (Box 3.14). Patients are usually monitored by CD4 counts and plasma viral load since these correlate well with clinical progress; at counts below 200/μL patients are at high risk

Box 3.14 Anti-retroviral agents

Reverse transcriptase inhibitors
• Abacavir (ABC) • Didanosine (ddI) • Emtricitabine • Lamivudine (3TC) • Stavudine (d4T) • Tenofovir (TFV) • Zalcitabine (ddC) • Zidovudine (AZT)

• Adefovir (ADV) • Delavirdine (DLV) • Efavirenz (EFV) • Nevirapine (NVP)

Protease inhibitors
• Amprenavir (APV) • Atazanavir (ATV) • Fosamprenavir • Indinavir (IDV) • Lopinavir (LPV) • Nelfinavir (NFV) • Ritonavir (RTV) • Saquinavir (SQV) • Tipravanir (TPV)

Fusion inhibitors
• Enfuvirtide

of *Pneumocystis carinii* infection, and at counts below 100/μL, CMV and *Mycobacterium avium-intracellulare* are more commonly present.

Management of co-morbid conditions There has been a growing recognition that many individuals who become HIV infected also have, or are vulnerable to, a host of co-morbid conditions, including other infectious diseases (e.g. fungal/viral infections, hepatitis, sexually transmitted infections [STIs], tuberculosis), substance abuse, mental illness and homelessness. The risks and the consequences of HIV infection for these individuals must be evaluated and addressed in the context of these other conditions:
■ Additional drug therapy may be required to manage the infections/tumours associated with HIV/AIDS. This may include anti-viral and anti-fungal therapy. ■ Social and psychological support – the positive diagnosis of HIV infection is often extremely disturbing for a patient and counselling is critical. Newly diagnosed HIV-positive patients often face the emotionally demanding task of communicating their test results to a partner and family members. In both gay and heterosexual couples, patients may feel extreme remorse over the possibility of having infected their partners. Conversely, patients may be angry about the likelihood that they were infected by their partners. Furthermore, the patient's immediate family will often have strong, conflicting reactions to the news of the patient's HIV test results. ■ Some patients testing positive may become increasingly depressed and suicidal and need close monitoring and long-term psychological support.

Prognosis HAART has significantly increased life quality and expectancy of HIV infected patients who receive it, so that HIV infection is nowadays considered a chronic illness. Vaccines are currently being developed but are as yet unsuccessful.

Oral findings

■ The majority of patients with HIV disease have head and neck and oral manifestations at some time ■ Oral lesions are most likely to appear when the CD4 cell count is low ■ Oral lesions are often controlled, at least temporarily, by anti-retroviral treatment ■ However, the anti-retroviral therapy may have adverse effects which present in the oral cavity: ● oral ulceration may be caused by abacavir, didanosine, zalcitabine and saquinavir ● circumoral paraesthesia has been reported with ritonavir and amprenavir ● increased human papillomavirus-associated warts with HAART ■ Oral features are now classified as strongly, less commonly or possibly, associated with HIV infection (Box 3.15).

Clinical findings, diagnosis and management of the main oral lesions are described in Table 3.72.

Dental management

Risk assessment ■ Dental treatment of persons with HIV/AIDS should be carried out with the standard precautions to prevent cross infection ■ Additional attention may need to be given to: ● the possibility, though small, of postoperative infection (especially in patients with neutropenia and/or profound lymphopenia) ● prolonged haemorrhage (mainly in patients with thrombocytopenia, or on some drugs such as ritonavir) ■ HIV does appear to have been transmitted within health care facilities on rare occasions; two prime dental examples are summarised: ● one dentist with HIV infection in Florida, USA appears to have transmitted HIV to at least six patients as a consequence of invasive dental procedures ● an outbreak of 14 cases of HIV infection was also discovered by chance in 1993 among haemodialysis patients at a hospital in Bucaramanga, Colombia, and seems most likely to have been transmitted by contaminated dental instruments ■ Many other studies, however, have shown no evidence of any transmission of HIV from HIV-infected dentists to patients ■ The chief occupational risk of acquiring HIV infection is as a result of injury by a sharp instrument,

Box 3.15 WHO Classification of oral lesions in HIV/AIDS

Group I: Lesions strongly associated with HIV infection
● Candidosis: erythematous, thrush (pseudomembranous) ● Hairy leukoplakia (EBV) ● Linear gingival erythema ● Necrotising ulcerative gingivitis ● HIV-periodontitis ● Kaposi's sarcoma ● Non-Hodgkin's lymphoma

Group II: Lesions less commonly associated with HIV infection:
● Atypical ulceration (oropharyngeal) ● idiopathic thrombocytopenic purpura ● Salivary gland diseases ● Dry mouth: unilateral or bilateral swelling of major salivary glands ● Viral infections (other than EBV): cytomegalovirus, Herpes simplex virus, Human papillomavirus (warty-like lesions: condyloma acuminatum, focal epithelial hyperplasia and verruca vulgaris), Varicella-zoster virus: herpes zoster and varicella ● Bacterial infections (*M.- avium-intracellulare, M. tuberculosis*) ● Melanotic hyperpigmentation

Group III: Lesions possibly associated with HIV infection
A miscellany of rare diseases

Table 3.72 The more common oral manifestations of HIV infection

Condition*	Features	Diagnosis	Management
Candidosis	White removable lesions or red lesions, typically in the palate, but anywhere	Clinical plus investigations; smear or rinse, culture, or biopsy	Antifungals
Hairy leukoplakia	White non-removable lesions almost invariably bilaterally on the tongue	Clinical plus investigations; cytology; DNA studies or biopsy	None usually
Periodontal disease	Linear gingival erythema, necrotising gingivitis or periodontitis	Clinical	Oral hygiene, plaque removal, chlorhexidine, metronidazole
Herpesvirus ulcers	Chronic ulcers anywhere but often on tongue, hard palate or gingivae. Zoster increased by HAART	Clinical plus investigations; cytology, EM, DNA studies or biopsy	Antivirals
Aphthous-like ulcers	Recurrent ulcers anywhere but especially on mobile mucosae	Clinical plus investigations; possibly biopsy	Corticosteroids or thalidomide or granulocyte colony stimulating factor
Papillomavirus infections	Warty lesions, increased by HAART	Clinical plus investigations; DNA studies possibly biopsy	Excise or remove with heat, laser, or cryoprobe, imiquimod or podophyllin
Salivary gland disease	Xerostomia and sometimes salivary gland enlargement	Clinical plus investigations; sialometry, possibly biopsy	Salivary substitutes and/or pilocarpine or cevimeline
Kaposi's sarcoma	Purple macules leading to nodules, seen mainly in the palate	Clinical plus investigations; biopsy	Chemotherapy, usually vinblastine, or laser or radiation
Lymphomas	Lump or ulcer in fauces or gingivae	Clinical plus investigations; biopsy	Chemotherapy or radiation or both

*HAART reduces many of these manifestations.

particularly a local anaesthetic needle which can contain a significant amount of contaminated body fluids. However, the risk of occupational transmission of HIV after needle-stick injuries appears to be far lower than the nearly 26% of persons who develop hepatitis B infection after an infected needle-stick injury, or the 10% who contract hepatitis C infection. Indeed, epidemiological studies have indicated that the average risk of HIV transmission after percutaneous exposure to HIV infected blood in health care settings is about 3 per 1000 injuries (0.3%).

Appropriate health care ■ There is a move towards normalisation and mainstreaming of oral health care provision ■ However, many HIV-infected individuals continue to have concerns about privacy; the additional stigma and social implications of their infection may prevent them from accessing general dental services – at least in their locality ■ It is therefore critical to ensure that there is a strict adherence to data protection and patient confidentiality – the patient should be reassured that any of their details will not be discussed, even with their physicians, unless permission is sought from the patient ■ Dental treatment may also be influenced by the long-term prognosis of the patient's medical conditions and the prior oral health status.

Pain and anxiety control **Analgesia** Bleeding can be aggravated by analgesics such as aspirin or other non-steroidal anti-inflammatory drugs such as indometacin. Codeine and acetaminophen are safer. The interaction between acetaminophen and zidovudine, inducing granulocytopenia, appears rarely to be clinically significant. **Local anaesthesia** Caution is advised to minimise the risk of needle-stick injury. There is a theoretical interaction of LA with protease inhibitors. **Conscious sedation** Protease inhibitors such as indinavir and nelfinavir can enhance benzodiazepine activity. **General anaesthesia** A comprehensive assessment in conjunction with the anaesthetist is critical. The patient's physician should be consulted and investigations undertaken to assess the risk of bleeding, infection, and whether there are any concurrent infections which would compromise respiration and/or the airway.

Treatment modification **Surgery** ■ Medical consultation is mandatory for symptomatic HIV-infected patients before any surgical procedure ■ Complications are less likely in symptomless HIV-infected persons ■ The prevalence of complications following dental extractions in HIV-infected persons overall is estimated at about 5%, similar to that achieved in HIV-negative patients. Most complications are mild (alveolitis and delayed healing) and easily treated. Postoperative bleeding is unusual, even in thrombocytopenic patients. ■ Patients with profound immunodeficiency (those with neutropenia and/or CD4 T lymphocyte count $<200 \times 10^6$/L) however, may require antibiotic cover before surgery or after maxillofacial injuries. Metronidazole, amoxicillin plus clavulanic acid, and clindamycin have been successfully administered. **Implantology** Implants are not contraindicated in patients with mild immuno-incompetence, although, to date, long-term series have not been published. **Endodontics** Endodontic treatment can usually be carried out without special precautions. **Periodontology** ■ Mechanical and chemical treatments of periodontitis are similar to those applied in HIV-negative patients; it may be prudent to test the tissue response to scaling in a few teeth before planning definitive treatment ■ Chlorhexidine is recommended during the maintenance phase ■ Frequent recall appointments for maintenance of periodontal health are required.

Drug use ■ Immunosuppression may inhibit suppressor T cells regulating IgE antibody synthesis and so enhance the sensitising potential of some drugs. HIV disease has become a major risk factor for adverse drug reactions: over half the patients with AIDS develop adverse reactions when treated with trimethoprim-sulphamethoxazole. The incidence of reactions to ampicillin is inversely proportional to CD4+ cell counts. Several other drugs have a higher than expected tendency to produce adverse reactions in HIV-infected patients. Most are mild-to-moderate skin eruptions, but the risk of anaphylaxis and even toxic epidermal necrolysis may also be enhanced in HIV infection. ■ Possible drug interactions with drugs used in oral health care are shown in Table 3.73.

Further reading ● Campo-Trapero J, Cano-Sanchez J, del Romero-Guerrero J, Moreno-Lopez L A, Cerero-Lapiedra R, Bascones-Martinez A 2003 Dental management of patients with human immunodeficiency virus. Quintessence Int 34:515–525 ● Diz Dios P 2002 Las lesiones orales en el Sida Infantil. In: Velasco E Odontoestomatología y SIDA. Publicaciones Médicas, Barcelona ● Diz Dios P, Scully C 2002 Adverse effects of antiretroviral therapies: focus on orofacial effects. Expert Opinions on Drug Safety 1:304–317 ● Diz Dios P, Vázquez García E, Fernández Feijoo J, Porter S R 1998 Tratamiento odontológico del paciente infectado por el virus de la inmunodeficiencia humana. Medicina Oral 3:222–229 ● Diz Dios P, Vázquez García E, Fernández Feijoo J 1998 Post-extraction complications in HIV-infected patients. J Dent Res 77:533–534 ● Diz Dios P, Fernández Feijoo J, Vázquez García E 1999 Tooth extraction in HIV sero-positive patients. Int Dent J 49:317–321 ● Diz Dios P, Ocampo Hermida A, Miralles Alvarez C, Limeres Posse J, Tomás Carmona I 2000 Changing prevalence of human immunodeficiency virus-associated oral lesions. Oral Surg Oral Med Oral Pathol Oral Radiol Endod 90:403–404 ● Patel A S, Glick M 2003 Oral manifestations associated with HIV infection: evaluation, assessment, and significance. Gen Dent 51:153–156

Table 3.73 **Possible drug interactions in HIV-infected patients**

Drug used in oral health care	May interact with	Possible consequence
Miconazole Fluconazole Itraconazole Ketoconazole	Terfenadine (astemizole and cisapride withdrawn because of interaction)	Arrhythmias and cardiotoxicity
	Anticoagulants	Anticoagulants potentiated
	Antacids	Impair absorption of the azole
	DDI	Impair absorption of the azole
	H2-antagonists	Impair absorption of the azole
	Omeprazole	Impair absorption of the azole
Benzodiazepines	Azoles Indinavir Ritonavir	All enhance sedation
Fluconazole	Rifabutin	Uveitis from rifabutin toxicity
Metronidazole	Ritonavir liquid	Disulphiram reaction

Table 3.74 **Key considerations for dental management in HIV/AIDS (see text)**

	Management modifications*	Comments/possible complications
Risk assessment	2	Prevent cross-infection; postoperative infection; prolonged haemorrhage
Appropriate dental care	2–4	Influenced by the long-term prognosis, the medical condition and the prior oral health status. Data protection; patient confidentiality
Pain and anxiety control		
– Local anaesthesia	1	
– Conscious sedation	2	Avoid benzodiazepines
– General anaesthesia	3/4	
Patient access and positioning		
– Access to dental office	0	
– Timing of treatment	0	
– Patient positioning	0	
Treatment modification		
– Oral surgery	3	Minimal complications; possibly antibiotic cover
– Implantology	3	
– Conservative/Endodontics	2	
– Fixed prosthetics	2	
– Removable prosthetics	2	
– Non-surgical periodontology	3	
– Surgical periodontology	3	
Hazardous and contraindicated drugs	2	Avoid aspirin and indometacin; multiple adverse drug reactions

*0 = No special considerations. 1 = Caution advised. 2 = Specialised medical advice recommended in some cases. 3 = Specialised medical advice mandatory. 4 = Only to be performed in hospital environment. 5 = Should be avoided.

HUNTINGTON'S CHOREA

Definition ■ Huntington's chorea is an inherited, chronic disease, characterised by progressive involuntary movements (chorea), emotional disturbances and dementia ■ The name 'chorea' comes from the Greek word for dance and refers to the characteristic and incessant quick, jerky and involuntary movements.

General aspects

Aetiopathogenesis Huntington's chorea (HC) is an autosomal dominant condition, with the responsible gene located on chromosome 4. The cerebral damage is due to atrophy of the caudate nucleus of the basal ganglia which shows decreased levels of gamma-aminobutyric acid (GABA).

Clinical presentation Signs and symptoms usually begin to appear in early to middle age, and may include: ■ involuntary, jerky movements of fingers, feet, arms, neck, trunk and face ■ hesitant, halting or slurred speech ■ wide, prancing gait ■ clumsiness or poor balance ■ personality changes (moodiness, paranoia) ■ intellectual deterioration (memory loss, inattention).

Diagnosis The diagnosis is suggested by: ■ family history – positive ■ clinical findings ■ EEG – abnormal ■ CT of brain lateral ventricles – 'wing of butterfly' image ■ growth hormone levels – increased ■ GABA levels – decreased.

However, it is now possible for individuals at risk for HC to undergo genetic testing, which detects the presence or absence of the genetic sequence that causes it. The decision of whether or not to undergo genetic testing is intensely personal, with many factors to consider. Genetic testing guidelines stress that the decision should only be made with informed consent, ensuring that the individual being tested fully understands the risks and benefits of genetic testing and can make an independent decision. Furthermore, the importance of counselling throughout the entire process is highlighted.

Treatment ■ Neuroleptics such as clonazepam, and antipsychotic drugs such as haloperidol and clozapine can help control chorea, violent outbursts and hallucinations ■ Lithium can help control extreme emotions and mood swings ■ Fluoxetine, setraline and nortriptyline can help control depression.

Prognosis ■ Progress of the disease is slow, but inexorable ■ Life is often ended by intercurrent infection, or sometimes suicide, since patients are often too well aware of the family history and poor prognosis.

Oral findings

There may be darting movements of the head and tongue, which increase as the disorder progresses.

Dental management

Risk assessment Involuntary movements may provoke injuries with sharp instruments during dental treatment.

Appropriate health care ■ Patient confidentiality is critical, as a positive diagnosis of HC has implications for the rest of the patient's family ■ Patients can often understand what they are being told and therefore every dental procedure should be previously explained to them ■ In the later

Table 3.75 **Key considerations for dental management in Huntington´s chorea (see text)**

	Management modifications*	Comments/possible complications
Risk assessment	2	Injuries with sharp instruments
Appropriate dental care	2–4	Early oral rehabilitation; communication difficulties; consent issues in advanced disease
Pain and anxiety control		
– Local anaesthesia	1	
– Conscious sedation	1/3/4	
– General anaesthesia	3/4	Exaggerated responses to sodium thiopentone and succinylcholine
Patient access and positioning		
– Access to dental office	1	Possibly wheelchair
– Timing of treatment	0	
– Patient positioning	1	Possibly wheelchair or bed-ridden
Treatment modification		
– Oral surgery	1/4	
– Implantology	5	
– Conservative/Endodontics	4/5	
– Fixed prosthetics	4/5	
– Removable prosthetics	1/5	
– Non-surgical periodontology	1/4/5	
– Surgical periodontology	1/4/5	
Hazardous and contraindicated drugs	0	

*0 = No special considerations. 1 = Caution advised. 2 = Specialised medical advice recommended in some cases. 3 = Specialised medical advice mandatory. 4 = Only to be performed in hospital environment. 5 = Should be avoided.

stages patients may be unable to respond, and this may give a false impression of the degree of dementia ■ Comprehensive oral rehabilitation is best completed as early as possible, since the patient's ability to cooperate during dental treatment diminishes with advancing disease. Consent may also become problematic in later stages of HC.

Patient access and positioning In advanced stages some patients may need to use a wheelchair or are bedbound.

Preventive dentistry ■ Oral hygiene may be impaired and worsened by medications that impair salivation ■ As the movements and dementia are progressive, preventive oral programmes involving family and caregivers are crucial.

Pain and anxiety control There are no contraindications regarding the use of LA. However, LA becomes increasingly difficult to administer safely as the disease progresses. Although conscious sedation may be of benefit, as the patient's condition further deteriorates, GA may become the only viable option.

Treatment modification ■ The chorea can make operative dentistry or the construction and wearing of prostheses difficult or virtually impossible ■ Due to the progressive character of the disease, complex treatment should not be planned.

Further reading ● Bradford H, Britto L R, Leal G, Katz J 2004 Endodontic treatment of a patient with Huntington's disease. J Endod 30:366–369 ● Cangemi C F Jr, Miller R J 1998 Huntington's disease: review and anesthetic case management. Anesth Prog 45:150–153 ● Kieser J, Jones G, Borlase G, MacFadyen E 1999 Dental treatment of patients with neurodegenerative disease. NZ Dent J 95:130–134.

HYDROCEPHALUS

Definition Hydrocephalus is a neurological condition that arises when there is: raised intracranial pressure due to an abnormal accumulation of cerebrospinal fluid (CSF) within the ventricles and/or subarachnoid space of the brain from an overproduction of CSF (choroid plexus papilloma) ■ an obstruction of flow of CSF or ■ a failure of the brain to reabsorb CSF.

Normal pressure hydrocephalus is when the ventricles are enlarged, but there is little or no rise in intracranial pressure.

General aspects

Aetiopathogenesis Hydrocephalus may be congenital or acquired. **Congenital** ■ Congenital hydrocephalus is often a part of other neurological conditions and congenital malformations, which include, from most to least common: ● Dandy–Walker syndrome ● neural tube defects ● spina bifida ● Chiari malformations ● vein of Galen malformations ● hydranencephaly ● craniosynostosis ● schizencephaly ● tracheoesophageal fistula ■ Hydrocephalus is also considered congenital when it is X-linked hydrocephalus, or its origin can be traced to a birth defect or brain malformation that causes a raised resistance to the drainage of CSF ■ It can be caused by TORCH syndrome from intrauterine infection with: ● **to**xoplasmosis ● **r**ubella ● **c**ytomegalovirus ● **h**erpes simplex ■ Hydrocephalus can be acquired later in life if there is a rise in the resistance to the drainage of CSF, such as obstruction caused by: ● brain tumour ● arachnoid cyst ● intracranial or intraventricular haemorrhage ● trauma to the head ● infections such as meningitis.

Clinical presentation ■ Signs include large head and bulky fontanelles ■ Complications include epilepsy, visual deficiency, spasticity and learning impairment.

Classification ■ Communicating hydrocephalus means that the site of raised resistance to CSF drainage resides outside of the ventricular system – in the subarachnoid space ■ Non-communicating, or obstructive, hydrocephalus is caused when there is an obstruction in the flow of CSF within the ventricular system of the brain, including the outlets of the fourth ventricle (the foramina of Luschka and Magendie). The most common place for the non-communicating CSF obstruction is in the aqueduct of Sylvius (also known as aqueductal stenosis). However, the obstruction can also occur in the outlets of the fourth ventricle and from the lateral ventricles into the third ventricle at the foramina of Monro.

Diagnosis ■ Head circumference – serial measurements show increase ■ Skull radiographs ■ CT – enlarged ventricles ■ Isotopic ventriculography.

Treatment ■ Hydrocephalus can be treated directly (by removing the cause of CSF obstruction or overproduction if one can be found) or indirectly by diverting the fluid build up to somewhere else, typically into another body cavity ('shunts') ■ There are three main types of shunt normally used:

- A *ventriculoperitoneal shunt* (V/P) diverts the CSF from the brain ventricles to the peritoneal cavity in the abdomen where the fluid is reabsorbed into the bloodstream. The one-way valve is placed next to the ventricle in the brain and the proximal catheter is placed in the ventricle while the distal catheter runs from the valve down to the peritoneal cavity. A catheter is an extremely narrow piece of tubing used for drainage purposes.
- A *ventriculoatrial shunt* (V/A) diverts CSF from the brain ventricles into the right atrium of the heart. Again, the valve rests next to the ventricle and one catheter is placed within the ventricle. The other catheter is placed into a vein in the neck and then carefully advanced into the right atrium, where the CSF enters the bloodstream.
- A *lumboperitoneal shunt* (L/P) is popularly used when the ventricles of the brain are too small to allow the placement of a V/P or V/A shunt. One catheter is placed in the low back (lumbar) area of the spine while the other end rests in the peritoneal cavity. As with V/P shunts, the shunted CSF then enters the bloodstream.

■ There are instances, usually as a result of head trauma, when excess CSF needs to be drained quickly in order to alleviate pressure upon the brain. This is accomplished via *external CSF drainage*. In cases such as this, CSF is drained from either the ventricles of the brain or the lumbar region of the spine into an external drainage and monitoring system. This is a short-term treatment only. ■ Shunt lengthening surgery may be needed as the child grows ■ Acetazolamide and furosemide may help lower CSF production.

Dental management

Risk assessment ■ The weight of the head may cause difficulties, especially in the anaesthetised patient ■ Other management difficulties may include: ● spina bifida (frequently associated) ● latex allergy

● epilepsy ● learning disability ● visual impairment ■ Infection of shunt – although rarely from a dental source – can be so devastating (e.g. acute renal failure) that antibiotic cover may need to be given before oral procedures that might produce bacteraemia ■ There are no reported cases of infective endocarditis occurring in association with V/A shunts.

Appropriate dental care ■ A V/A shunt is often viewed as higher risk for infection following bacteraemic dental procedures, as it is in direct communication with blood in the right atrium, but there is no scientific evidence to support this assumption ■ However, the neurosurgeon should be consulted in all cases.

Pain and anxiety control **Local anaesthesia/conscious sedation** Although there are no contraindications regarding the use of LA and conscious sedation, the cause of the hydrocephalus should be determined,

Table 3.76 **Key considerations for dental management in hydrocephalus (see text)**

	Management modifications*	Comments/possible complications
Risk assessment	2	Latex allergy, epilepsy, learning disability, etc.
Appropriate dental care	1/4	Influenced by the underlying disease; antibiotic cover
Pain and anxiety control		
– Local anaesthesia	1	
– Conscious sedation	2	
– General anaesthesia	3/4	Associated conditions/ complications
Patient access and positioning		
– Access to dental office	1	Consider cause of hydrocephalus
– Timing of treatment	1	
– Patient positioning	1	
Treatment modification		
– Oral surgery	2	May require antibiotic cover
– Implantology	2	
– Conservative/Endodontics	1	
– Fixed prosthetics	1	
– Removable prosthetics	1	
– Non-surgical periodontology	2	May require antibiotic cover
– Surgical periodontology	2	
Hazardous and contraindicated drugs	0	

*0 = No special considerations. 1 = Caution advised. 2 = Specialised medical advice recommended in some cases. 3 = Specialised medical advice mandatory. 4 = Only to be performed in hospital environment. 5 = Should be avoided.

as this may impact on the feasibility of these techniques.

General anaesthesia A thorough preoperative assessment in conjunction with the anaesthetist is essential. The neurosurgeon/physician should be consulted, not only in terms of the need for antibiotic cover, but also because hydrocephalus is often associated with other conditions such as spina bifida, meningitis, encephalitis or brain haemorrhage. Furthermore, congenital diaphragmatic hernia has been reported in patients with hydrocephalus. It carries a high mortality rate, despite intensive perioperative care. Postoperative recovery depends on the degree of pulmonary hypertension and pulmonary hypoplasia.

Further reading ● Helpin M L, Rosenberg H M, Sayany Z, Sanford R A 1998 Antibiotic prophylaxis in dental patients with ventriculo-peritoneal shunts: a pilot study. ASDC J Dent Child 65:244–247 ● Pirttiniemi P, Poikela A, Huggare J, Lopponen T 2004 Dental maturation in children with shunt-treated hydrocephalus. Cleft Palate Craniofac J 41:651–654.

HYPERALDOSTERONISM

Definition Hyperaldosteronism is a syndrome associated with adrenal aldosterone overproduction. Aldosterone increases sodium retention in distal renal tubules, and potassium secretion.

General aspects

Aetiopathogenesis ■ Conn's syndrome (adrenocortical adenoma) is the main cause ■ Other causes include: ● adrenocortical hyperplasia ● adrenal carcinoma ● glucocorticoid-remediable aldosteronism (abnormal control by ACTH).

Clinical presentation Excess aldosterone results in hypokalaemia and alkalosis. ■ Hypokalaemia is responsible for most clinical findings including: ● hypertension (usually without associated complications) ● headache ● muscular weakness and possibly paralysis ■ Alkalosis may produce tetany.

Classification ■ In primary hyperaldosteronism there are increased plasma aldosterone and reduced plasma renin levels ■ Secondary hyperaldosteronism is a consequence of renin–angiotensin system activation, seen in renal, cardiac and hepatic failure. In these patients there is hypokalaemia but no hypertension.

Diagnosis ■ Plasma potassium – reduced ■ Plasma sodium – often raised ■ Plasma aldosterone – raised ■ Plasma renin – reduced ■ CT/MRI.

Treatment ■ Spironolactone ■ Surgery.

Dental management

Risk assessment ■ In the untreated patient, hypertension and muscle weakness are the main complications ■ If bilateral adrenalectomy has been carried out, the patient is at risk from collapse during dental treatment and therefore requires corticosteroid cover.

Table 3.77 **Key considerations for dental management in hyperaldosteronism (see text)**

	Management modifications*	Comments/possible complications
Risk assessment	2	Hypertension; muscle weakness
Appropriate dental care	2	Possibly corticosteroid cover
Pain and anxiety control		
– Local anaesthesia	1	
– Conscious sedation	1	
– General anaesthesia	3/4	Avoid muscle relaxants
Patient access and positioning		
– Access to dental office	1	
– Timing of treatment	1	
– Patient positioning	1	
Treatment modification		
– Oral surgery	1	
– Implantology	1	
– Conservative/Endodontics	1	
– Fixed prosthetics	1	
– Removable prosthetics	1	
– Non-surgical periodontology	1	
– Surgical periodontology	1	
Hazardous and contraindicated drugs	0	

*0 = No special considerations. 1 = Caution advised. 2 = Specialised medical advice recommended in some cases. 3 = Specialised medical advice mandatory. 4 = Only to be performed in hospital environment. 5 = Should be avoided.

Pain and anxiety control **Local anaesthesia** LA should be undertaken with caution in view of the systemic complications of hyperaldosteronism. **Conscious sedation** Conscious sedation should be undertaken with caution in view of the systemic complications of hyperaldosteronism. **General anaesthesia** Competitive muscle relaxants should be used with restraint, as they can cause profound paralysis.

Further reading • Greenwood M, Meechan J G 2003 General medicine and surgery for dental practitioners. Part 6: The endocrine system. Br Dent J 195:129–133.

HYPERPARATHYROIDISM

Definition Hyperparathyroidism is parathyroid hormone (PTH) overproduction, which leads to increased calcium absorption from the gastrointestinal tract, renal calcium resorption, and mobilisation of calcium from bones (osteoclastic resorption).

General aspects

Aetiopathogenesis ■ *Primary* hyperparathyroidism is usually caused by parathyroid adenoma or hyperplasia, with autonomous secretion of PTH ■ *Secondary* hyperparathyroidism is caused by hypocalcaemia in renal failure or vitamin D deficiency, resulting in raised PTH ■ *Tertiary* hyperparathyroidism occurs when the parathyroids become autonomous after secondary hyperparathyroidism.

Clinical presentation Excess PTH results in hypercalcaemia, which presents (Fig. 3.21) as: ■ General: polydipsia, polyuria, weight loss ■ Renal: colic, haematuria, back pain, polyuria ■ Cardiovascular:

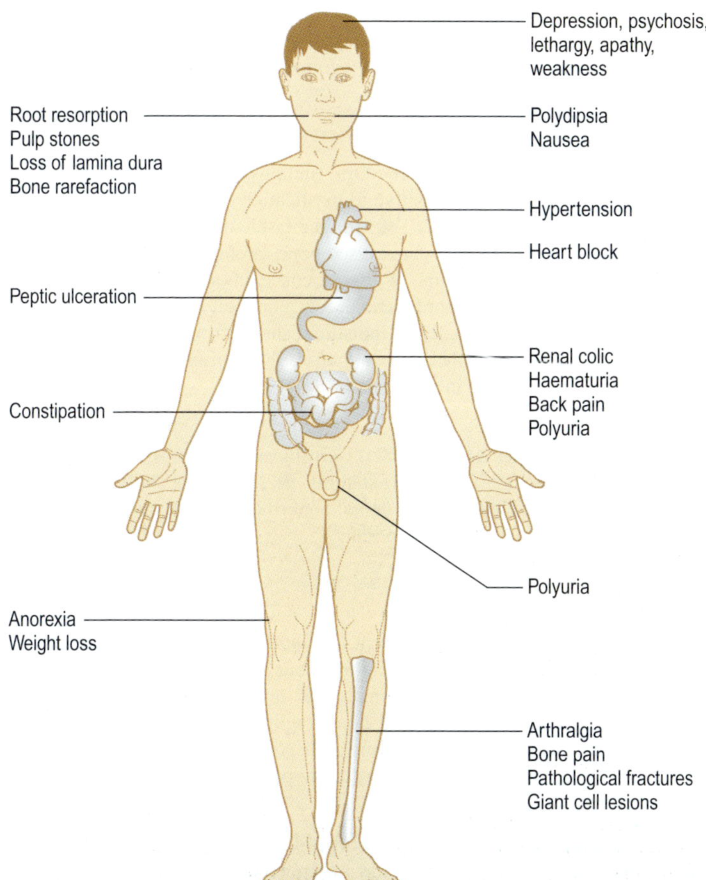

Figure 3.21 **Clinical presentation of hyperparathyroidism**

hypertension, heart block ■ Musculoskeletal: arthralgia, bone pain, pathological fractures, giant cell lesions (rare) ■ Gastrointestinal: anorexia, nausea, dyspepsia, constipation, peptic ulceration ■ Neurological: depression (Sagliken syndrome), lethargy, apathy, weakness, psychosis.

Occasionally signs of pluriglandular disease are present: ■ MEA (multiple endocrine adenopathy) I (diabetes or Cushing's syndrome) ■ MEA II or III (phaeochromocytoma).

Diagnosis Diagnosis of primary hyperparathyroidism is confirmed by: ■ blood analysis ● plasma calcium – raised ● plasma phosphate – reduced ● plasma alkaline phosphatase – raised ● plasma PTH – raised ■ radioisotope scan ■ CT.

Treatment ■ Lowering the plasma calcium level by diuresis ■ Mithramycin ■ Calcitonin ■ Surgery.

Prognosis Severe hypercalcaemia may result in arrhythmia, bronchospasm, convulsions, lethargy, stupor, and finally coma and death due to tetany.

Oral findings

Primary hyperparathyroidism Oral findings are late and uncommon, and include: ■ Teeth ● sensitive to mastication ● root resorption ● pulp stones ■ Sialolithiasis ■ Tongue fasciculations ■ Bone ● loss of the lamina dura ● generalised bone rarefaction (ground-glass appearance) ● jaw bone pain ● loss of cortical bone of the inferior mandibular border and mandibular canal ● giant cell lesions (brown tumours) are rare but histologically indistinguishable from central giant cell granulomas of the jaws. If, therefore, a giant cell lesion is found, particularly in a middle-aged patient or in a patient with renal failure, parathyroid function should be investigated.

Secondary hyperparathyroidism Orofacial findings seen in chronic renal failure may include: ■ short stature ■ significant skull, maxillary and mandibular bone changes ■ dental abnormalities ■ soft and innocuous tumoural tissues in the mouth.

Dental management

Risk assessment Dental treatment in hyperparathyroidism can be often performed without special precautions but it may be complicated by: ■ hypertension ■ cardiac arrhythmias ■ renal disease ■ peptic ulcer ■ sensitivity to muscle relaxants ■ bone fragility ■ pluriglandular disease; MEA I (diabetes or Cushing's syndrome); MEA II or III (phaeochromocytoma) ■ hepatitis B or C in secondary or tertiary hyperparathyroidism, resulting from renal dialysis.

Pain and anxiety control **Local anaesthesia** LA should be undertaken with caution in view of the systemic complications of hyperparathyroidism. **Conscious sedation** Conscious sedation should be undertaken with caution in view of the systemic complications of

Table 3.78 **Key considerations for dental management in hyperparathyroidism (see text)**

	Management modifications*	Comments/possible complications
Risk assessment	2	Hypertension; arrhythmias; renal disease; bone fragility
Pain and anxiety control		
– Local anaesthesia	1	
– Conscious sedation	1	
– General anaesthesia	3/4	Avoid muscle relaxants
Patient access and positioning		
– Access to dental office	0	
– Timing of treatment	0	
– Patient positioning	0	
Treatment modification		
– Oral surgery	2	Brown tumours; bone fractures
– Implantology	2	
– Conservative/Endodontics	1	
– Fixed prosthetics	1	
– Removable prosthetics	1	
– Non-surgical periodontology	1	
– Surgical periodontology	1	
Imaging	1	Ground-glass appearance; loss of cortical bone and lamina dura; brown tumours
Hazardous and contraindicated drugs	2	Select drugs carefully in patients with renal disease

*0 = No special considerations. 1 = Caution advised. 2 = Specialised medical advice recommended in some cases. 3 = Specialised medical advice mandatory. 4 = Only to be performed in hospital environment. 5 = Should be avoided.

hyperparathyroidism. **General anaesthesia** GA should be undertaken with caution in view of the systemic complications of hyperparathyroidism. Muscle relaxants should be avoided.

Treatment modification **Surgery** Brown tumours need not necessarily always be removed, particularly where the risk of bone fracture is high.

Further Reading

• Aggunlu L, Akpek S, Coskun B 2004 Leontiasis ossea in a patient with hyperparathyroidism secondary to chronic renal failure. Pediatr Radiol 34:630–632 • Sagliker Y, Balal M, Sagliker Ozkaynak P et al 2004 Sagliker syndrome: uglifying human face appearance in late and severe secondary hyperparathyroidism in chronic renal failure. Semin Nephrol 24:449–455 • Solt D B 1991 The pathogenesis, oral manifestations, and implications for dentistry of metabolic bone disease. Curr Opin Dent 1:783–791.

HYPERTENSION

Definition Hypertension is defined as blood pressure consistently over 140/90 mmHg (systolic/diastolic).

General aspects

Aetiopathogenesis ■ The cause of primary hypertension (essential hypertension) (95% of all hypertension) remains unknown, but inheritance and environmental factors have been implicated ■ Secondary hypertension is often due to renal disease. Endocrine conditions such as hyperaldosteronism or phaeochromocytoma may also be implicated in some patients.

Clinical presentation ■ Most hypertension is asymptomatic ■ Symptoms in advanced hypertension may include headache, blurred vision, tinnitus, fatigue and dizziness (Box 3.16) ■ Systolic hypertension is a main risk factor in cardiac ischaemia and strokes ■ Malignant hypertension is severely raised blood pressure (BP) (>200/>130 mmHg) which causes bilateral retinal haemorrhage and exudates ■ Hypertension can lead to complications related to arteriosclerosis, retinal damage, left ventricular hypertrophy, proteinuria and renal failure.

Classification Hypertension may be divided into the following categories (Table 3.79): ■ borderline, mild (stage 1) ■ moderate (stage 2) ■ severe (stage 3).

Diagnosis Blood pressure estimation by sphygmomanometry (two to three separate readings at rest).

Treatment ■ Reduce weight ■ Low-salt diet ■ No smoking ■ Reduce alcohol ■ Diuretic (e.g. thiazide-bendrofluazide) ■ Beta-blocker (e.g. atenolol) or ACE inhibitor (e.g. captopril) ■ Statins ■ Aspirin.

Prognosis With prolonged or severe hypertension, angina, myocardial infarct or stroke may occur.

Oral findings

■ Although there are no recognised oral manifestations of hypertension, facial palsy is an occasional complication of malignant hypertension ■ Antihypertensive drugs can sometimes cause orofacial side effects such

Box 3.16 Features of hypertension

Symptoms (advanced hypertension)
● Headaches ● Visual problems ● Tinnitus ● Dizziness ● Angina

Signs
● Hypertension on testing ● Retinal changes ● Left ventricular hypertrophy ● Proteinuria ● Haematuria

Table 3.79 **Hypertension – ASA (American Society of Anesthesiologists) grading and dental management considerations**

Blood pressure mmHg (systolic and diastolic)	ASA grade	Hypertension stage	Key considerations
< 140 and < 90	I	–	Routine dental care
140–159 and 90–99	II	1	Recheck BP, before starting dental care Routine dental care
160–179 and 95–109	III	2	Recheck BP, before starting Medical advice before routine dental care Restrict vasoconstrictors Conscious sedation may help
> 180 and > 110	IV	3	Recheck BP after 5 min quiet rest Only emergency dental care until BP controlled

as xerostomia, salivary gland swelling or pain, lichenoid reactions, erythema multiforme, angio-oedema, gingival hyperplasia, sore mouth or paraesthesia ■ Clonidine, in particular, can cause xerostomia.

Dental management

Risk assessment ■ Ideally, the blood pressure should be controlled before elective dental treatment ■ If the patient indicates that their blood pressure has been persistently high and no further medical management is planned, the opinion of a physician should be sought first before commencing dental treatment. In these cases, continuous BP monitoring is indicated and, if it rises, management includes: ● discontinue dental treatment ● place patient in supine position ● allow the patient to rest ● re-check BP after 5 minutes ● if the BP is consistently high and severe, the patient may be given furosemide (40 mg) or captopril (25 mg) orally (sublingual nifedipine is no longer recommended) ● if there is no improvement, call for medical assistance. ■ The management of hypertensive patients may also be complicated by the underlying disease or other problems such as cardiac or renal failure.

Appropriate health care Dental care should be modified in relation to the severity of the hypertension (Table 3.79).

Pain and anxiety control It is important to avoid anxiety and pain, since endogenous epinephrine released in response to pain or fear may induce hypertension or arrhythmias. **Local anaesthesia** ■ Preoperative reassurance is important ■ Blood pressure tends to rise during oral surgery under LA, and epinephrine theoretically can contribute to this but this is usually of little practical importance ■ Under most circumstances the use of epinephrine in combination with LA is not contraindicated in the hypertensive patient unless the systolic pressure is over 200 mmHg and/or the diastolic is over 115 mmHg ■ Epinephrine-containing LA should not be administered to patients taking beta-blockers, since interactions between epinephrine and the beta-blocking agent may induce hypertension and cardiovascular complications ■ Lidocaine should be used with caution in patients taking beta-blockers. **Conscious sedation** ■ Conscious sedation can usually be used safely, although this does depend on the underlying disease and the presence of any long-term complications of hypertension ■ Sedation with 10 mg temazepam, or 6–8 mg diazepam may be helpful ■ Avoid opioids. **General anaesthesia** ■ All antihypertensive drugs are potentiated by GA agents and can produce hypotension – this is especially the case for barbiturates and opioids ■ However, antihypertensive drugs should not be stopped when a GA is given, since the risks of cerebrovascular accidents and cardiovascular instability that result from withdrawal and rebound hypertension outweigh the dangers of drug interactions, which to some extent are predictable and manageable by an expert anaesthetist ■ Hypertension may be a contraindication to GA if complicated by: ● cardiac failure ● coronary or cerebral artery insufficiency ● renal insufficiency ■ Chronic administration of some diuretics such as furosemide may lead to potassium deficiency; potassium levels should therefore be checked preoperatively in order to avoid arrhythmias and increased sensitivity to muscle relaxants such as curare, gallamine and pancuronium ■ Intravenous barbiturates in particular can be dangerous in patients on antihypertensive therapy, but halothane, enflurane and isoflurane may also cause hypotension in patients on beta-blockers.

Patient access and positioning **Timing of treatment** ■ Patients with stable hypertension may receive dental care in short, minimally stressful appointments ■ Recent evidence indicates that endogenous epinephrine levels peak during morning hours and adverse cardiac events are most likely in the early morning, so late morning appointments are recommended. **Patient positioning** Raising the patient suddenly from the supine position may cause postural hypotension and loss of consciousness if the patient is using antihypertensive drugs such as thiazides or furosemide, or the calcium-channel blockers.

Treatment modification **Fixed prosthetics and conservation** Gingival retraction cords containing epinephrine should be avoided.

Drug use ■ Systemic corticosteroids may raise the blood pressure and antihypertensive treatment may have to be adjusted accordingly ■ Some non-steroidal anti-inflammatory drugs (indometacin, ibuprofen and naproxen) can reduce the efficacy of antihypertensive agents ■ Patients administered aspirin to prevent thrombosis may have a bleeding tendency.

Further reading
● Merin R L 2004 Hypertension guidelines. J Am Dent Assoc 135:1220–1222 ● Miyawaki T, Nishimura F, Kohjitani A et al 2004 Prevalence of blood pressure levels and hypertension-related diseases in Japanese dental patients. Community Dent Health 21:134–137.

Table 3.80 **Key considerations for dental management in hypertension (see text)**

	Management modifications*	Comments/possible complications
Risk assessment	2/3	Influenced by hypertension severity
Pain and anxiety control		
– Local anaesthesia	2	Caution with epinephrine and lidocaine
– Conscious sedation	1	Avoid opioids
– General anaesthesia	3–5	Hypotension; rebound hypertension; arrhythmias; avoid barbiturates, opioids, muscle relaxants, halothane and isofluorane
Patient access and positioning		
– Access to dental office	0	
– Timing of treatment	1	Late morning
– Patient positioning	1	Postural hypotension
Treatment modification		
– Oral surgery	2	
– Implantology	2	
– Conservative/Endodontics	2	
– Fixed prosthetics	2	Avoid gingival retraction cords containing epinephrine
– Removable prosthetics	1	
– Non-surgical periodontology	2	
– Surgical periodontology	2	
Hazardous and contraindicated drugs	2	Avoid indometacin, steroids, ibuprofen and naproxen; some patients are on aspirin

*0 = No special considerations. 1 = Caution advised. 2 = Specialised medical advice recommended in some cases. 3 = Specialised medical advice mandatory. 4 = Only to be performed in hospital environment. 5 = Should be avoided.

HYPERTHYROIDISM

Definition Hyperthyroidism is defined as raised thyroid hormone (T3 and T4) blood levels.

General aspects

Aetiopathogenesis Hyperthyroidism is due to thyroid overactivity (leading to low thyroid stimulating hormone –TSH) because of: ■ Graves' disease: caused by inappropriate immune system activation that targets the thyroid gland and causes overproduction of thyroid hormones (risk factors are being a woman over 20 years old, although the disorder may occur at any age and may affect men) ■ toxic goitre ■ toxic thyroid adenoma.

Clinical presentation ■ Thyroid hyperactivity mimics epinephrine excess, with: ● raised pulse ● tremor ● dislike of heat ● irritability and anxiety ● hypertension ■ Hyperthyroidism may also be associated with (Fig. 3.22): ● eyelid lag ● exophthalmos or proptosis ● thyroid swelling/lump ● warm, moist and erythematous skin ● increased appetite ● diarrhoea.

Diagnosis ■ Serum T3 and T4 levels raised ■ Serum TSH reduced.

Treatment ■ Control symptoms with: ● beta-blockers such as propranolol or nadolol ■ Treat hyperthyroidism with: ● antithyroid drugs (carbimazole or propylthiouracil, and methimazole) ● radioiodine ● surgery.

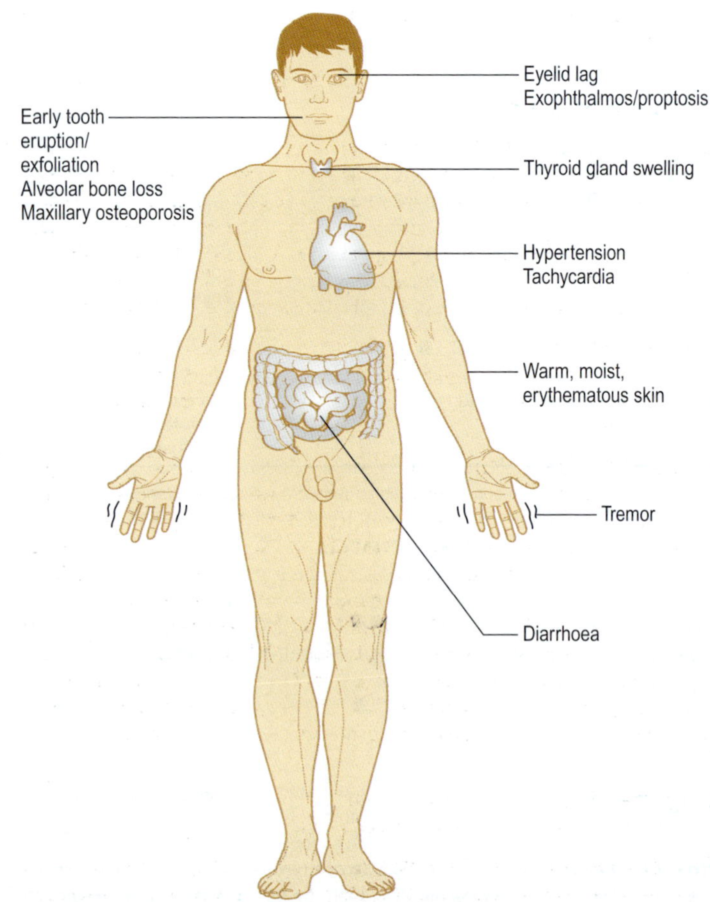

Figure 3.22 **Clinical presentation of hyperthyroidism**

Prognosis The severity of hyperthyroidism depends on: ■ the amount and duration of hormone excess ■ age ■ complications. Thyrotoxic crisis or thyroid storm is a severe condition which starts with extreme anxiety, nausea, vomiting and abdominal pain; then fever, sweating, tachycardia and pulmonary oedema; finally stupor, coma and occasionally death.

Oral findings

■ Early tooth eruption and early exfoliation of the primary teeth have been described ■ Alveolar bone osteoporosis ■ Increased caries and periodontal disease in patients with high carbohydrate consumption (to satisfy caloric requirements) ■ Medical treatment of hyperthyroidism with carbimazole occasionally leads to agranulocytosis – which may cause oral or oropharyngeal ulceration ■ Ectopic thyroid tissue located on the foramen caecum of the tongue is called lingual thyroid, and in some cases may be the only active thyroid tissue present.

Dental management

Risk assessment ■ These patients may be difficult to manage as a result of heightened anxiety and irritability. The sympathetic overactivity may lead to fainting. ■ A thyroid storm may be provoked during dental treatment by the stress, or by epinephrine, infection or traumatic surgery. Such patients must immediately be admitted to hospital. ■ A blood cell count with differential and bleeding tests should be performed regularly in patients on propylthiouracil due to the risk of lymphopenia and bleeding tendency.

Appropriate health care ■ Behavioural control and techniques to allay anxiety are essential in patients with untreated hyperthyroidism. ■ Definitive dental treatment should be delayed until the patient has been rendered euthyroid.

Pain and anxiety control **Local anaesthesia** The risks of giving epinephrine-containing LA in moderate amounts are more theoretical than real. If there is concern, prilocaine with felypressin can be given, but is not known to be safer. **Conscious sedation** ■ Sedation is desirable since anxiety may precipitate a thyroid crisis ■ Nitrous oxide, which is rapidly controllable, is probably safest for dental sedation ■ Benzodiazepines may potentiate antithyroid drugs and are thus contraindicated ■ Antihistamines such as hydroxyzine may also be useful. **General anaesthesia** ■ The hyperthyroid patient is especially at risk from GA because of the risk of precipitating dangerous arrhythmias ■ After hyperthyroidism treatment, the patient is at risk from hypothyroidism – this must be borne in mind if a GA is required.

Drug use ■ Benzodiazepines should be avoided. ■ Povidone-iodine and similar compounds are best avoided (iodine is taken up by the thyroid).

Further reading
● Biron C R 1996 Patients with thyroid dysfunctions require risk management before dental procedures. RDH 16:42–44, 60 ● Gortzak R A, Asscheman H 1996 Hyperthyroidism and dental treatment. Ned Tijdschr Tandheelkd 103:511–513.

Table 3.81 Key considerations for dental management in hyperthyroidism (see text)

	Management modifications*	Comments/possible complications
Risk assessment	2	Thyroid storm; fainting; possibly lymphopenia and bleeding tendency
Appropriate dental care	2	Behaviour control; delay elective dental treatment until the patient rendered euthyroid
Pain and anxiety control		
– Local anaesthesia	1	Reduce epinephrine dose
– Conscious sedation	1	Avoid benzodiazepines
– General anaesthesia	3/4	Arrhythmias
Patient access and positioning		
– Access to dental office	0	
– Timing of treatment	0	
– Patient positioning	0	
Treatment modification		
– Oral surgery	2	
– Implantology	2	
– Conservative/Endodontics	1	
– Fixed prosthetics	1	
– Removable prosthetics	1	
– Non-surgical periodontology	2	
– Surgical periodontology	2	
Imaging	1	Alveolar osteoporosis
Hazardous and contraindicated drugs	2	Avoid benzodiazepines and povidone-iodine

*0 = No special considerations. 1 = Caution advised. 2 = Specialised medical advice recommended in some cases. 3 = Specialised medical advice mandatory. 4 = Only to be performed in hospital environment. 5 = Should be avoided.

HYPOCHONDRIASIS

Definition Hypochondriacal neurosis is an excessive preoccupation with physical symptoms or bodily functions, in which minute details are related incessantly, with fear of disease or strong belief in having disease due to false interpretation of a trivial symptom.

General aspects

Clinical presentation Hypochondriacal neurosis is sometimes referred to as 'illness as a way of life' and features include: ■ the medical history is often presented in great detail ■ absence of organic disease or physiological disturbance ■ unwarranted fear or idea persisting despite reassurances

■ clinically significant distress. Most patients are depressed and some are deluded. Minor degrees of hypochondriasis, however, are common, especially among the elderly.

Diagnosis Diagnosis, in a patient with suggestive clinical manifestations, is made by exclusion of organic disease by physical examination and laboratory results.

Treatment Reassurance and supportive care are needed; antidepressant drugs may help. Unnecessary surgery must be avoided.

Oral findings

The common oral symptoms are: ■ dry or burning mouth ■ disturbed taste ■ oral or facial pain.

Table 3.82 **Key considerations for dental management in hypochondriasis (see text)**

	Management modifications*	Comments/possible complications
Risk assessment	2	Recognition of hypochondriasis
Appropriate dental care	2	Eliminate organic cause for complaints; sympathetic handling; consider psychiatric consultation
Pain and anxiety control		
– Local anaesthesia	1	
– Conscious sedation	1	
– General anaesthesia	3/4	
Patient access and positioning		
– Access to dental office	0	
– Timing of treatment	0	
– Patient positioning	0	
Treatment modification		
– Oral surgery	1	
– Implantology	1/5	Individualised evaluation
– Conservative/Endodontics	1	
– Fixed prosthetics	1	
– Removable prosthetics	1	
– Non-surgical periodontology	1	
– Surgical periodontology	1	
Hazardous and contraindicated drugs	1	Avoid acetaminophen and erythromycin in patients on antidepressants

*0 = No special considerations. 1 = Caution advised. 2 = Specialised medical advice recommended in some cases. 3 = Specialised medical advice mandatory. 4 = Only to be performed in hospital environment. 5 = Should be avoided.

Dental management

Appropriate health care ■ Listen to the patient's story – which may be written in detail ('maladie du petit papier') ■ Eliminate any organic cause ■ Consider a psychiatric consultation.

Pain and anxiety control **Local anaesthesia** LA should be undertaken with caution in view of the patient's propensity to display symptoms. **Conscious sedation** Conscious sedation should be undertaken with caution in view of the patient's propensity to display symptoms. **General anaesthesia** Caution must be exercised, and advice obtained from the patient's medical practitioner, to ensure that the patient is not undergoing a GA, with all the risks involved, needlessly.

Further reading ● Boning J 1990 Psychosomatic and psychopathological aspects in dental-orofacial medicine with special reference to old age. Z Gerontol 23:318–321 ● Macfarlane T V, Kincey J, Worthington H V 2002 The association between psychological factors and oro-facial pain: a community-based study. Eur J Pain 6:427–434 ● Scully C 1993 La maladie du petit papier. Br Dent J 175:289–292 ● Weiner A A, Sheehan D V 1988 Differentiating anxiety-panic disorders from psychologic dental anxiety. Dent Clin North Am 32:823–840.

HYPOPARATHYROIDISM

Definition ■ Hypoparathyroidism is parathyroid hormone (PTH) underproduction ■ This leads to hypocalcaemia and hyperphosphataemia, with an increase in muscular contractility.

General aspects

Aetiopathogenesis ■ The most frequent cause of hypoparathyroidism is thyroidectomy, but this is relatively transient and resolves when the remaining parathyroid tissue undergoes compensatory hyperplasia ■ Rare cases of idiopathic hypoparathyroidism are congenital (e.g. DiGeorge or CATCH 22 syndrome).

Clinical presentation ■ Low plasma calcium leads to muscle and nerve irritability: ● tetany is the classical feature (Fig. 3.23), with facial twitching (Chvostek's sign – contracture of the facial muscles upon tapping over the facial nerve) ● carpopedal spasms (Trousseau's sign; contracture of the hand and fingers [main d'accoucheur – obstetrician's hand] on occluding the arm with a cuff) ● numbness and tingling of arms and legs ● laryngeal stridor ■ Rare cases of idiopathic (congenital) hypoparathyroidism may be associated with CATCH 22, and other endocrine defects, especially hypoadrenocorticism. Multiple autoantibodies may be present. Features include: ● cataracts ● calcification of the basal ganglia ● oral changes/defects of the teeth (see later) ● occasionally, chronic mucocutaneous candidosis. ■ Pseudohypoparathyroidism, characterised by normal or raised PTH secretion but unresponsive tissue receptors, has clinical features similar to

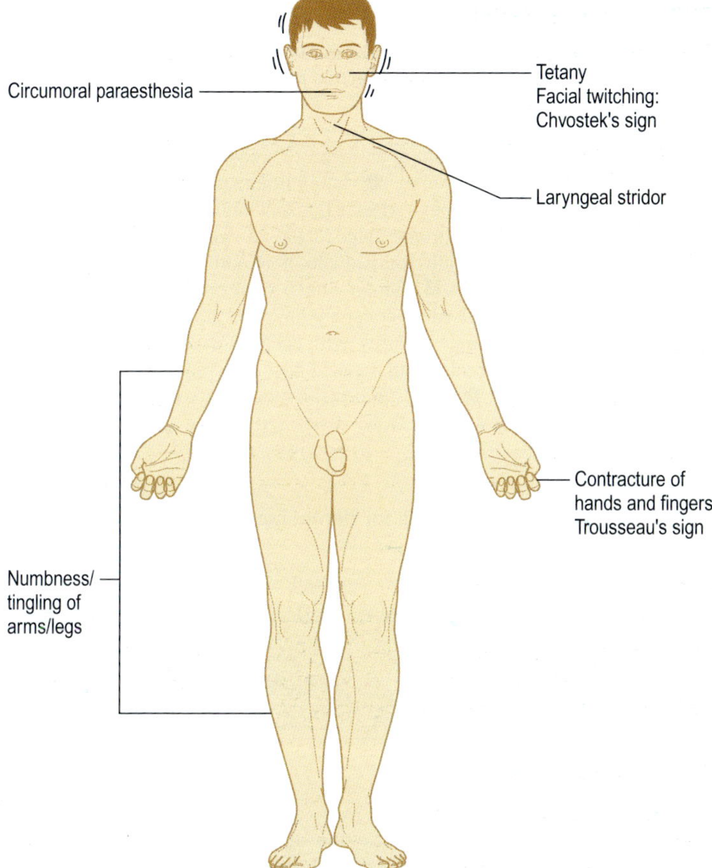

Figure 3.23 **Clinical features of hypoparathyroidism**

idiopathic hypoparathyroidism. A similar appearance in patients with normal biochemistry is termed pseudo-pseudohypoparathyroidism: ● patients have a liability to develop cataracts ● they are short in stature and have small fingers and toes ● no dental defects are present.

Diagnosis ■ Blood analysis: ● plasma calcium – reduced ● plasma phosphate – raised ● PTH stimulation test – reduced response.

Treatment ■ Replacement therapy includes vitamin D and calcium supplements ■ A low phosphate diet is recommended.

Prognosis Severe complications include seizures, cardiac arrhythmia and bronchospasm.

Oral findings

■ Oral manifestations seen in idiopathic (congenital) hypoparathyroidism may include: ● enamel hypoplasia (which predisposes to caries) ● shortened roots ● dentine dysplasia ● delayed eruption ● impacted teeth ● hypodontia ● mandibular exostosis ■ Chronic mucocutaneous candidosis which can be resistant to antimycotic treatment may be seen in candida-endocrinopathy syndrome ■ **A**utoimmune **p**oly**e**ndocrinopathy-**c**andidosis-**e**ctodermal **d**ystrophy (APECED) is an autosomal recessive disease which presents with chronic mucocutaneous candidosis and dental abnormalities due to hypoparathyroidism and often adrenocortical and gonadal failure are common ■ Sanjad–Sakati syndrome is an autosomal recessive disorder characterised by congenital hypoparathyroidism, severe growth failure and dysmorphic features, with deep set eyes, microcephaly, thin lips, depressed nasal bridge with beaked nose, external ear anomalies and learning difficulties ■ In postpubertal hypoparathyroidism there may be: ● circumoral paraesthesia ● Chvostek's sign.

Table 3.83 **Key considerations for dental management in hypoparathyroidism (see text)**

	Management modifications*	Comments/possible complications
Risk assessment	2	Tetany; seizures; psychiatric problems; endocrinopathies; arrhythmias
Appropriate dental care	2–4	Influenced by calcium levels
Pain and anxiety control		
– Local anaesthesia	1	
– Conscious sedation	1	
– General anaesthesia	3/4	
Patient access and positioning		
– Access to dental office	0	
– Timing of treatment	0	
– Patient positioning	0	
Treatment modification		
– Oral surgery	1	
– Implantology	1	Poor osseointegration?
– Conservative/Endodontics	1	
– Fixed prosthetics	1	
– Removable prosthetics	1	
– Non-surgical periodontology	1	
– Surgical periodontology	1	
Hazardous and contraindicated drugs	0	

*0 = No special considerations. 1 = Caution advised. 2 = Specialised medical advice recommended in some cases. 3 = Specialised medical advice mandatory. 4 = Only to be performed in hospital environment. 5 = Should be avoided.

Dental management

Risk assessment Dental management may be complicated by:
- tetany
- seizures
- psychiatric problems or learning disability
- hypoadrenocorticism, diabetes mellitus or other endocrinopathies
- arrhythmias
- there may be facial paraesthesia and Chvostek's sign.

Appropriate health care ■ Patients with calcium levels below 8 mg/100 mL should be treated in a hospital environment and receive only emergency dental care ■ Patients whose calcium hypoparathyroidism is controlled may receive routine dental care.

Pain and anxiety control **Local anaesthesia** LA should be undertaken with caution in view of the systemic complications of hypoparathyroidism. **Conscious sedation** Conscious sedation should be undertaken with caution in view of the systemic complications of hypoparathyroidism, particularly laryngeal stridor. **General anaesthesia** GA should be undertaken with caution in view of the systemic complications of hypoparathyroidism and specialist advice from the patient's physician should be sought.

Further reading
• Ahonen P, Myllarniemi S, Sipila I, Perheentupa J 1990 Clinical variation of autoimmune polyendocrinopathy-candidiasis-ectodermal dystrophy (APECED) in a series of 68 patients. N Engl J Med 322:1829–1836
• Al-Malik M I 2004 The dentofacial features of Sanjad–Sakati syndrome: a case report. Int J Paediatr Dent 14:136–140
• Porter S R, Eveson J W, Scully C 1995 Enamel hypoplasia secondary to candidiasis endocrinopathy syndrome: case report. Pediatr Dent 17:216–219
• Porter S R, Scully C 1986 Candidosis endocrinopathy syndrome. Oral Surg Oral Med Oral Pathol 61:573–578
• Walls A W, Soames J V 1993 Dental manifestations of autoimmune hypoparathyroidism. Oral Surg Oral Med Oral Pathol 75:452–454.

HYPOPITUITARISM (DWARFISM)

Definition Hypopituitarism is defined as a complete or partial loss of production of the anterior pituitary hormones:
- adrenocorticotrophic hormone (ACTH)
- follicle-stimulating hormone (FSH)
- luteinising hormone (LH)
- prolactin
- growth hormone (GH)
- thyroid stimulating hormone (TSH)
- melanocyte-stimulating hormone (MSH).

General aspects

Aetiopathogenesis ■ Main cause is pituitary surgery or irradiation ■ Rarer causes include disease in/around pituitary: • tumours (craniopharyngioma) • infections • trauma • haemorrhage.

Clinical presentation ■ Weakness, weight loss, hypotension (from lack of ACTH) ■ Oligomenorrhoea, loss of libido, infertility, hypogonadism (FSH, LH, prolactin) ■ Obesity, weakness (GH) ■ Constipation, mood change (TSH) (Fig. 3.24).

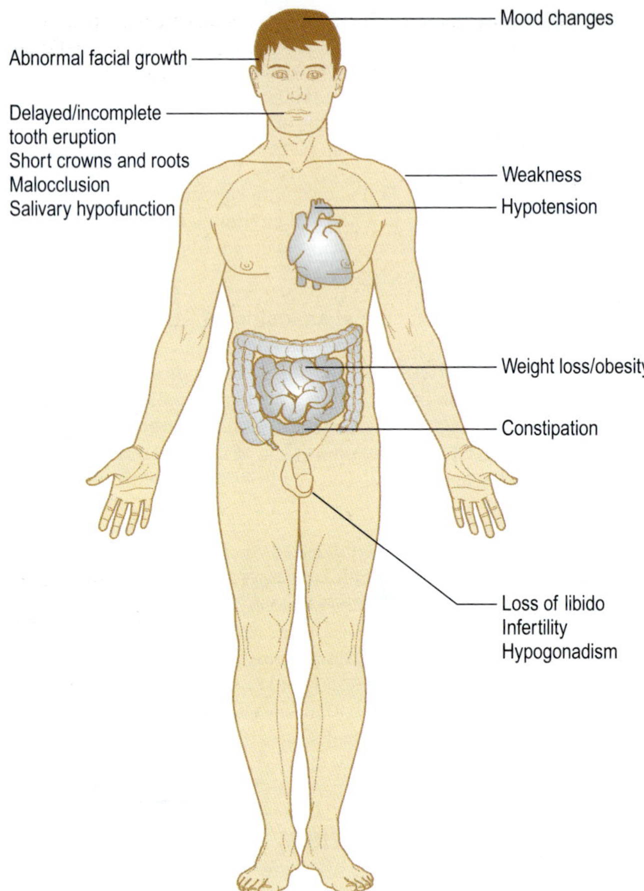

Figure 3.24 **Hyopopituitarism**

Diagnosis ■ Hormone assays and stimulation tests ■ CT/MRI.

Treatment Hormone replacement.

Oral findings

■ Abnormal facial growth: lean, with facial widths, facial heights and mandibular size significantly smaller than in controls ■ Delayed and incomplete tooth eruption ■ Short tooth crowns and roots ■ Crowding and malocclusion ■ Salivary hypofunction (increased risk of caries and periodontal disease) ■ Johanson–Blizzard syndrome is a rare autosomal recessive disorder characterised by aplasia of the alae nasi, aplasia cutis, dental anomalies, postnatal growth retardation and pancreatic exocrine aplasia. Endocrinological dysfunctions, such as growth hormone deficiency, hypothyroidism, and diabetes mellitus, complicate this syndrome.

Dental management

Risk assessment ■ Patients are at risk from adrenal crisis and hypopituitary coma ■ The management of hypopituitary coma includes:
● 200 mg hydrocortisone sodium succinate (IV) ● oxygen by face mask
● call for medical assistance.

Pain and anxiety control **Local anaesthesia** LA should be undertaken with caution in view of the multiple systemic complications of hypopituitarism. **Conscious sedation** Sedatives should be avoided in view of the multiple systemic complications of hypopituitarism, and the risk of respiratory depression. Where unavoidable, conscious sedation should only be undertaken with specialist advice. **General anaesthesia** GA should be avoided if at all possible, in view of the multiple systemic complications of

Table 3.84 **Key considerations for dental management in hypopituitarism (see text)**

	Management modifications*	Comments/possible complications
Risk assessment	2	Adrenal crisis; hypopituitary coma
Appropriate dental care	2	
Pain and anxiety control		
– Local anaesthesia	1	
– Conscious sedation	3/4	Avoid sedatives
– General anaesthesia	3/4	Hypopituitary coma
Patient access and positioning		
– Access to dental office	0	
– Timing of treatment	0	
– Patient positioning	1	Postural hypotension
Treatment modification		
– Oral surgery	1	
– Implantology	1	
– Conservative/Endodontics	1	
– Fixed prosthetics	1	
– Removable prosthetics	1	
– Non-surgical periodontology	1	Frequent recall
– Surgical periodontology	1	
– Orthodontics	1	Early treatment
– Paediatric dentistry	1	Fluoride supplement
Hazardous and contraindicated drugs	1	Some patients are on corticosteroids

*0 = No special considerations. 1 = Caution advised. 2 = Specialised medical advice recommended in some cases. 3 = Specialised medical advice mandatory. 4 = Only to be performed in hospital environment. 5 = Should be avoided.

hypopituitarism, and the risk of hypopituitary coma, which can be precipitated by sedatives or hypnotics or GA.

Patient access and positioning **Patient positioning** The patient is at risk of postural hypotension, and thus best not treated supine.

Treatment modification **Periodontology** Frequent recall is important in patients with dental crowding and salivary hypofunction. **Orthodontics** Early orthopaedic and orthodontic treatment of malocclusion, often related to small dental arches, has been recommended. **Paediatric dentistry** Dietary control and fluoride supplement is mandatory in patients with hyposalivation.

Drug use Some patients with hypoadrenalism are on corticosteroids.

Further reading ● Kjellberg H, Beiring M, Albertsson Wikland K 2000 Craniofacial morphology, dental occlusion, tooth eruption, and dental maturity in boys of short stature with or without growth hormone deficiency. Eur J Oral Sci 108:359–367 ● Krekmanova L, Carlstedt-Duke J, Marcus C, Dahllof G 1999 Dental maturity in children of short stature – a two-year longitudinal study of growth hormone substitution. Acta Odontol Scand 57:93–96 ● Pirinen S, Majurin A, Lenko H L, Koski K 1994 Craniofacial features in patients with deficient and excessive growth hormone. J Craniofac Genet Dev Biol 14:144–152.

HYPOTHYROIDISM

Definition Hypothyroidism is a deficiency of thyroid hormone. In infants and young children it is called cretinism whereas in the adult it is termed myxoedema.

General aspects

Aetiopathogenesis The most common causes of thyroid underactivity include: ■ previous treatment of thyroid disease (surgery or radiotherapy) ■ spontaneous primary thyroid atrophy (autoimmune) ■ drugs (e.g. amiodarone, lithium).

Clinical presentation ■ Usual findings in cretinism include: ● somnolence ● hypothermia ● feeding problems ● delayed physical and mental development ■ Common signs and symptoms of hypothyroidism: ● weight gain ● dislike of cold ● tiredness/lethargy ● constipation ● hoarse voice ● depression/dementia ● bradycardia ■ Other associated features: ● hypotension and hypoadrenocorticism may be associated with hypothyroidism, leading to a diminished cardiac output and bradycardia ● anaemia or ischaemic heart disease are often complications ● occasional additional problems include acquired von Willebrand disease, hypopituitarism and other autoimmune disorders such as Sjögren's syndrome.

Diagnosis ■ Serum T4 – low ■ Serum TSH – usually raised ■ Thyroid autoantibodies.

Treatment Thyroxine (thyroid hormone replacement).

Prognosis ■ Delay in cretinism diagnosis may result in cerebral deficits ■ Without treatment the hyperthyroid patient can progress to myxoedematous coma (heart failure, hypoventilation, hypothermia, seizures and lack of consciousness).

Oral findings

■ Oral findings in cretinism are common: • large and protruded tongue • swollen lips • enamel hypoplasia • delayed eruption • mouth breathing • mandibular retrusion and malocclusion (Angle class II) ■ Oral findings in myxoedema are often related to mucoprotein accumulation and include: • enlarged tongue • thick lips • mouth breathing • gingivitis and rampant caries are not unusual • husky voice.

Dental management

Risk assessment ■ The main danger is of precipitating myxoedematous coma by the use of sedatives (including diazepam or midazolam), opioid analgesics (including codeine), and other tranquillisers or general anaesthetics – these should therefore either be avoided or given in low dose ■ Myxoedematous coma may also be precipitated by stress, infection or traumatic surgery, especially in the elderly ■ The presence of any associated disorders such as hypotension or hypoadrenocorticism may further complicate management.

Appropriate health care Definitive dental treatment should be delayed until the patient has been rendered euthyroid.

Preventive dentistry Caries and periodontal disease prophylaxis are mandatory to prevent the consequences of mouth breathing and gingival swelling.

Pain and anxiety control **Local anaesthesia** Local anaesthesia is preferable to GA. **Conscious sedation** The respiratory centre in hypothyroidism is hypersensitive to drugs such as opioids or sedatives. Nitrous oxide, which is rapidly controllable, is probably safer than benzodiazepines for sedation. **General anaesthesia** GA, if unavoidable, should be delayed if possible until thyroxine has been started.

Treatment modification **Orthodontics** Early orthodontic evaluation to prevent malocclusion is mandatory.

Drug use Benzodiazepines and opioids are best avoided. Povidone-iodine and similar compounds are best avoided.

Further reading • Attard N J, Zarb G A 2002 A study of dental implants in medically treated hypothyroid patients. Clin Implant Dent Relat Res 4:220–231 • Attivissimo L A, Lichtman S M, Klein I 1995 Acquired von Willebrand's syndrome causing a hemorrhagic diathesis in a patient with hypothyroidism. Thyroid 5:399–401 • August M, Wang J, Plante D, Wang C C 1996 Complications associated with therapeutic neck radiation. J Oral Maxillofac Surg 54:1409–1415 • Biron C R 1996 Patients with thyroid dysfunctions require risk management before dental procedures. RDH 16:42–44, 60.

Table 3.85 **Key considerations for dental management in hypothyroidism (see text)**

	Management modifications*	Comments/possible complications
Risk assessment	2	Myxoedematous coma; hypotension; anaemia; ischaemic heart disease
Appropriate dental care	2	Delay elective dental treatment until the patient rendered euthyroid
Pain and anxiety control		
– Local anaesthesia	1	
– Conscious sedation	1	Avoid benzodiazepines and opioids
– General anaesthesia	3/4	
Patient access and positioning		
– Access to dental office	0	
– Timing of treatment	0	
– Patient positioning	0	
Treatment modification		
– Oral surgery	2	Rarely, acquired von Willebrand disease can cause bleeding tendency
– Implantology	2	
– Conservative/Endodontics	1	
– Fixed prosthetics	1	
– Removable prosthetics	1	
– Non-surgical periodontology	2	
– Surgical periodontology	2	
Hazardous and contraindicated drugs	2	Avoid benzodiazepines, opioids and povidone-iodine

*0 = No special considerations. 1 = Caution advised. 2 = Specialised medical advice recommended in some cases. 3 = Specialised medical advice mandatory. 4 = Only to be performed in hospital environment. 5 = Should be avoided.

IMMUNODEFICIENCIES (PRIMARY)

Definition Primary immunodeficiencies are a group of rare congenital immune system defects that result in an increased susceptibility to infections.

General aspects

Aetiopathogenesis Primary immune deficiencies are genetically determined or the result of development anomalies.

Classification Primary immunodeficiencies are classified based on the predominant immune defect: B cell defects, T and B cell defects, complement and phagocyte defects (Box 3.17).

Clinical presentation ■ B lymphocyte deficiency results mainly in: ● recurrent pyogenic infections involving inner ear, respiratory tract and skin – pneumococci, meningococci and *Haemophilus influenzae* are often responsible ● eczema and allergies ● increased incidence of malignancies, particularly lymphomas ■ T lymphocyte deficiency results mainly in: ● serious or life-threatening fungal, viral and mycobacterial infections within the first months of life, especially pneumonia, meningitis, and sepsis ● viral infections such as herpes simplex and cytomegalovirus ● fungal infections, especially by *Candida* spp ■ Complement deficiencies

Box 3.17 Main categories of primary immunodeficiencies

Predominant B cell defects
- IgA deficiency (the most common primary immune defect)
- Transient hypogammaglobulinaemia of infancy
- X-linked infantile hypogammaglobulinaemia (XLA: Bruton syndrome)
- Non-X-linked hyper IgM syndrome
- X-linked hyper IgM syndrome
- Common variable immunodeficiency
- Hypogammaglobulinaemia after intrauterine viral infections, e.g. rubella
- Wiskott–Aldrich syndrome
- IgG2 subclass deficiency

T and B cell defects
- Congenital thymic aplasia (Di George syndrome)
- Severe combined immunodeficiency
- Deficiencies of MHC class II, CD3, ZAP-70 or TAP-2
- Immunodeficiency with ataxia telangiectasia
- Late onset immunodeficiency

Complement deficiencies
- Complement deficiencies C1, C2 or C4
- C1, C3 or C5 deficiencies
- C1 esterase inhibitor deficiency

Granulocyte defects
- Interferon-gamma receptor (IFNGR) deficiency
- Cyclical neutropenia
- Chronic granulomatous disease
- Myeloperoxidase deficiency
- Chediak–Higashi syndrome
- Leucocyte adhesion defect (LAD) 1
- LAD defect 2
- Papillon–Lefevre syndrome
- Job's syndrome
- Hyperimmunoglobulinaemia E (HIE)
- Glycogen storage disease b
- Schwachman syndrome (lazy leucocyte syndrome)

result mainly in: ● autoimmune disease, especially lupus erythematosus ● increased susceptibility to meningococcal and gonococcal infections ● swelling of face and neck and airway obstruction in hereditary angio-oedema only ■ Granulocyte defects result mainly in: ● bacterial respiratory and skin infections, especially by *Staphylococcus aureus*, *Pseudomonas* spp and *Serratia* spp ● lymph node and hepatic bacterial abscesses ● fungal infections by *Candida* spp and *Aspergillus*.

Diagnosis ■ Recurrent or severe infections ■ Full blood picture ■ Lymphocyte count ■ T and B lymphocyte count and subtypes ■ Specific serum immunoglobulins and antibody profile ■ Delayed hypersensitivity skin tests ■ Levels and activity of serum complement fractions.

Treatment ■ B cell defects: gammaglobulin (contraindicated in IgA deficiency) ■ T cell defect: fetal thymus transplantation ■ T and B cell defects: bone marrow transplantation ■ Granulocyte defects: granulocyte colony stimulating factor (G-CSF).

Prognosis Severe primary immune deficiencies cause early death, usually from pneumonia.

Oral findings

■ B cell defects: ● sinusitis ● cervical lymph node enlargement ● enlarged tonsils ● oral ulcers ● enamel hypoplasia ■ T and B cell defects: ● sinusitis ● oral ulcers ● chronic candidosis ● herpetic infections ■ Complement deficiency: ● facial swelling in C1 esterase deficiency (hereditary angio-oedema) ■ Granulocyte defects: ● cervical lymph node enlargement ● oral ulcers ● chronic candidosis ● enamel hypoplasia ● periodontitis.

Dental management

Risk assessment Medical consultation is recommended before any dental procedure to discuss: ■ general health status and prognosis ■ drug intake and potential drug interactions ■ most appropriate time and location where dental treatment should be carried out ■ need for antimicrobial prophylaxis.

Appropriate health care Although local policies/advice from the responsible physician may vary, in general: ■ no dental operative treatment should be performed in patients with serum gamma-globulin levels below 20 mg/100 mL ■ antibiotic prophylaxis is indicated before any operative procedure likely to be associated with bleeding in patients with neutrophil counts between 500 and 1000 cells/mL ■ patients with neutrophil counts < 500 cells/mL should be treated in a hospital environment.

Pain and anxiety control **Local anaesthesia** LA should be undertaken with caution. A preoperative rinse for one minute with chlorhexidine mouthwash (0.2%) is advisable. **Conscious sedation** Conscious sedation should be undertaken with caution. It must be ensured that respiratory function is not compromised by concurrent infection, prior to the administration of sedative agents. **General anaesthesia** GA should be undertaken with caution in view of the systemic complications of immunosuppression and the increased risk of perioperative morbidity. Specialist advice from the patient's physician should be sought.

Preventive dentistry Instructing patients (and their families) in oral hygiene, use of antimicrobial rinses and regular plaque control is the mainstay of dental management to reduce oral infections.

Treatment modification **Surgery** ■ Patients with gamma-globulin deficiency need a 100–200 mg/kg dose (intramuscular) of immune globulin

Table 3.86 **Key considerations for dental management in primary immunodeficiencies (see text)**

	Management modifications*	Comments/possible complications
Risk assessment	3	Evaluate general health status, prognosis, drug intake, and appropriate location for dental treatment
Appropriate dental care	3/4	Delay elective dental care with gamma-globulin levels < 20 mg/100 mL; possibly antibiotic prophylaxis
Pain and anxiety control		
– Local anaesthesia	1	Chlorhexidine rinse
– Conscious sedation	1	Pulmonary function
– General anaesthesia	3/4	
Patient access and positioning		
– Access to dental office	1	
– Timing of treatment	2	
– Patient positioning	1	
Treatment modification		
– Oral surgery	3/4	Immune globulin supplementation; chlorhexidine; antibiotic cover; possibly G-CSF
– Implantology	3–5	See oral surgery
– Conservative/Endodontics	3	
– Fixed prosthetics	3	
– Removable prosthetics	3	
– Non-surgical periodontology	3–5	
– Surgical periodontology	3–5	
Hazardous and contraindicated drugs	2	Antibiotic resistance

*0 = No special considerations. 1 = Caution advised. 2 = Specialised medical advice recommended in some cases. 3 = Specialised medical advice mandatory. 4 = Only to be performed in hospital environment. 5 = Should be avoided.

the day before surgery ■ Chlorhexidine mouthwashes are recommended pre- and postoperatively ■ Oral surgery, periodontal scaling and implant insertion have successfully been performed in neutropenic patients after G-CSF therapy (0.5 × 10^6 U/kg/day). **Drug use** ■ Penicillins are the antibiotics of choice (macrolides in penicillin-allergic patients) ■ In bacterial infections resistant to therapy, an antibiotic susceptibility test is mandatory ■ Oral candidosis is best treated with nystatin, fluconazole or itraconazole ■ Herpes simplex infections can be treated with aciclovir or valaciclovir.

Further reading ● Diz Dios P, Ocampo Hermida A, Fernández Feijoo J 2002 Alteraciones cuantitativas y funcionales de los neutrófilos. Medicina Oral 7:206–221 ● Porter S R, Scully C 1993 Orofacial manifestations in primary immunodeficiencies involving IgA deficiency. J Oral Pathol Med 22: 117–119 ● Porter S R, Scully C 1993 Orofacial manifestations in primary immunodeficiencies: T lymphocyte defects. J Oral Pathol Med 22:308–309 ● Porter S R, Scully C 1993 Orofacial manifestations in primary immunodeficiencies: polymorphonuclear leucocyte defects. J Oral Pathol Med 22:310–311 ● Scully C, Porter S R 1993 Orofacial manifestations in primary immunodeficiencies: common variable immunodeficiencies. J Oral Pathol Med 22:157–158.

IMMUNOSUPPRESSIVE TREATMENT

Definition ■ Following organ or bone marrow transplantation, all patients are placed on immunosuppressive drugs to prevent rejection ■ The goals of immunosuppressive therapy are to: ● prevent acute or chronic rejection ● minimise drug toxicity ● minimise rates of infection and malignancy ● achieve the highest possible rates of patient and graft survival ■ These medications are usually started in the operating room and are continued thereafter ■ The current high graft survival rate follows the introduction of effective immunosuppression with azathioprine, ciclosporin, OKT3 monoclonal antibodies, daclizumab, and immunosuppressives such as mycophenolate mofetil ■ The advent of newer immunosuppressants, such as tacrolimus and interleukin (IL)-2 receptor blockers, has paved the way for further growth in this field.

General aspects

Mechanism of action ■ The actions of immunosuppressive drugs are complex and by no means fully understood, but most of them predominantly affect cell-mediated responses and autoantibody production more strongly than normal antibody production ■ Others, such as azathioprine, cyclophosphamide and chlorambucil, are cytotoxic to a range of cells, including some immunocytes, so they are far less specific.

Classification Two broad groups of immunosuppressive agents exist: intravenous induction/anti-rejection agents and maintenance immunotherapy agents. **Induction immunotherapy** This consists of intensive treatment with potent intravenous drugs, such as OKT3, for several days after transplantation. It is not commonly used after transplantation, although the recent introduction of the newer IL-2 receptor-blocking antibody preparations, daclizumab and basiliximab, may change this approach in the future.

Maintenance immunosuppression This is usually based on a calcineurin inhibitor (i.e. ciclosporin or tacrolimus), sirolimus, and/or corticosteroids. These are sometimes combined with newer antimetabolites (e.g. mycophenolate mofetil) or antiproliferative agents (e.g. rapamycin) with the goal of decreasing corticosteroid and/or calcineurin inhibitor use. ■ *Ciclosporin* is a highly lipid-soluble drug that is metabolised in the liver by cytochrome P-450 enzymes (CYP3A4). Inhibitors of the cytochrome P-450 hepatic microsomal enzyme system increase or decrease its clearance. ■ *Tacrolimus* is a macrolide antibiotic similar to ciclosporin. It inhibits IL-2, interferon- gamma, and IL-3 production; transferrin and IL-2 receptor expression; mixed lymphocyte reactions; and cytotoxic T generation. Tacrolimus is metabolised by the same cytochrome P-450 system as ciclosporin. ■ *Sirolimus* is a non-calcineurin inhibiting immunosuppressant that inhibits lymphocyte proliferation ■ *Corticosteroids* may decrease inflammation by reversing increased capillary permeability and suppressing PMN activity ■ *Azathioprine* is metabolised by the enzyme thiopurine methyl transferase (TPMT) to mercaptopurine, which acts as purine analogue that interacts with DNA and inhibits lymphocyte cell division, and may cause myelosuppression and hepatotoxicity ■ *Mycophenolate mofetil* is a second-line immunosuppressive agent that may be used as an alternative to azathioprine in solid organ transplantation, acting via selective inhibition of T and B cell proliferation.

Complications ■ Immunosuppressive therapy results in patients being significantly immunocompromised and at risk from infections, particularly viral, fungal, mycobacterial and protozoal ■ Drug toxicity is common: ● the most important toxicities are related to corticosteroids ● azathioprine increases the risk of myelosuppression ● ciclosporin toxicity can manifest with hypertension, tremor, hypertrichosis, gingival swelling, hepatotoxicity, and nephrotoxicity with hyperkalaemia and/or renal tubular acidosis ● tacrolimus toxicity manifests as nephrotoxicity, neurotoxicity, cardiomyopathy and hyperglycaemia ● sirolimus may cause hyperlipidaemia ● rapamycin has been associated with cytopenias and hyperlipidaemia ■ Immunosuppressed patients are also liable to neoplasms, at least some of which are virally-related: Kaposi's sarcoma (HHV-8), lymphomas (EBV) and squamous cell carcinomas of the skin, anogenital region and the lip (HPV).

Oral findings

■ Oral candidosis may be persistent in the immunosuppressed patient. Topical antifungal preparations of nystatin, amphotericin or miconazole are usually effective where there is no evidence of disseminated spread. ■ Viral infections such as herpes simplex or zoster, cytomegalovirus, and Epstein–Barr virus can be prevented, deferred or ameliorated by prophylactic low dose antivirals. Carriage of hepatitis viruses is common, and patients should be kept away from sources of infection. ■ Oral bacteria are an important source of bacteraemias. Rarely dental infections may spread, with serious complications such as cavernous sinus thrombosis or metastatic infections. Mixed bacterial plaques may develop on the oral mucosa, which may respond to the appropriate antibiotic and possibly to an aqueous chlorhexidine (0.2%) mouthwash. Some patients carry enterococci in these plaques. ■ Routine cancer surveillance is mandatory to assure rapid diagnosis and treatment of any malignancy ■ Ciclosporin may cause gingival swelling.

Dental management

Risk assessment In patients who are iatrogenically immunosuppressed, there is an increased risk of oral infections and extra-oral bacterial spread.

Appropriate health care A medical consultation is mandatory before invasive procedures, but only severely immunosuppressed patients need be treated in a hospital. There may be a need for antimicrobial prophylaxis.

Pain and anxiety control **Local anaesthesia** LA should be undertaken with caution. A preoperative rinse for one minute with chlorhexidine mouthwash (0.2%) is advisable. **Conscious sedation** Conscious sedation should be undertaken with caution. It must be ensured that respiratory function is not compromised by concurrent infection, prior to the administration of sedative agents. Benzodiazepines (e.g. diazepam) have been successfully administered in patients on immunosuppressive therapy. **General anaesthesia** GA should be undertaken with caution in view of the systemic complications of immunosuppression and the increased risk of perioperative morbidity. Specialist advice from the patient's physician should be sought.

Preventive dentistry Instructing the patient in oral hygiene, use of antimicrobial rinses and early elimination of any oral infection is the mainstay of dental management.

Treatment modification **Surgery** Medical advice is mandatory. Although the British Society for Antimicrobial Chemotherapy (BSAC) does not recommend antimicrobial cover for immunosuppressed patients (in contrast to AHA), it is advisable to discuss the planned procedure and need for antimicrobials with the patient's specialist physician. Some patients may need steroid cover.

Drug use ■ Ciclosporin levels/toxicity may alter with drugs such as: carbamazepine, isoniazid, itraconazole, ketoconazole, fluconazole, amphotericin B, azithromycin, erythromycin, aminoglycosides, clarithromycin and aciclovir ■ Tacrolimus levels/toxicity may increase with clotrimazole, itraconazole, ketoconazole, fluconazole, erythromycin, clarithromycin and methylprednisolone. Tacrolimus levels may decrease with carbamazepine.

Further reading ● Akintoye S O, Brennan M T, Graber C J et al 2002 A retrospective investigation of advanced periodontal disease as a risk factor for septicaemia in hematopoietic stem cell and bone marrow transplant recipients. Oral Surg Oral Med Oral Pathol Oral Radiol Endod 94:581–588 ● Papas A S, Clark R E, Martuscelli G, O'Loughlin K T,

Table 3.87 **Key considerations for dental management in immunosuppressive treatment (see text)**

	Management modifications*	Comments/possible complications
Risk assessment	3	Oral and extraoral infections
Appropriate dental care	3/4	Consider antimicrobial prophylaxis and steroid cover
Pain and anxiety control		
– Local anaesthesia	1	Chlorhexidine rinse
– Conscious sedation	1	Respiratory function
– General anaesthesia	3/4	
Patient access and positioning		
– Access to dental office	0	
– Timing of treatment	0	
– Patient positioning	0	
Treatment modification		
– Oral surgery	3/4	Chlorhexidine; antibiotic cover
– Implantology	3/4	
– Conservative/Endodontics	2	
– Fixed prosthetics	2	
– Removable prosthetics	2	
– Non-surgical periodontology	3/4	Chlorhexidine; antibiotic cover
– Surgical periodontology	3/4	
Hazardous and contraindicated drugs	2	Avoid drugs which may increase the immunosuppressive agents' levels/toxicity

*0 = No special considerations. 1 = Caution advised. 2 = Specialised medical advice recommended in some cases. 3 = Specialised medical advice mandatory. 4 = Only to be performed in hospital environment. 5 = Should be avoided.

Johansen E, Miller K B 2003 A prospective, randomised trial for the prevention of mucositis in patients undergoing hematopoietic stem cell transplantation. Bone Marrow Transplant 31:705–712 ● Rolland S L, Seymour R A, Wilkins B S, Parry G, Thomason J M 2004 Post-transplant lymphoproliferative disorders presenting as gingival overgrowth in patients immunosuppressed with ciclosporin. J Clin Periodontol 31:581–585.

INFECTIOUS DISEASES

General aspects

Background ■ Infectious agents are especially important because of the increased risk of cross-infection among immunosuppressed and medically compromised patients ■ To prevent cross-infection, in 1976 the American Dental Association published some recommendations ('universal precautions' – now termed 'standard precautions') which have been periodically modified and updated, especially after the onset of the HIV epidemic, and have been published widely ■ The British Dental Association Advice Sheet A12 on infection control in dentistry, summarises current UK practice ■ The key to using these precautions is *risk assessment*, both of the possible exposure to blood/saliva and body fluids, and the risk of the substance containing harmful organisms. This is in order to protect health care workers and patients from the transmission of blood-borne pathogens and to minimise the spread of infection.

Aetiopathogenesis The microorganisms potentially involved in transmission in health care facilities are mainly bacterial, fungal or viral. Transmission is by direct contact with contaminated mucosa or blood and body secretions, aerosols or air drops, or dental instruments – particularly by percutaneous (needle-stick or sharps) injury.

Clinical presentation Clinical findings related to infections are detailed in Tables 3.89–3.91.

Classification Based on the risk of occupational transmission, a new classification has been proposed which classifies the most common microorganisms into classes I to V (Table 3.88). The diseases caused by prions could represent a new class (VI) due to their resistance to conventional disinfection methods (see Creutzfeldt–Jakob disease).

Diagnosis ■ Clinical findings ■ Specific cultures and microbiological identification.

Treatment Treatment of the main infections that can have implications in dentistry is detailed in Tables 3.89–3.91.

Further reading ● Bedi R, Scully C 2002 Tropical oral health. In: Cook G C, Zumla A (ed) Manson's Tropical diseases, 21st edn. W B Saunders, Edinburgh, p515–531 ● Diz Dios P, Limeres Posse J 2005 Enfermedades infecciosas. Hepatitis. In: Bullón P, Machuca G (eds) La atención odontológica de pacientes médicamente comprometidos. Normon SA, Madrid ● Lavine S R, Drumm J W, Keating L K 2004 Safeguarding the health of dental professionals. J Am Dent Assoc 135:84–89 ● Li R W, Leung K W, Sun F C, Samaranayake L P 2004 Severe Acute Respiratory Syndrome (SARS) and the GDP. Part I: Epidemiology, virology, pathology and general health issues. Br Dent J 97:77–80 ● Limeres Posse J, Tomás Carmona I, Fernández Feijoo J, Martínez Vázquez C, Castro Iglesias A, Diz Dios P 2003 Abscesos cerebrales de origen oral. Rev Neurol 37:201–206 ● Power J 2004 Old bugs and new: classical and emerging pathogens – relevance to dental practice. J Ir Dent Assoc 50:79–80 ● Scott C M, Flint S R 2005 Oral syphilis – re-emergence of an old disease with oral manifestations. Int J Oral Maxillofac Surg 34:58–63.

Table 3.88 **Classes I–V for microorganisms based on the risk of occupational transmission**

Class	Vaccine available	Occupational risk above that in community	Prevalence in the community	Other characteristics	Microorganisms
I	Yes	Virtually none	Low		*Rubella virus* *Measles virus* *Clostridium tetani* *Corynebacterium diphtheriae* *Poliovirus* *Influenza virus*
II	No	Low	Low		*Neisseria gonorrhoeae* *Treponema pallidum* *Staphylococcus* spp *Streptococcus* spp *Candida* spp
III	No	Yes	High		*Herpes simplex* *Varicella zoster* *Cytomegalovirus* *Epstein–Barr* *Herpes 6* *Herpes 7* *Herpes 8*
IV	No (except HBV)	Yes	Low	High morbidity/mortality	*HBV* *HCV* *HIV*
V	No	Yes	Low	Resistant strains; air transmission	*Mycobacterium tuberculosis*

Table 3.89 **Bacterial infections with occasional implications in dentistry**

Infecting organism	Main features	Orofacial lesions	Treatment
Bacillus anthracis	Anthrax	Painful or ulcerated swellings mainly on palate	Penicillin
Brucella melitensis, suis and *abortus*	Brucellosis	Rare infections or cranial nerve palsies	Tetracycline with streptomycin
Clostridium perfringens (Cl. welchii), sporogenes, oedematiens and *septicum*	Gas gangrene	Gas gangrene	Antitoxin Penicillin
Mycobacterium tuberculosis	Tuberculosis	Ulceration	Antibiotics
Mycoplasma hominis and *pneumoniae*	Pneumonia	Rare infections or cranial nerve palsies? Reiter's syndrome	Tetracyclines
Neisseria gonorrhoea	Urethritis (gonorrhoea)	Stomatitis	Penicillin
Neisseria meningitidis	Meningitis	Petechiae Occasionally: herpes labialis Facial palsy	Penicillin
Salmonella typhi, paratyphi, choleraesuis and *enteritidis*	Typhoid and paratyphoid fever	Occasional infections	Co-trimoxazole Ampicillin
Streptococcus pyogenes	Acute pharyngitis Cellulitis Scarlet fever Erysipelas	Peritonsillar abscess Cellulitis Palatal punctiform erythema or petechiae Raspberry tongue	Penicillin
Treponema pallidum	Syphilis	Ulcers or mucous patches	Penicillin

Table 3.90 **Viral infections with occasional implications in dentistry**

Infecting organism	Main features	Orofacial lesions	Treatment
Coxsackie viruses	± rash	Ulcers	Symptomatic
Cytomegalovirus	Glandular fever	Ulcers	Ganciclovir Foscarnet Valganciclovir
ECHO viruses	± rash	Ulcers	Symptomatic
Epstein-Barr virus	Glandular fever	Ulcers Hairy leukoplakia Lymphomas Petechiae	Aciclovir Ganciclovir
Hepatitis viruses	See Hepatitis		
Herpes simplex virus	Stomatitis or genital infection Recurrent lesions at mucocutaneous junctions	Ulcers Ulcers	Aciclovir Penciclovir Aciclovir Valaciclovir
Herpes varicella virus	Chickenpox (varicella) Zoster (shingles)	Ulcers Ulcers	Aciclovir Valaciclovir Famciclovir Valaciclovir
HIV	See HIV/AIDS		
Human herpesvirus-8	Kaposi's sarcoma	Kaposi's sarcoma	Symptomatic
Influenza virus	Respiratory infection	–	Amantadine Oseltamivir Rimantadine Zanamivir
Measles virus	Exanthem	Koplick's spots	Symptomatic
Mumps virus	Sialadenitis	Sialadenitis	Symptomatic
Respiratory syncytial virus	Respiratory infection	–	Symptomatic
Rhinoviruses	Common cold	–	Symptomatic
Rubella virus	Exanthem	Petechiae	Symptomatic

Table 3.91 **Fungal infections with occasional implications in dentistry**

Disease	Organism	Source	Main endemic areas	Main features	Prognosis and treatment*
Aspergillosis	*Aspergillus fumigatus* *Aspergillus flavus* *Aspergillus niger* Others	Ubiquitous	Worldwide	Allergic bronchopulmonary Pulmonary disseminated aspergilloma	Variable
Blastomycosis	*Blastomyces dermatitidis*	Soil	Mississippi and Ohio valleys in USA, Canada, North Africa and Venezuela	Cavitary pulmonary Disseminated Others	Often good, except in disseminated form
Candidosis	*Candida albicans* *Candida tropicalis* *Candida glabrata* *Candida parapsilosis* *Candida krusei* *Candida lusitaniae* *Candida kefyr* *Candida guilliermondii* *Candida dubliniensis*	Ubiquitous	Worldwide	Oral and mucocutaneous lesions	Often good, except in disseminated forms

Table 3.91 **Fungal infections with occasional implications in dentistry—cont'd**

Disease	Organism	Source	Main endemic areas	Main features	Prognosis and treatment*
Coccidioidomycosis	*Coccidiodes immitis*	Soil	Southwestern USA, Mexico, Latin America	Acute pulmonary Disseminated Chronic pulmonary Meningitis	Often good, except in disseminated or meningeal form
Cryptococcosis	*Cryptococcus neoformans*	Soil, pigeon droppings	Worldwide	Pneumonia Meningitis Disseminated Cryptococcoma	Poor in disseminated form
Histoplasmosis	*Histoplasma capsulatum*	Soil, bird and bat droppings	Mississippi and Ohio valleys in USA, Latin America, Africa, India, Far East, Australia	Benign pulmonary Disseminated Chronic pulmonary Cutaneous	Often good, except in disseminated form
Mucormycosis	Mucor, Rhizopus and Absidia	Ubiquitous	Worldwide	Rhinocerebral Pulmonary Gastrointestinal	Variable

Table 3.91 **Fungal infections with occasional implications in dentistry—cont'd**

Disease	Organism	Source	Main endemic areas	Main features	Prognosis and treatment*
Paracoccidioidomycosis (South American blastomycosis)	*Paracoccidioides brasiliensis*	Soil	South America, esp. Brazil	Pulmonary Disseminated	Good in young patients
Pneumocystosis	*Pneumocystis carinii*	Ubiquitous	Worldwide	Pulmonary Disseminated	Variable
Sporotrichosis	*Sporothrix schenkii*	Associated with thorny plants, wood, sphagnum moss	Worldwide	Lymphocutaneous Localised cutaneous Pulmonary Disseminated	Good

*Apart from candidosis, the rest require systemic treatment with fluconazole or another azole (e.g. ketoconazole, miconazole, itraconazole, voriconazole), or amphotericin. Candidosis may respond to topical antifungals (nystatin, amphotericin or an azole).

INHALANT ABUSE

Definition Inhalants are breathable chemical vapours that produce psychoactive effects. Inhalants fall into the following categories: ■ solvents ■ nitrites ■ gases.

General aspects

Pathogenesis When inhalants enter the brain, they are particularly attracted to fatty tissues. Because myelin is a fat, it becomes quickly damaged or even destroyed, interfering with the rapid flow of messages from one nerve to another.

Clinical presentation ■ Findings that may indicate a drug addiction problem are as for amphetamine/LSD/MDMA abuse. However, most solvent abusers are children. ■ Chronic misuse of inhalants can impair memory and concentration and cases of permanent damage to brain, liver or kidneys have been reported ■ Signs of solvent misuse include slurred speech, euphoria, anorexia and a circumoral rash (glue sniffers); jaundice may be seen and the pulse may be irregular ■ Other common signs are: ● breath may smell of acetone or glue ● drug-abuse associated diseases: neuropathies.

Classification The most common inhalants of misuse are shown in Table 3.92.

Adverse effects of solvent abuse **Nitrous oxide** ■ Nitrous oxide induces impaired consciousness with a sense of dissociation and often of exhilaration (laughing gas) ■ Addiction to nitrous oxide, however, is an occupational hazard of anaesthetists and dental staff ■ Chronic misuse of nitrous oxide can lead to interference with vitamin B_{12} metabolism and neuropathy. **Specific chemicals** ■ Respiratory damage, anaemia, lead poisoning and cranial nerve palsies can follow chronic misuse of petrol/gasoline ■ A syndrome of mental handicap, hypotonia, scaphocephaly and high malar bones has also been reported in children of mothers who inhaled petrol during pregnancy (fetal gasoline/petrol syndrome) ■ Hearing

Table 3.92 **Common inhalant drugs of misuse and the possible consequences**

Drug class	Risks from misuse	Examples
Solvents	Liver and kidney damage Respiratory damage	Paint thinners Degreasers Petrol, glues
Nitrites	Blood oxygen depletion	Cyclohexyl, amyl and butyl nitrite
Gases	Neuropathies	Household aerosol propellants Butane Propane Medical anaesthetic gases such as nitrous oxide, halothane, ether and chloroform

loss – toluene (paint sprays, glues, dewaxers) and trichloroethylene (cleaning fluids, correction fluids) ■ Peripheral neuropathies or limb spasms – hexane (glues, gasoline/petrol) and nitrous oxide (whipping cream, gas cylinders) ■ Central nervous system damage – toluene (paint sprays, glues, dewaxers) ■ Bone marrow damage – benzene (gasoline/petrol) ■ Serious but potentially reversible effects include: ● liver and kidney damage – toluene-containing substances and chlorinated hydrocarbons (correction fluids, dry-cleaning fluids) ● blood oxygen depletion – organic nitrites ('poppers', 'bold' and 'rush') and methylene chloride (varnish removers, paint thinners).

Severe adverse effects ■ Inhalant misuse is increasingly common and has led to many deaths of children and young adults (Sudden Sniffing Death Syndrome) ■ Sniffing highly concentrated amounts of the chemicals in solvents or aerosol sprays can directly induce hypoxia, cardiac arrhythmias and sometimes sudden death, liver damage and neurological damage and delusions – this is especially common from the misuse of fluorocarbons and butane-type gases ■ High concentrations of inhalants also cause death from suffocation by displacing oxygen in the lungs and then in the central nervous system so that breathing ceases. Deliberately inhaling from a paper or plastic bag or in a closed area greatly increases the chances of suffocation.

Withdrawal and treatment ■ Toxic chemicals from inhalants stay in the body for weeks. Because of this, when chronic abusers stop using inhalants they may feel the effects of withdrawal for weeks. During withdrawal from inhalants, a person may have: ● excess sweating ● constant headaches ● nervousness ● hand tremors. ■ Inhalant abuse is a difficult form of substance abuse to treat. It is best to recognise and start treatment before the problem becomes a habit. Parents and educators need to be able to recognise the signs of inhalant abuse, especially because most abusers do not seek treatment on their own. ■ Treatment for inhalant abusers is usually long-term, sometimes as long as 2 years. It must address the many social problems most inhalant abusers have and involves: ● support of the child's family ● moving the child away from unhealthy friendships with other abusers ● teaching and fostering better coping skills ● building self-esteem and self-confidence ● helping the child adjust to school or another learning setting.

Oral findings

■ 'Huffer rash' – erythematous 'frost bite' eruption on the face and oral mucosa ■ Oral/airway burns ■ Nausea, vomiting may cause dental erosion ■ Neglected oral hygiene may lead to caries and periodontal disease ■ Many may be smokers, and have signs of this (e.g. staining).

Dental management

Risk assessment ■ Recognition of individuals who may be abusing drugs is critical ■ Behavioural problems or drug interactions may interfere with dental treatment ■ Recognition of the social issues often associated with solvent abuse is essential, to ensure that support is offered and treatment is tailored to the individual.

Table 3.93 **Key considerations for dental management in inhalant abuse (see text)**

	Management modifications*	Comments/possible complications
Risk assessment	2	Drug abuser recognition; abnormal behaviour; drug interactions; associated social issues
Appropriate dental care	2	Control behaviour; appropriate analgesia
Pain and anxiety control		
– Local anaesthesia	2	Painful mucosa
– Conscious sedation	3/4	Avoid opioids
– General anaesthesia	3/4	Avoid halothane, ketamine, suxamethonium, barbiturates and opioids; resistance to GA
Patient access and positioning		
– Access to dental office	0	
– Timing of treatment	1	
– Patient positioning	0	
Treatment modification		
– Oral surgery	1	
– Implantology	1/5	Neglected oral hygiene; periodontitis; heavy smokers
– Conservative/Endodontics	1	
– Fixed prosthetics	1/5	Neglected oral hygiene; heavy smokers
– Removable prosthetics	1	
– Non-surgical periodontology	1	
– Surgical periodontology	1/5	Neglected oral hygiene; heavy smokers
Hazardous and contraindicated drugs	1	Avoid opioids

*0 = No special considerations. 1 = Caution advised. 2 = Specialised medical advice recommended in some cases. 3 = Specialised medical advice mandatory. 4 = Only to be performed in hospital environment. 5 = Should be avoided.

Pain and anxiety control **Local anaesthesia** LA may be used but with caution as solvent use may make the patient uncooperative and agitated. Furthermore, the oral mucosa may be painful due to erythema/burns. **Conscious sedation** Opioid use should be avoided and benzodiazepines should not be used in patients actively abusing and with decreased levels of consciousness. **General anaesthesia** A thorough preoperative assessment in conjunction with the anaesthetist is essential. Oral/nasal/pharyngeal burns may compromise the airway. Oral or tracheal intubation should be considered in any patient with significantly decreased level of consciousness or inability to protect the airway. Social support is required and appropriate discharge arrangements care need to be confirmed.

Further reading ● van der Bijl P 2003 Substance abuse – concerns in dentistry: an overview. S Afr Dent J 58:382–385 ● Cornelius J R, Clark D B, Weyant R et al 2004 Dental abnormalities in children of fathers with substance use disorders. Addict Behav 29(5):979–982 ● Sandler N A 2001 Patients who abuse drugs. Oral Surg Oral Med Oral Pathol Oral Radiol Endod 91:12–14.

ISCHAEMIC HEART DISEASE

Definition Ischaemic (coronary) heart disease (IHD or CHD) is the result of progressive myocardial ischaemia due to persistently reduced coronary blood flow.

General aspects

Aetiopathogenesis ■ The major contributory factors to IHD are: ● atherosclerosis (also termed atheroma or arteriosclerosis) ● hypertension ■ Atherosclerosis is a disease linked to smoking, lack of exercise, hypertension and hyperlipidaemia (Box 3.18), caused by the accumulation of lipids in artery walls ■ IHD leads to angina pectoris (pain arising from the myocardial oxygen demand exceeding the supply) or to myocardial infarction, which, if severe, causes acute failure of the whole circulation, loss of cerebral blood supply and often death ■ Myocardial infarction (MI) is mainly caused by rupture of an atheromatous plaque but sometimes results from emboli, coronary arterial spasm or vasculitis.

Clinical presentation

The first signs of IHD are usually the dramatic complications of angina pectoris or MI, often without warning or history of heart disease.

Angina ■ Angina is characterised by retrosternal chest pain or discomfort (tightness, heaviness), which may radiate to the arms, shoulders and neck ■ Stable or classic angina is characterised by pain that is predictably brought on by exercise or emotional upset and relieved by rest; symptoms that have not changed in the last two months; responds to nitroglycerine ■ Unstable angina is characterised by a decreased threshold of precipitants such that pain may occur at rest, and a recent increase in severity or frequency of pain; the response to nitroglycerine is unpredictable ■ Of particular concern are those patients who have 'silent angina'. These individuals comprise up to 25% of patients with significant coronary artery disease. They have no symptoms at all, even though they clearly lack adequate blood and oxygen supply to the heart muscle, and have the same risk of heart attack as those with symptoms of angina. The lack of symptoms could be due to psychological factors that persistently inhibit the perception of pain. Autonomic neuropathy involving cardiac afferent nerves is the most likely explanation of the high incidence of silent ischaemia in diabetic patients.

Box 3.18 Risk and protective factors for ischaemic heart disease

Primary risk factors
● High LDL (low density lipoprotein) ● Hypertension ● Smoking

Secondary risk factors
● Low HDL (high density lipoprotein) ● Diabetes ● Obesity ● Family history of CHD ● Physical inactivity ● Type A personality ● Gout ● Ethnic (Asians) ● Male gender ● Increasing age ● Low social class ● High homocysteine levels ● Chronic renal failure

Unclear effects
● Low dietary fibre ● Hard water ● High plasma fibrinogen ● Raised blood factor VII ● Raised lipoprotein levels

Protective factors
● Increased HDL:LDL ratio ● Exercise ● Moderate red wine or alcohol

Myocardial infarction ■ Acute myocardial infarction is characterised by varying degrees of chest pain, sweating, weakness, nausea, vomiting and arrhythmias, sometimes causing loss of consciousness ■ MI differs from angina in that: ● it causes more severe and persistent chest pain (>20 min) ● pain is not controlled by rest ● it leads to irreversible cardiac damage or sudden death (cardiac arrest) ■ Risk of postoperative re-infarction after a previous MI is: ● 35% after 0–3 months ● 15% after 3–6 months ● 4% after more than 6 months.

Diagnosis Diagnosis of IHD is generally from the history, but confirmed by: ■ ECG ● angina: the ECG trace is normal, or shows ST depression, flat or inverted T waves ● MI: ECG shows hyperacute T waves and ST elevation within the first few hours; within 24 h the T waves become inverted as the ST elevation begins to resolve. Pathological Q waves may be present ■ Exercise ECG – this is also usually carried out in order to increase stress to the patient's heart and reveal the ECG changes in angina ■ Coronary arteriography (angiography) – shows arterial stenosis or occlusion ■ Thallium scan – confirms decreased perfusion ■ Cardiac enzymes – increase in the serum levels. In MI, plasma troponin rises within 6 hours and other serum cardiac enzymes (creatine kinase, aspartate transaminase, lactic dehydrogenase), rise over 12–36 h.

Treatment **Lifestyle changes** The most effective way to treat patients with IHD is to implement lifestyle changes, namely: ■ reducing: ● stress and tension ● smoking ● alcohol ● salt ● animal fats ● body weight ■ increasing: ● exercise ● fruits and vegetables ● omega 3 oils (fish). **Drugs** ■ Anticoagulant/antiplatelet drugs (aspirin, clopidogrel, ticlopidine, warfarin) to inhibit clotting ■ Beta-blockers (atenolol, metoprolol, propranolol) to lower the blood pressure ■ Angiotensin converting enzyme (ACE) inhibitors (captopril, enalapril, fosinopril, lisinopril, ramipril), to lower peripheral resistance and cardiac workload ■ Statins to lower lipid levels ■ During attacks of angina, or before anticipated physical activity or stress, use of nitroglycerine (glyceryl trinitrate) 0.3–0.6 mg sublingually may treat or prevent pain; long-acting nitrates (isosorbide dinitrate) may help prevent anginal attacks. **Surgical management of IHD** Includes angioplasty, stents and coronary artery bypass graft (CABG; 'cabbage'). **Treatment of MI** ■ Aspirin ■ Morphine ■ Oxygen ■ Beta-blocker (e.g. metoprolol) ■ Bypass graft.

Prognosis Cardiovascular diseases kill more persons than all other diseases combined. Unstable angina is also known as pre-infarction angina. Collateral circulation may re-route blood in mild myocardial damage; but in large MI sudden death may result. Severe complications of MI usually involve thromboembolism and decreased cardiac output.

Oral findings

■ Angina is a rare cause of pain in the mandible, teeth or other oral tissues ■ Patients with IHD appear to have more severe dental caries and periodontal disease than the general population, but whether these infections bear any causative relationship to the heart disease, or whether they share some aetiological factor, remains uncertain ■ Drugs used in the care of patients with angina may cause oral adverse effects such as lichenoid lesions (calcium channel blockers), gingival swelling (calcium channel blockers), angioedema (ACE inhibitors) or ulcers (nicorandil).

Dental management

Risk assessment ■ Dental procedures, or drugs, can affect blood pressure and can precipitate angina, or possibly even provoke MI – reactions which appear to be largely related to the catecholamine (epinephrine/norepinephrine) release because of anxiety or pain ■ Changes in heart rate and blood pressure can be seen even before the administration of a dental LA injection ('white coat syndrome'), during tooth extraction and even when epinephrine-impregnated gingival retraction cords are used, but most of all when the patient experiences any pain ■ Dental care should therefore be carried out with minimal anxiety, and monitoring of oxygen saturation (by pulse oximetry), blood pressure and pulse ■ Perioperative monitoring with a three-lead ECG is also helpful, particularly in those patients who are unstable with dyspnoea on minimal exertion, cyanosis, frequent angina or a recent infarct ■ Preoperative glyceryl trinitrate and oral sedation are advised ■ Ready access to medical help, oxygen and nitroglycerine is crucial.

■ If a patient with a history of angina experiences chest pain in the dental surgery: ● dental treatment must be stopped ● place the patient upright ● give glyceryl trinitrate (GTN) 0.5 mg sublingually ● give oxygen 5 L/min ● monitor vital signs ● the pain should be relieved within 5 minutes; the patient should then rest and be accompanied home; and the medical practitioner advised ● if chest pain is *not* relieved, a further dose of GTN should be given ● MI is a possible cause and medical help should be summoned ● pain that persists after three doses of nitroglycerine given every 5 minutes; that lasts more than 15–20 minutes; or that is associated with nausea, vomiting, syncope, or hypertension is highly suggestive of MI ● if pain persists for 10 minutes, the patient should continue oxygen at 10–15 L/min, chew 300 mg of aspirin, and an intravenous cannula should be inserted; in addition, nitrous oxide/oxygen inhalation or 5–10 mg of morphine sulphate given intravenously may be useful to relieve pain and anxiety ● remain alert throughout for signs of cardiac arrest (i.e. no pulse, loss of consciousness); commence basic life support if these signs are detected and attach the automated external defibrillator.

Appropriate health care ■ The most important aspect is to consider how well the patient's heart is compensated, and the exact dental intervention that is contemplated ■ A stable cardiac patient receiving atraumatic treatment under local anaesthesia should be manageable in dental practice ■ A cardiac patient who requires complex surgery or needs a general anaesthetic and is unstable with dyspnoea on minimal exertion, cyanosis, frequent angina or a recent infarct, requires dental treatment in hospital. **Stable angina** ■ For anything other than routine dental treatment under local anaesthesia, the physician should be consulted and consideration should be given to any other complicating factors such as beta-blocker therapy, hypertension or cardiac failure; other medication should not be interfered with ■ Before dental treatment, patients with stable angina should be reassured and sedation considered to further allay anxiety (e.g. oral diazepam 5 mg) ■ Prophylactic administration of 0.3–0.6 mg GTN may be indicated if the patient has angina more than once a week. It should be noted that some patients may suffer from headaches and/or polyuria after GTN use, and may be reluctant to use their GTN prophylactically if they are largely asymptomatic. **Unstable angina** ■ Both emergency and elective dental care should be deferred until a physician has been consulted, because of the risk of postoperative chest pain, arrhythmias or MI ■ Preoperative 0.5 mg GTN sublingually or by inhalation should be used, together with relative analgesia monitored by pulse oximetry, and local analgesia ■ Such patients are best cared for in a hospital environment, particularly as there may be an indication for coronary vasodilators to be given intravenously. Other medication should not be interfered with. **Post-angioplasty** Elective dental care should be deferred for 6 months; emergency dental care should be in a hospital setting.

Patients with bypass grafts ■ Do not require antibiotic cover against infective endocarditis ■ Although there is research evidence to suggest that epinephrine-containing LA may precipitate arrhythmias, in clinical practice it is given using a careful LA technique with an aspirating syringe, without any notable problems.

Patients with vascular stents that are successfully engrafted
■ Do not require antibiotic cover against infective endocarditis but it may be prudent to provide antibiotic coverage if emergency dental treatment is required during the first 6 weeks postoperatively. Elective dental care should

be deferred. ■ May be on long-term anticoagulant medication and therefore appropriate action is required.

Pain and anxiety control **Local anaesthesia** ■ Epinephrine-containing LA should not be administered to patients taking beta-blockers, since interactions between epinephrine and the beta-blocking agent may induce hypertension and cardiovascular complications ■ Mepivacaine 3% is preferable to lidocaine for use in patients taking beta-blockers. **Conscious sedation** ■ Conscious sedation should be deferred for at least 6 months in patients with recent MI, recent onset angina, unstable angina or recent development of bundle branch block. After this period, if required in these patients, it should be given in hospital. ■ Conscious sedation rarely needs to be modified in other patients but extra care is needed ■ Premedication may be warranted in order to reduce anxiety levels, for example, diazepam, temazepam or nitrous oxide may be used ■ Benzodiazepines can increase the effect of digoxin. **General anaesthesia** GA should be deferred for at least 6 months in patients with recent MI, recent onset angina, unstable angina or recent development of bundle branch block and, in any case, it must be given in hospital. Intravenous barbiturates are particularly dangerous.

Patient access and positioning **Timing of treatment** Endogenous epinephrine levels peak during morning hours and adverse cardiac events are most likely in the early morning, so late morning or early afternoon appointments are recommended. **Patient positioning** It is potentially dangerous to lay any cardiac patient supine during dental treatment. Antihypertensive drugs may lead to orthostatic hypotension, so the back of the reclined dental chair should only be raised upright slowly and in stages.

Drug use ■ Many cardiac patients are also on aspirin or other antiplatelet drugs, or are otherwise anticoagulated with a resultant bleeding tendency. If possible, it is prudent to defer surgery until the drug effect has abated. However, when the patients are on these drugs long-term, local measures such as suturing, placement of packs or tranexamic acid are useful. ■ NSAIDs such as indometacin and ibuprofen, if used for more than 3 weeks, can impair the effect of beta-blockers and ACE inhibitors ■ Antimicrobial drugs can affect the function of cardiac drugs: ● a number of antibiotics, but not penicillin or tetracycline, increase the effect of warfarin ● ampicillin, in prolonged use, reduces serum levels of atenolol ● erythromycin and tetracycline can induce digitalis toxicity by reducing gut breakdown ● azole antifungals and macrolide antibiotics such as erythromycin and clarithromycin interact with statins to increase muscle damage (rhabdomyolysis).

Further reading ● Chapman P J 2002 Chest pain in the dental surgery: a brief review and practical points in diagnosis and management. Aust Dent J 47:259–261 ● Niwa H, Sato Y, Matsuura H 2000 Safety of dental treatment in patients with previously diagnosed acute myocardial infarction or unstable angina pectoris. Oral Surg Oral Med Oral Pathol Oral Radiol Endod 89:35–41 ● Seymour R A 2003 Dentistry and the medically compromised patient. Surgeon 1:207–214.

Table 3.94 **Key considerations for dental management in ischaemic heart disease (see text)**

	Management modifications*	Comments/possible complications
Risk assessment	2/3	Angina; MI; hypertension
Appropriate dental care	2–4	Evaluate type of IHD and dental intervention; sedation; preoperative glyceryl trinitrate
Pain and anxiety control		
– Local anaesthesia	2	Avoid lidocaine and epinephrine
– Conscious sedation	3/4	Delay 6 months after MI and other conditions
– General anaesthesia	3/4	Delay 6 months after MI and other conditions; avoid barbiturates
Patient access and positioning		
– Access to dental office	0	
– Timing of treatment	1	Late morning or early afternoon
– Patient positioning	1	Upright position; orthostatic hypotension
Treatment modification		
– Oral surgery	3	
– Implantology	3	
– Conservative/Endodontics	2	
– Fixed prosthetics	2	
– Removable prosthetics	2	
– Non-surgical periodontology	3	
– Surgical periodontology	3	
Hazardous and contraindicated drugs	2	Some patients are on anticoagulants; avoid NSAID usage for more than 3 weeks; avoid antimicrobials which affect other drugs

*0 = No special considerations. 1 = Caution advised. 2 = Specialised medical advice recommended in some cases. 3 = Specialised medical advice mandatory. 4 = Only to be performed in hospital environment. 5 = Should be avoided.

LEARNING IMPAIRMENT

Definition ■ The term learning disability or impairment is a label ■ It is used as a convenience in discussion and for planning services ■ Every person described as having a learning disability is a person first ■ The term itself was widely adopted in the UK following a speech in 1996 to Mencap by Stephen Dorrell, the then Secretary for Health ■ Many who have the label prefer the term 'people with learning difficulties' – this is the term used by *People First*, an international advocacy organisation ■ Learning disability or impairment is a term often used when a person has certain limitations in mental functioning (cognition) and in skills such as communicating, taking care of him or herself, and sociability ■ However, in the USA, the same term usually is used to denote specific learning impairments such as dyslexia, rather than impaired cognition ■ Learning impairment affects as many as 3 out of every 100 people: about 2% of the population have a mild learning disability and about 0.35% of the population have a severe learning disability.

General aspects

Aetiopathogenesis ■ Learning impairment is frequently the result of brain damage of many types, to such a degree that medical treatment, special care and/or training is needed ■ Causes of learning impairment are usually unknown but include: • genetic conditions (e.g. Down syndrome, fragile X syndrome, phenylketonuria) • pregnancy problems (e.g. fetal alcohol syndrome or rubella infection) • birth problems (e.g. during labour and birth) • post-natal problems (e.g. whooping cough, measles, meningitis, head trauma, extreme malnutrition or poisons like lead or mercury).

Clinical presentation ■ Children with learning impairment often take longer to learn to speak, walk, and take care of their personal needs such as dressing or eating, and may also have difficulty: • remembering things • solving problems • thinking logically • seeing the consequences of their actions • understanding social rules • understanding the need and how to pay for things ■ Brain damage may also cause physical impairments, and epilepsy, visual defects, hearing, speech or behavioural disorders ■ Craniofacial deformities, cardiac or other defects may be present in various syndromes ■ Other problems that may be increased in persons with learning impairment may include: • psychiatric disorders • hyperkinesis and stereotyped movements • feeding difficulties • pica (the ingestion of inedible substances) • sexual abuse.

Classification ■ Intelligence is not a unitary characteristic; it should be assessed on the basis of a large number of different skills ■ Although the general tendency is for all these skills to develop to a similar level in each individual, there can be large discrepancies, especially in persons who have learning impairment (e.g. individuals with autistic spectrum disorder) ■ This presents problems when determining the diagnostic category in which a person with learning impairment should be classified ■ The diagnostic category chosen should therefore be based on global assessments of ability and not on any single area of specific impairment or skill ■ The IQ levels (based on the intelligence quotient, IQ) are provided as a guide and should not be applied rigidly, as they are arbitrary divisions of a complex continuum, and cannot be defined with absolute precision (Table 3.95).

Diagnosis Diagnosis is established based on multiple factors such as clinical presentation, intelligence quotient (which represents the quotient between chronological age and mental age), and learning skills.

Treatment Learning impairment is so varied in severity and character, and possible underlying cause, that generalisations about care cannot really be justified, but: ■ Many patients can be cared for adequately at home by committed parents or guardians ■ Support care workers and respite care are critical to ensure that full-time carers are assisted in their role ■ Where care at home is not possible, sheltered accommodation and care in the community are alternatives ■ Special educational and vocational training are required ■ Drugs to limit hyperactivity may sometimes be useful; some patients respond to sedative agents such as haloperidol ■ Complications may result from: ● prolonged medication with sedatives, tranquillisers or anticonvulsants ● over-indulgence, with consequent obesity and its sequelae ● physical, sexual or drug abuse.

Oral findings

There are no specific oral manifestations attributed to learning disability but there are significant oral health differences by behaviour group, age, and oral healthcare/dental support: ■ People with learning disability tend to have

Table 3.95 **Learning impairment**

Category of impairment	IQ (average IQ in the population is 100)	Clinical features
Borderline patients	70–84	
Mild	50–69	Frequently live at home Hold conversations Full independence in self-care Practical domestic skills Basic reading/writing
Moderate	35–49	Limited language Need help with self-care Simple practical work (with supervision) Usually fully mobile
Severe	< 35	Often totally dependent on others for care Use words/gestures for basic needs Activities need to be supervised Work only in very structured/sheltered setting Impairments in movement are common

fewer filled teeth than in the normal population of similar age, but more teeth are decayed and missing. Although root caries is not a significant problem, oral hygiene and periodontal disease are. ■ Age-adjusted CPITN scores significantly differ by behavioural group. Those with severe physical and learning disability have the highest CPITN 3 category mean score. ■ Self-mutilation may involve the oral or orofacial tissues, as in Lesch–Nyhan syndrome where the lips or tongue may be chewed almost to destruction. Rarely, oral self-mutilation is accidental in patients with congenital indifference to pain, including Riley–Day syndrome (familial dysautonomia). ■ Oral ulcers are a common finding. Although in many cases the aetiology remains unknown, some predisposing factors have been identified, including: stress or anxiety, neuroleptic drug-induced immunodeficiency, oral infections, some respiratory and digestive disorders, and vitamin and folic acid deficiencies. ■ Drooling is not uncommon from poor orofacial muscle control.

Dental management

Risk assessment ■ Although in many cases judicious use of behavioural techniques and anxiety management may result in adequate cooperation for dental procedures to be undertaken, sometimes patients lack cooperation, and may exhibit aggressive, antagonistic behaviour ■ Unexpected movements may provoke injuries with sharp instruments.

Appropriate health care ■ Informed consent is a fraught issue in patients with learning disability and requires careful assessment ■ Many people with learning disability are amenable to treatment in the dental surgery (Fig. 3.25), although more time may be required – up to one-third may require sedation or a general anaesthetic ■ A greater proportion of people with learning disability require special facilities or an escort nurse to facilitate dental treatment than those who are psychiatrically ill ■ Communication can be difficult with some patients, particularly if the individual has associated visual or hearing impairment ■ Communicating with the patient who has mild learning disability can be aided if dental staff: • minimise distractions • use short explanations • use simple language • use 'tell–show–do' • use positive reinforcement • use verbal praise • take more time to present information • teach activities rather than concepts • encourage consistency ■ When communicating with the patient who has severe learning disability: • use short simple explanations • repeat instructions • practice oral hygiene procedures with the patient and carer • use positive reinforcement.

Pain and anxiety control **Local anaesthesia** Lip biting after LA is a common problem. **Conscious sedation** CS is a very useful adjunct to enable dental treatment to be provided. However, consent issues must be carefully assessed. **General anaesthesia** People with severe learning disability can usually be safely managed under GA for dental treatment, with minimal morbidity and without extensive preoperative investigations. Intraoperative complications are uncommon, but may include non-fatal ventricular arrhythmia, slight fall in blood pressure or hypertension (greater than 20% of preoperative value), laryngospasm and minor airway problems

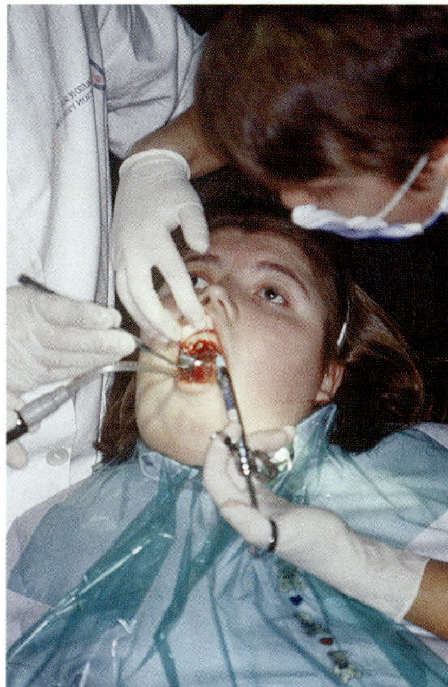

Figure 3.25 **An individual with learning impairment accepting dental treatment under local analgesia**

resulting in a desaturation of oxygen to a level below 85%. Every attempt should be made to minimise the frequency of these GAs, and to acclimatise the patient to accept at least an oral examination without GA.

Patient access and positioning **Access to dental surgery** Since the third part of the UK Disability and Discrimination Act became law, access to facilities has dramatically improved. However, there is still some reluctance from clinicians to provide care. In view of this, many patients are seen by specialist services either in the community dental services, or within hospital-based units.

Treatment modification **Preventive dentistry** ■ Poor oral hygiene is the most common problem in patients with learning impairment, and it is frequently impossible for these patients to improve their level of plaque control because of lack of understanding or motivation, or limitations imposed by associated physical handicaps or other disabilities ■ In individuals with more severe learning disability, electric toothbrushes may be easier to use and more effective ■ Significant plaque reduction can be maintained with the use of aqueous chlorhexidine spray, solutions and gels ■ High fluoride toothpastes may also be used but care should be taken that excessive amounts are not swallowed. **Fixed prosthetics and conservation** ■ Routine conservative dental treatment should be carried out wherever possible to preserve the teeth ■ For this purpose, LA (if necessary supplemented with intravenous or inhalational sedation) is preferable and is usually satisfactory. **Removable prosthetics** ■ Patients with learning disability are often rendered prematurely edentulous ■ Dentures may not be practical if patients are incapable of managing them and clinical prosthetic work is unfeasible ■ Impression-taking is facilitated by using a viscous material (such as composition or a putty-type material), which, if the patient objects violently, can be readily removed without leaving unset material in the

Table 3.96 **Key considerations for dental management in learning disability (see text)**

	Management modifications*	Comments/possible complications
Risk assessment	2	Unpredictable, occasionally aggressive behaviour; injuries from sharp instruments
Appropriate dental care	2/4	Informed consent; special facilities
Pain and anxiety control		
– Local anaesthesia	1	Control lip biting
– Conscious sedation	2/4	
– General anaesthesia	3/4	Arrhythmia; hypo- or hypertension; laryngospasm
Patient access and positioning		
– Access to dental office	2	Limited access; clinician reluctance
– Timing of treatment	0	
– Patient positioning	0	
Treatment modification		
– Preventive dentistry	2/4	Electric toothbrushes; chlorhexidine
– Oral surgery	2/4/5	Poor cooperation
– Implantology	2/4	Neglected oral hygiene; parafunctions
– Conservative/Endodontics	2/4	
– Fixed prosthetics	2/4/5	
– Removable prosthetics	2/4	Use viscous impression material; possibly a mouth prop; mark dentures
– Non-surgical periodontology	2/4	
– Surgical periodontology	2/5	
Imaging	2	Poor cooperation
Hazardous and contraindicated drugs	1	Some patients receive sedatives

*0 = No special considerations. 1 = Caution advised. 2 = Specialised medical advice recommended in some cases. 3 = Specialised medical advice mandatory. 4 = Only to be performed in hospital environment. 5 = Should be avoided.

oropharynx ■ If patients will not keep their mouths open, a mouth prop on alternate sides and sectional impressions may overcome the difficulty. In patients with severe cerebral palsy, stridor can be caused by a bite block in the mouth. Those patients who have more severe learning impairment tend to have a deterioration of breathing function when using a bite block. ■ Registration of occlusal records can be very problematic, but with patience can usually be effected ■ Dentures should be marked with the patient's name typed onto a paper strip. This can be added to the fitting surface at flasking and covered with clear acrylic before processing.

Periodontology ■ Regular, routine scaling usually improves the gingival state considerably. If there are cardiac defects, antibiotic cover may be indicated. ■ Other factors contributing to periodontal disease include gingival swelling caused by phenytoin or by one of the genetic syndromes, where gingivectomy may sometimes be justifiable.

Further reading ● Bedi R, Champion J, Horn R 2001 Attitudes of the dental team to the provision of care for people with learning disabilities. Spec Care Dentist 21:147–152 ● Blomqvist M, Holmberg K, Fernell E, Dahllof G 2004 A retrospective study of dental behavior management problems in children with attention and learning problems. Eur J Oral Sci 112:406–411 ● Stanfield M, Scully C, Davison M F, Porter S 2003 Oral healthcare of clients with learning disability: changes following relocation from hospital to community. Br Dent J 194:271–277 ● Tomás Carmona I, Diz Dios P, Limeres Posse J, Ocampo Hermida M T, Vázquez García E, Fernández Feijoo J 2000 Ulceras orales en discapacitados psíquicos. Archivos de Odontoestomatología 16:551–558 ● Waldman H B, Perlman S P 2004 Children with attention deficit disorder and learning disability: findings from the First National Study. J Dent Child (Chic) 71:101–104

● http://www.bsdh.org.uk/guidelines/longstay.pdf
● http://www.bsdh.org.uk/guidelines/mcntal.pdf
● http://www.bsdh.org.uk/guidelines/Dianatru.pdf
● http://www.ldbook.co.uk

LEUKAEMIAS

Definition Leukaemia is a malignant proliferation of haematopoietic tissue that progressively displaces normal blood-forming elements of the bone marrow.

General aspects

Aetiopathogenesis The cause of leukaemia remains unknown but some predisposing factors have been implicated, such as: ■ chromosomal abnormalities ■ immunodeficiency states ■ exposure to toxic chemicals ■ cytotoxic drugs ■ ionising radiation ■ some viruses ■ most patients with chronic myeloid leukaemia have hybrid chromosomes formed between chromosome 22 and 9 (Philadelphia chromosome).

Clinical presentation The most common findings in leukaemias include: ■ malaise and weakness, as a consequence of bone marrow failure causing anaemia ■ thrombocytopenia, leading to bleeding ■ leucocyte defects, predisposing to opportunistic infections. When disease progresses, leukaemic tissue may infiltrate gingivae, testes, liver, spleen, lymph nodes, ears and CNS.

Classification Leukaemias are classified according to the predominant cell type (lymphoid and myeloid cells) and the degree of maturity that the cells display. Acute or chronic types reflect the clinical course (Table 3.97).

Diagnosis ■ White blood cells count with differential ■ Bone marrow biopsy ■ Cytogenetics.

Treatment ■ Chemotherapy: ● busulfan ● cyclophosphamide ● daunorubicin ● doxorubicin ● mitomycin ● cytarabine

Table 3.97 **Classification of leukaemias**

Type of leukaemia	Variant	Characteristics
Acute lymphoblastic (ALL)	Homogeneous small blast type Heterogeneous blast type Homogeneous large blast type	Predominantly affects children – peak incidence 4–5 years CNS involvement No pre-leukaemic phase 2–12 years >60% cure rate with chemotherapy Adults 20% cure rate
Acute non-lymphoblastic (predominantly AML)	Myeloblastic without differentiation Myeloblastic with differentiation Hypergranular promyelocytic Acute myelomonocytic Monocytic Erythroleukaemia Megakaryoblastic	Predominantly affects adults – peak incidence young adults/middle age CNS involvement unusual 30% cure rate with chemotherapy 15% resistant disease
Chronic lymphoid (CLL)	Lymphocytic Sezary syndrome Hairy cell Prolymphocytic T-cell	~25% of all leukaemias Most common in elderly M:F = 2:1 Deranged apoptosis – CLL cells survive for abnormally long time and accumulate
Chronic myeloid (CML)	Granulocytic Atypical granulocytic Juvenile Myelomonocytic Eosinophilic	< 20% of all leukaemias Median age of onset 40–50 years Males slightly more commonly Progressive splenomegaly Leucocytosis Marrow hypercellularity > 90% have Philadelphia chromosome – 'balanced translocation' between chromosomes 9 and 22

● hydroxyurea (hydroxycarbamide) ● mercaptopurine ● methotrexate ● thioguanine ■ Alpha interferon ■ Haemopoietic stem cell transplant.

Prognosis ■ Acute lymphoblastic leukaemia has the best prognosis, especially in children under 10 years old ■ In half of patients with acute non-lymphoblastic leukaemia, treatment produces temporary remission ■ In chronic leukaemia, death occurs usually within 3–5 years.

Oral findings

Oropharyngeal lesions can be the presenting complaint in over 10% of cases of acute leukaemia:

■ *Oral bleeding and petechiae* are typical manifestations. Severe bleeding from the mouth, particularly from the gingival margin, may occur because of the thrombocytopenia, and needs treatment with desmopressin, or occasionally platelet transfusion. Gentle oral hygiene measures should control gingivitis that, otherwise, aggravates the bleeding.

■ *Herpetic oral and perioral infections* are common and troublesome, including varicella-zoster infections. They should be treated vigorously with aciclovir. Varicella-zoster (and measles viruses) can also cause encephalitis or pneumonia. Prophylactic aciclovir has greatly reduced the incidence, morbidity and mortality from herpetic infections, including those secondary to bone marrow transplants.

■ *Candidosis* is particularly common in the oral cavity and the paranasal sinuses, usually caused by *Candida albicans*. Prophylactic antifungal therapy, such as nystatin mouthwashes or pastilles, or amphotericin lozenges, is therefore indicated. Fluconazole-resistant candidal species and a rising number of cases of infection with *Candida krusei* are seen.

■ *Aspergillosis* or *mucormycosis* can involve the maxillary antrum and be invasive.

■ *Bacterial infections* with Gram-negative species occasionally cause oral lesions that can be a major source of septicaemia or metastatic infections in leukaemic patients. Lesions tend to become infected with *Pseudomonas*, *Serratia*, *Klebsiella*, *Enterobacter*, *Proteus* and *Escherichia*, or with *Candida* or *Aspergillus*. In severely immunosuppressed patients, over 50% of systemic infections result from oropharyngeal microorganisms. Microbiological investigations, with care to obtain specimens for anaerobic culture, are essential to enable appropriate antimicrobial therapy to be given.

■ *Gingival swelling* is secondary to infiltration of the gingival tissue with leukaemia cells. It is most commonly seen with the AML subtypes acute monocytic leukaemia (M5) (66.7%), acute myelomonocytic leukaemia (M4) (18.5%), and acute myelocytic leukaemia (M1, M2) (3.7%).

■ Other oral findings which may be present are: ● mucosal pallor ● mucosal or gingival ulceration ● pericoronitis ● cervical lymphadenopathy ● tonsillar swelling ● paraesthesia (particularly of the lower lip) ● extrusion of teeth ● painful swellings over the mandible and of the parotid (Mikulicz syndrome) ● bone changes – seen on radiography these may include destruction of the crypts of developing teeth, thinning or disappearance of the lamina dura, especially in the premolar and molar regions, and loss of the alveolar crestal bone; bone destruction near the apices of mandibular posterior teeth may also be seen; these bone changes may be reversible with chemotherapy ● many of the cytotoxic drugs can precipitate mucositis, sometimes with ulceration.

Dental management

Risk assessment The main dental management problems in leukaemia are as follows: ■ Bleeding tendency ■ Increased susceptibility to infection. The patient may be in isolation, such as in a laminar flow room, when strict asepsis is indicated. Antimicrobial cover is needed for any surgery, particularly for those with indwelling atrial catheters ■ Anaemia ■ Hepatitis B or C and HIV infection ■ Corticosteroid treatment ■ Other factors, such as disseminated intravascular coagulopathy, complications of bone marrow transplantation, or interaction between methotrexate and nitrous oxide (largely theoretical).

Appropriate health care ■ Dental treatment should only be carried out after close consultation with the oncologist/physician, as it may be affected by various aspects of leukaemia management and the patient's probable life expectancy ■ Oral health care principles are summarised in Box 3.19.

Pain and anxiety control **Local anaesthesia** Regional local anaesthetic injections may be contraindicated if there is a severe haemorrhagic tendency. A preoperative chlorhexidine rinse is recommended, as this will reduce the risk of inoculating the patient with oral pathogens. **Conscious sedation** Nitrous oxide, which interferes with vitamin B_{12} and hence folate metabolism, should be avoided if the patient is being treated with methotrexate, since the toxic effects of the latter may be exacerbated. **General anaesthesia** Anaemia may be a contraindication to general anaesthesia; intravenous sedation or relative analgesia may be used as alternatives.

Box 3.19 Synopsis of principles of oral health care in leukaemia

Pre-chemotherapy
● Assessment ● Treatment planning ● Remove teeth with a poor prognosis ● Stabilise caries ● Dietary advice ● Start fluoride prophylaxis ● Oral hygiene advice ● Start chlorhexidine prophylaxis

During induction chemotherapy
● Continue preventive oral health care ● Antifungal prophylaxis (nystatin) ● Antiviral prophylaxis (aciclovir or valaciclovir)

During remission
● Continue preventive oral health care

Long term
● Continue preventive oral health care ● Monitor craniofacial and dental development

Treatment modification **Preventive dentistry** Meticulous oral hygiene should be carefully maintained, with regular frequent warm aqueous chlorhexidine mouth rinses and the use of a soft nylon toothbrush. Fluoride mouthwash and/or supplements should also be implemented. **Surgery** ■ Surgery should be deferred (except for emergencies such as fractures, haemorrhage, potential airway obstruction or dangerous sepsis) until a remission phase ■ Full blood and platelet counts should be checked before surgery; desmopressin, platelet infusions or blood may be needed preoperatively. Tranexamic mouthwash may also be used to control postoperative

Table 3.98 **Key considerations for dental management in leukaemia (see text)**

	Management modifications*	Comments/possible complications
Risk assessment	3	Bleeding tendency; bacterial infections; anaemia; HCV, HBV and HIV infection
Appropriate dental care	3/4	Stage of disease life expectancy
Pain and anxiety control		
– Local anaesthesia	2	Avoid regional block; use chlorhexidine rinse
– Conscious sedation	2	Methotrexate interacts with nitrous oxide
– General anaesthesia	3–5	Avoid in severe anaemia
Patient access and positioning		
– Access to dental office	1	Coordinate with oncologist
– Timing of treatment	1	Coordinate with oncologist
– Patient positioning	0	
Treatment modification		
– Oral surgery	3–5	Delay until remission phase; full blood count; antibiotic cover; do not pack sockets
– Implantology	3–5	See oral surgery
– Conservative/Endodontics	3/5	
– Fixed prosthetics	3/5	
– Removable prosthetics	3	
– Non-surgical periodontology	3–5	See oral surgery
– Surgical periodontology	3–5	See oral surgery
– Orthodontics	3	Remove bands
– Paediatric dentistry	3	Remove mobile primary teeth
Hazardous and contraindicated drugs	2	Avoid aspirin and NSAIDs; some patients receive corticosteroids

*0 = No special considerations. 1 = Caution advised. 2 = Specialised medical advice recommended in some cases. 3 = Specialised medical advice mandatory. 4 = Only to be performed in hospital environment. 5 = Should be avoided.

bleeding ■ Sockets should not be packed, as this appears to predispose to infection. Absorbable Vicryl rapide or polyglycolic acid sutures (Dexon) are preferred. ■ Antibiotics are given until the surgical wound has healed, to reduce the risk of osteomyelitis or septicaemia; penicillin is the antibiotic of choice. **Periodontology** ■ Full blood and platelet counts should be checked before scaling and periodontal surgery. Desmopressin, platelet infusions or blood may be needed preoperatively. ■ Teeth with periodontal pockets > 7 mm should be extracted before chemotherapy. **Orthodontics** Orthodontic bands and appliances that contribute to poor oral hygiene or mucosal irritation should be removed before chemotherapy. **Paediatric dentistry** Mobile primary teeth should normally be removed before starting chemotherapy.

Drug use Aspirin and NSAIDs should not be given, since they can aggravate bleeding.

Further reading

● Ayers K M, Colquhoun A N 2000 Leukaemia in children. Part II – Dental care of the leukaemic child, including management of oral side effects of cancer treatment. NZ Dent J 96:141–146 ● Parisi E, Draznin J, Stoopler E, Schuster S J, Porter D, Sollecito T P 2002 Acute myelogenous leukemia: advances and limitations of treatment. Oral Surg Oral Med Oral Pathol Oral Radiol Endod 93:257–263 ● Raut A, Huryn J M, Hwang F R, Zlotolow I M 2001 Sequelae and complications related to dental extractions in patients with hematologic malignancies and the impact on medical outcome. Oral Surg Oral Med Oral Pathol Oral Radiol Endod 92:49–55.

LIVER CIRRHOSIS

Definition Cirrhosis is an irreversible loss of normal liver structure due to necrosis and fibrosis, which results in a reduced number of hepatocytes and in impaired liver function.

General aspects

Aetiopathogenesis Cirrhosis is mainly caused by alcohol, viral hepatitis B and C, and haemochromatosis. Other known causes include biliary obstruction, chemicals, congestive heart failure or immune-mediated damage. However, 30% of cases are cryptogenic (cause unknown).

Clinical presentation ■ May be asymptomatic ■ Clinical signs/symptoms (Fig. 3.26) include: ● skin signs – jaundice, leuconychia, clubbing, palmar erythema, Dupuytren's contracture, spider naevi ● gynaecomastia or testicular atrophy ■ Later signs include: ● bleeding ● oesophageal varices ● ascites ● peritonitis ● encephalopathy ● hepatorenal syndrome ● liver cancer.

Classification Based on its aetiology, three clinical types have been defined: ■ nutritional (alcohol abuse) ■ biliary (biliary obstruction) ■ post-necrotic (viral infection or toxins).

Diagnosis ■ Liver function tests – abnormal ■ Serum albumin – reduced ■ Prothrombin time – increased ■ Hepatitis virus serology ■ Autoantibodies ■ Liver ultrasound.

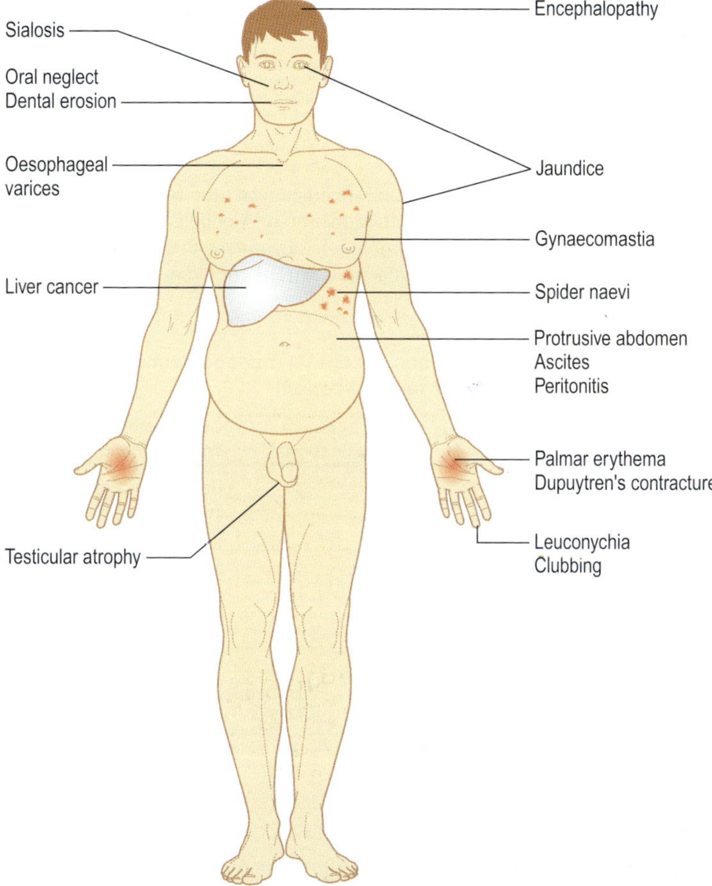

Figure 3.26 **Clinical presentation of liver cirrhosis**

Treatment ■ Low protein and low salt diet ■ Avoid alcohol and drugs ■ Interferon alpha ■ Liver transplantation.

Prognosis ■ There is an increased risk of liver cancer (hepatocellular carcinoma) ■ Most patients die in 5–10 years ■ In developed countries, cirrhosis is the third most common cause of death among adults.

Oral findings

■ Liver cirrhosis patients often show neglected dental status from poor oral hygiene and poor dental care related to alcohol abuse and neglect ■ Some patients have sialosis and parotid enlargement ■ Tooth erosion can be a consequence of gastric regurgitation ■ An association between liver cirrhosis and oral carcinoma has been proposed.

Dental management

See Liver failure.

Risk assessment Routine dental treatment can usually be carried out, although alcoholism may influence treatment (see Alcoholism). Spontaneous bacterial peritonitis is a potential problem in cirrhosis with ascites. Though most infections are with normal gut aerobic bacteria or Gram-positive bacteria,

Table 3.99 **Key considerations for dental management in liver cirrhosis (see text and Liver failure section)**

	Management modifications*	Comments/possible complications
Risk assessment	2	Underlying disease; impaired haemostasis; bacterial peritonitis
Appropriate dental care	2	Antibiotic prophylaxis; avoid hepatotoxic drugs
Pain and anxiety control		
– Local anaesthesia	1	Avoid lidocaine
– Conscious sedation	2	Avoid intravenous benzodiazepine
– General anaesthesia	3/4	Avoid halothane
Patient access and positioning		
– Access to dental office	0	
– Timing of treatment	0	
– Patient positioning	0	
Treatment modification		
– Oral surgery	3	Bleeding tendency; underlying disease; poor wound healing; liability to peritonitis
– Implantology	3/5	Avoid in alcoholism
– Conservative/Endodontics	2	
– Fixed prosthetics	2	
– Removable prosthetics	1	
– Non-surgical periodontology	3/5	See oral surgery
– Surgical periodontology	3/5	See oral surgery
Hazardous and contraindicated drugs	2	Avoid aspirin, NSAIDs, erythromycin estolate, tetracyclines and ketoconazole

*0 = No special considerations. 1 = Caution advised. 2 = Specialised medical advice recommended in some cases. 3 = Specialised medical advice mandatory. 4 = Only to be performed in hospital environment. 5 = Should be avoided.

invasive dental or oral surgical procedures may increase the risk and, since the mortality approaches 30%, antibiotic prophylaxis may be considered, in consultation with the patient's hepatologist. Amoxicillin orally 2–3 g, with metronidazole one hour preoperatively are recommended, or imipenem intravenously.

Appropriate health care ■ The physician should be contacted if surgery, GA or drug therapy are needed ■ Before any surgical procedure, check haemostatic function.

Pain and anxiety control **Local anaesthesia** Local anaesthesia is preferred. Articaine is preferred to lidocaine, as it differs from other amide local anaesthetics in that 90–95% is metabolised in the blood and only 5–10% in the liver. **Conscious sedation** Relative analgesia with nitrous oxide/oxygen is preferable to intravenous sedation with a benzodiazepine. **General anaesthesia** Halothane is contraindicated as it can be hepatotoxic.

Treatment modification **Surgery** Surgery is hazardous, particularly in view of the bleeding tendency, but also because of any accompanying diabetes, anaemia, drug therapy, HCV or HBV carriage or infection, poor wound healing and a liability to peritonitis.

Drug use Aspirin and NSAIDs, erythromycin estolate, tetracyclines, ketoconazole and other hepatically metabolised drugs should be avoided. Acetaminophen may be used but in reduced dosage.

Further reading ● Golla K, Epstein J B, Cabay R J 2004 Liver disease: current perspectives on medical and dental management. Oral Surg Oral Med Oral Pathol Oral Radiol Endod 98:516–521 ● Lodi G, Porter SR, Scully C 1998 Hepatitis C virus infection: Review and implications for the dentist. Oral Surg Oral Med Oral Pathol Oral Radiol Endod 86:8–22.

LIVER FAILURE

General aspects

Background ■ Failure of normal liver functions affects the metabolism of drugs and toxins, and production of blood coagulation factors ■ *Impaired drug detoxification and excretion* means that the effects of drugs are increased but not entirely predictable; factors determining the response include the type and severity of the liver damage, as well as any induction of hepatic drug-metabolising enzymes by previous medication ■ *Malabsorption of fats* causes malabsorption of fat-soluble vitamins such as vitamin K and this, with depressed synthesis of plasma proteins (including most clotting factors), is the main cause of a bleeding tendency.

Aetiopathogenesis Liver damage is usually caused mainly by:
■ infections (e.g. viral hepatitis) ■ drugs (e.g. alcohol, halothane, acetaminophen/paracetamol and many others) ■ other conditions (see Liver cirrhosis).

Clinical presentation Features include: ■ jaundice ■ tremor ■ halitosis (hepatic fetor) ■ encephalopathy (mood/behaviour change, progressing to drowsiness, confusion and coma).

Diagnosis ■ Liver function tests – abnormal ■ Prothrombin time (and INR) – increased ■ Blood glucose – reduced ■ EEG – abnormal ■ Abdominal ultrasound.

Treatment ■ Dextrose IV ■ Restrict protein intake ■ Transplant if possible.

Dental management

Risk assessment ■ There may be alcoholism, autoimmune disease, hepatitis B, C or D antigen carriage or diabetes ■ Patients with parenchymal liver disease have impaired haemostasis and can therefore present serious problems if invasive procedures (e.g. surgery or periodontal scaling) are needed.

Appropriate dental care ■ A prothrombin time is indicated before any procedure likely to result in bleeding. If the prothrombin time is prolonged, vitamin K 10mg parenterally should be given daily for several days preoperatively in an attempt to improve haemostatic function. If there is an inadequate response as shown by the prothrombin time, a transfusion of fresh blood or plasma may be required. ■ Drugs used in dentistry that, in varying degrees, are hepatotoxic and should be avoided include: tetracyclines, erythromycin estolate, halothane and aspirin. Alternative drugs are shown in Table 3.100.

Pain and anxiety control **Analgesia** ■ NSAIDs should not be used ■ Analgesia is best achieved with paracetamol/acetaminophen or codeine used in lower than normal doses. **Local anaesthesia** Local anaesthesia is safe if given in normal doses – prilocaine or articaine more so than lidocaine. **Conscious sedation** Brain metabolism is abnormal and becomes more sensitive to drugs. Encephalopathy or coma can thus be precipitated by sedatives, hypnotics, tranquillisers or opioids. Relative analgesia with nitrous oxide is preferable to intravenous sedation with a benzodiazepine. Midazolam doses, if used for sedation, should be reduced. **General anaesthesia** ■ Premedication with opioids must be avoided ■ Drugs (particularly the barbiturates, such as thiopentone) liable to cause respiratory depression are especially dangerous ■ Nitrous oxide with pethidine or phenoperidine appears to be suitable for anaesthesia but it is essential to avoid hypoxia ■ Halothane can cause hepatitis, which may follow a single exposure in 1 in 35000 cases among the general population, but is more common when anaesthetics are given repeatedly at intervals of less than 3 months, in middle-aged females, and in the obese. In consequence, isoflurane, sevoflurane or desflurane are preferable to halothane. However, desflurane should be used in lower than normal doses. ■ Suxamethonium is best avoided since the impaired cholinesterase activity in liver disease causes increased sensitivity to this neuromuscular blocker.

Drug use ■ Aspirin and most other NSAIDs such as indometacin should be avoided because they aggravate the haemorrhagic tendency and because

Table 3.100 **Drugs contraindicated and alternatives in patients with liver disease**

	Drugs contraindicated	Alternatives
Analgesics	Aspirin Codeine Indometacin Mefenamic acid Meperidine* NSAIDs Opioids Paracetamol/acetaminophen*	Codeine Hydrocodone Oxycodone
Antimicrobials	Aminoglycosides Azithromycin Azole antifungals (miconazole, fluconazole, ketoconazole, itraconazole) Clarithromycin* Clindamycin* Co-amoxiclav* Co-trimoxazole Doxycycline Erythromycin estolate Metronidazole* Roxithromycin Talampicillin Tetracycline	Amoxicillin Ampicillin Cephalosporins Erythromycin stearate Imipenem Minocycline Nystatin Penicillins
Antidepressants	Monoamine oxidase inhibitors	SSRIs Tricyclics*
Muscle relaxants	Suxamethonium	Atracurium Cisatracurium Pancuronium Vecuronium
Local anaesthetics	Lidocaine*	Articaine Prilocaine
Anaesthetics	Halothane Thiopentone	Desflurane Isoflurane Sevoflurane
Central nervous system depressants	Barbiturates Diazepam* Midazolam* Phenothiazines Propofol*	Lorazepam* Oxazepam* Pethidine*
Corticosteroids	Prednisone	Prednisolone

Table 3.100 **Drugs contraindicated and alternatives in patients with liver disease—cont'd**

	Drugs contraindicated	Alternatives
Others	Anticoagulants Anticonvulsants Biguanides Carbamazepine Diuretics Liquid paraffin Lomotil Methyldopa Oral contraceptives	

*Or use in lower doses than normal.

of the risk of gastric haemorrhage in those patients with portal hypertension or those with peptic ulcers ■ Aminoglycosides are best avoided altogether, as impaired liver metabolism may increase their nephrotoxicity ■ The nephrotoxicity of vancomycin may also be increased ■ There is a risk of liver damage from tetracyclines but only if massive doses are given ■ Erythromycin estolate is potentially hepatotoxic but the effect is reversible when the drug is stopped; erythromycin stearate is not hepatotoxic ■ Broad-spectrum antibiotics (at least in theory) may further reduce vitamin K availability by destroying the gut flora ■ Antimicrobials that can safely be used in normal doses include penicillins, cephalexin, cefazolin, erythromycin stearate, minocycline and imipenem; clindamycin and metronidazole can be used in lower than normal doses, but should be avoided in end-stage liver disease ■ The dosages of many drugs may need to be reduced due to impaired metabolism (see, for example, British National Formulary).

Further reading ● Douglas L R, Douglass J B, Sieck J O, Smith P J 1998 Oral management of the patient with end-stage liver disease and the liver transplant patient. Oral Surg Oral Med Oral Pathol Oral Radiol Endod 86:55–64 ● Lockhart P B, Gibson J, Pond S H, Leitch J 2003 Dental management considerations for the patient with an acquired coagulopathy. Part 1: Coagulopathies from systemic disease. Br Dent J 195:439–445.

LIVER TRANSPLANTATION

Definition ■ Liver transplantation is the surgical replacement of a diseased liver with a healthy one, used typically for treatment of end-stage liver disease (e.g. from biliary atresia, metabolic disease or malignancy) ■ Usually the liver is obtained from a cadaveric or brain-dead donor ■ Due to the shortage of donor organs, the use of reduced size, split, and living-related donor liver tissue is being advocated.

General aspects

Treatment All liver transplant recipients require life-long immunosuppression to prevent a T-cell alloimmune rejection response.

Prognosis ■ Liver transplant recipients may be susceptible to recurrence of their original disease; the rate of developing cirrhosis in the transplant at 5 years can approach 25% ■ The 1-year survival after transplantation is around 80%; of these, 90% survive 5 years and 85% for 10 years.

Table 3.101 **Key considerations for dental management in liver failure (see text)**

	Management modifications*	Comments/possible complications
Risk assessment	2	Underlying disease; impaired haemostasis
Appropriate dental care	2	Bleeding tests; preoperative vitamin K; avoid hepatotoxic drugs
Pain and anxiety control		
– Local anaesthesia	1	Avoid lidocaine
– Conscious sedation	2	Avoid intravenous benzodiazepine
– General anaesthesia	3/4	Avoid barbiturates, opioids, halothane and suxamethonium
Patient access and positioning		
– Access to dental office	0	
– Timing of treatment	0	
– Patient positioning	0	
Treatment modification		
– Oral surgery	3	Bleeding tendency; underlying disease
– Implantology	3/5	Avoid in alcoholism
– Conservative/Endodontics	2	
– Fixed prosthetics	2	
– Removable prosthetics	1	
– Non-surgical periodontology	3/5	See oral surgery
– Surgical periodontology	3/5	See oral surgery
Hazardous and contraindicated drugs	2	Avoid aspirin, NSAIDs, erythromycin estolate, tetracyclines and some other antimicrobials (see Table 3.100)

*0 = No special considerations. 1 = Caution advised. 2 = Specialised medical advice recommended in some cases. 3 = Specialised medical advice mandatory. 4 = Only to be performed in hospital environment. 5 = Should be avoided.

Oral findings

■ Children needing liver transplants may have delayed tooth eruption and discoloured and hypoplastic teeth ■ Neglected oral health status has been observed in some series in both children and adults waiting for a liver transplantation ■ Gingival swelling may be seen in patients on ciclosporin or some other drugs.

Dental management

Risk assessment ■ Bacterial sepsis is the most common cause of death occurring during the first postoperative months. In consequence, a full preventive oral health care programme should be instituted. ■ Some patients may be on anticoagulants.

Table 3.102 **Key considerations for dental management in liver transplantation (see text and Transplantation section)**

	Management modifications*	Comments/possible complications
Risk assessment	2	Bacterial sepsis; bleeding due to anticoagulants; pre-existing disease
Appropriate dental care	2	Postpone elective care for 6 months; antibiotic prophylaxis
Pain and anxiety control		
– Local anaesthesia	1	
– Conscious sedation	2	Avoid sedatives
– General anaesthesia	4/5	
Patient access and positioning		
– Access to dental office	0	
– Timing of treatment	0	
– Patient positioning	0	
Treatment modification		
– Oral surgery	2	Bleeding; infection
– Implantology	2	Bleeding; infection
– Conservative/Endodontics	1	
– Fixed prosthetics	1	
– Removable prosthetics	0	
– Non-surgical periodontology	2	Bleeding; infection
– Surgical periodontology	2	Bleeding; infection
Hazardous and contraindicated drugs	2	Avoid sedatives, aspirin and drugs interfering with ciclosporin

*0 = No special considerations. 1 = Caution advised. 2 = Specialised medical advice recommended in some cases. 3 = Specialised medical advice mandatory. 4 = Only to be performed in hospital environment. 5 = Should be avoided.

Appropriate health care ■ A meticulous pre-surgery oral assessment is required and dental treatment undertaken with particular attention to establishing optimal oral hygiene and eradicating sources of potential infection; dental treatment should be completed before surgery ■ Elective dental care is best deferred until after 6 months post-transplantation ■ Invasive dental treatment should only be carried out after medical consultation and having in mind the bleeding tendency, any infectious risk and, in some cases, impaired drug metabolism ■ Antibiotic prophylaxis for spontaneous bacterial peritonitis should be discussed with the responsible physician before any invasive dental procedure peri- and post-transplantation.

Pain and anxiety control **Local anaesthesia** Caution should be exercised when providing LA, as there may be an associated bleeding/infection risk. **Conscious sedation** Sedatives should be avoided due to impaired drug metabolism. **General anaesthesia** GA should be avoided due to the risks associated with impaired drug metabolism, bleeding and infection – all of which can contribute to significant postoperative morbidity.

Further reading ● Douglas L R, Douglass J B, Sieck J O, Smith P J 1998 Oral management of the patient with end-stage liver disease and the liver transplant patient. Oral Surg Oral Med Oral Pathol Oral Radiol Endod 86:55–64 ● Sheehy E C, Roberts G J, Beighton D, O'Brien G 2000 Oral health in children undergoing liver transplantation. Int J Paediatr Dent 10:109–119 ● Seow W K, Shepherd R W, Ong T H 1991 Oral changes associated with end-stage liver disease and liver transplantation: implications for dental management. ASDC J Dent Child. 58:474–480.

LUNG TRANSPLANTATION

Definition ■ Patients with end-stage pulmonary disease may be considered for potential lung transplantation ■ The lung for a lung transplant usually comes from a brain-dead organ donor.

General aspects

Treatment ■ All transplant recipients require life-long immunosuppression to prevent a T-cell immune rejection response ■ Most centres use a combination of ciclosporin, azathioprine and glucocorticoids.

Prognosis ■ Early graft failure following lung transplantation presents as diffuse alveolar damage due to reimplantation oedema, reperfusion oedema, primary graft failure, or allograft dysfunction ■ Inhaled nitric oxide modulates pulmonary vascular tone via smooth muscle relaxation and can improve ventilation/perfusion and oxygenation in diseased lungs.

Oral findings

■ Dry mouth and progressive periodontal disease due to mouth breathing are common in patients awaiting lung transplantation ■ Gingival swelling may be seen in patients on ciclosporin.

Dental management

Appropriate health care ■ A meticulous pre-surgery oral assessment is required and dental treatment undertaken with particular attention to establishing optimal oral hygiene and eradicating sources of potential infection; dental treatment should be completed before surgery ■ For 6 months after surgery, elective dental care is best deferred ■ If surgical treatment is needed during that period, antibiotic prophylaxis is probably warranted.

Pain and anxiety control **Local anaesthesia** Caution should be exercised when providing LA – a preoperative chlorhexidine rinse is recommended as this will reduce the risk of inoculating the patient with oral pathogens. **Conscious sedation** Sedatives should be avoided as they may compromise respiratory function. **General anaesthesia** GA should be avoided due to the risks of significant postoperative morbidity.

Drug use Most patients are on corticosteroids.

Table 3.103 **Key considerations for dental management in lung transplantation (see text and Transplantation section)**

	Management modifications*	Comments/possible complications
Risk assessment	2	Infections
Appropriate dental care	2	Postpone 6 months elective care; antibiotic cover; possibly corticosteroid supplementation
Pain and anxiety control		
– Local anaesthesia	1	
– Conscious sedation	2	Avoid sedatives
– General anaesthesia	4/5	
Patient access and positioning		
– Access to dental office	0	
– Timing of treatment	0	
– Patient positioning	0	
Treatment modification		
– Oral surgery	2	Infection
– Implantology	2	Infection
– Conservative/Endodontics	1	
– Fixed prosthetics	1	
– Removable prosthetics	0	
– Non-surgical periodontology	2	Infection
– Surgical periodontology	2	Infection
Hazardous and contraindicated drugs	2	Avoid drugs interfering with ciclosporin; some patients are on corticosteroids

*0 = No special considerations. 1 = Caution advised. 2 = Specialised medical advice recommended in some cases. 3 = Specialised medical advice mandatory. 4 = Only to be performed in hospital environment. 5 = Should be avoided.

Further reading ● al-Sarheed M, Angeletou A, Ashley P F, Lucas V S, Whitehead B, Roberts G J 2000 An investigation of the oral status and reported oral care of children with heart and heart–lung transplants. Int J Paediatr Dent 10:298–305 ● Kilpatrick N M, Weintraub R G, Lucas J O, Shipp A, Byrt T, Wilkinson J L 1997 Gingival overgrowth in pediatric heart and heart–lung transplant recipients. J Heart Lung Transplant 16:1231–1237.

LUPUS ERYTHEMATOSUS

Definition Systemic lupus erythematosus (SLE) is a multi-system connective tissue disease characterised by antinuclear antibodies (ANA) directed against double-strand DNA.

General aspects

Aetiopathogenesis SLE is considered to have a genetic basis, with a defect in immune regulation, possibly virally-induced. Antigen–antibody complexes are deposited in blood vessels and trigger vasculitis by their activation of complement.

Clinical presentation ■ The main features (Fig. 3.27) are: ● musculoskeletal (myopathy, myalgia, arthritis) ● cutaneous (malar rash, alopecia, Raynaud's phenomena) ● renal (proteinuria, nephritis) features are prominent ■ Other features include ● mouth – ulcers ● pulmonary – pleurisy (pleuritis) ● blood – pancytopenia ● fever ● lymphadenopathy ● CNS – various manifestations ● cardiac – myocarditis which leads to cardiac failure; there is a higher risk of infarction and a characteristic (Libman–Sacks) sterile endocarditis which renders the patient susceptible to infective endocarditis ● women who have SLE can pass antibodies across the placenta which can lead to fetal heart block.

Classification Lupus can be categorised into three groups: ■ systemic lupus erythematosus – involves multiple organs and tissues ■ discoid lupus erythematosus – cutaneous variant with few, if any, systemic manifestations ■ drug-induced systemic lupus erythematosus – usually causes only mild-to-moderate symptoms; drugs implicated are especially procainamide, hydralazine, gold, d-penicillamine, isoniazid and phenytoin.

Diagnosis The American College of Rheumatology diagnostic criteria for SLE are based on the presence of at least four of the following: ■ malar rash (photosensitive) ■ discoid rash ■ photosensitivity ■ oral ulcers ■ arthritis ■ serositis (pleuritis or pericarditis) ■ renal disorder (persistent proteinuria or cellular casts) ■ neurological disorder (seizures or psychosis) ■ haematologic disorder (anaemia, leukopenia or lymphopenia on two or more occasions, thrombocytopenia) ■ immunological disorder (positive LE cell preparation, anti-DNA or anti-Sm, false-positive VDRL).

Treatment ■ Avoid sun exposure ■ Drugs: ● NSAIDs ● hydroxychloroquine ● immunosuppression (corticosteroids, methotrexate, azathioprine).

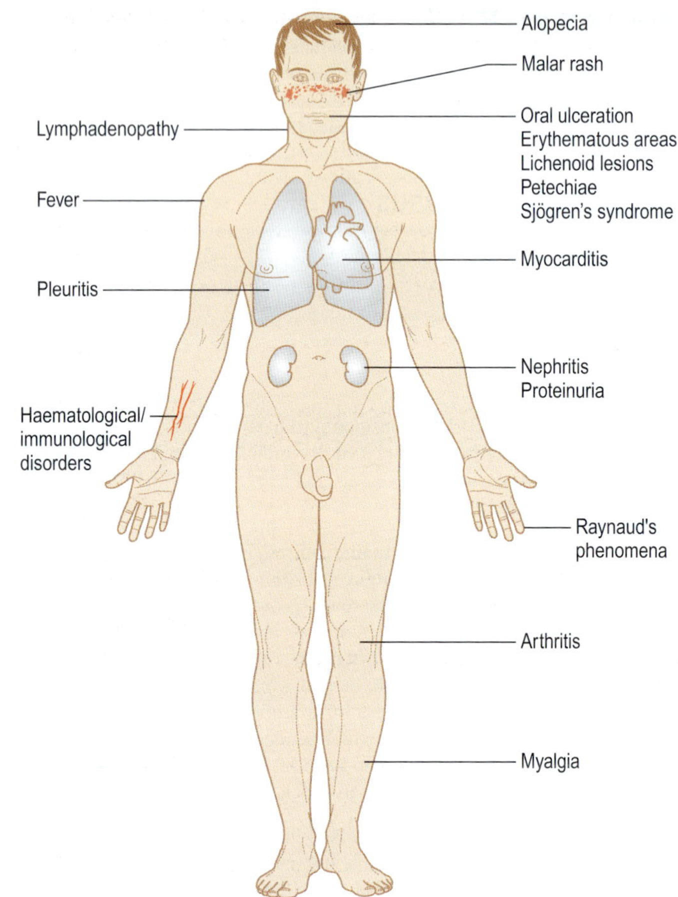

Figure 3.27 **Clinical presentation of lupus erythematosus**

Prognosis The most severe complications include lupus nephritis, pericarditis and central nervous system involvement – all of which indicate a poor prognosis.

Oral findings

SLE may be complicated by: ■ Oral lesions, which typically consist of erythematous areas, erosions or white patches fairly symmetrically distributed. These may be seen in 10–20% of patients with SLE but are rarely an early feature. The lesions often resemble those of oral lichen planus. Slit-like ulcers may also be seen near the gingival margins. ■ Sjögren's syndrome in 10–30% of cases ■ Lichenoid oral lesions or occasionally oral hyperpigmentation from the antimalarials sometimes used to control SLE ■ Petechiae related to thrombocytopenia ■ TMJ dysfunction with condylar deformation. ■ Discoid lupus erythematosus can sometimes lead to lip carcinoma.

Dental management

Risk assessment ■ SLE is a multi-system disease, and as such it may be associated with significant complications, including renal disease, anaemia, leucopenia or lymphopenia ■ Surgery may exacerbate the symptoms of SLE ■ Patients are susceptible to cardiac failure and to infective endocarditis if there has been Libman–Sacks endocarditis – due to the valvular damage. Antibiotics are recommended prophylactically before invasive dental

Table 3.104 **Key considerations for dental management in lupus erythematosus (see text)**

	Management modifications*	Comments/possible complications
Risk assessment	2	Multi-system disease; SLE symptoms exacerbation; infective endocarditis; bleeding tendency
Appropriate dental care	2/4	Bleeding tests; antibiotic prophylaxis; avoid elective dental care during active phases of SLE
Pain and anxiety control		
– Local anaesthesia	0	
– Conscious sedation	1	
– General anaesthesia	3/4	Pulmonary disease
Patient access and positioning		
– Access to dental office	0	
– Timing of treatment	0	
– Patient positioning	0	
Treatment modification		
– Oral surgery	2	Bleeding tests; consider need for antibiotic prophylaxis
– Implantology	2	See oral surgery
– Conservative/Endodontics	1	
– Fixed prosthetics	1	
– Removable prosthetics	1	
– Non-surgical periodontology	2	See oral surgery
– Surgical periodontology	2	See oral surgery
Hazardous and contraindicated drugs	2	Avoid tetracyclines and penicillin; some patients receive corticosteroids or immunosuppressives

*0 = No special considerations. 1 = Caution advised. 2 = Specialised medical advice recommended in some cases. 3 = Specialised medical advice mandatory. 4 = Only to be performed in hospital environment. 5 = Should be avoided.

procedures ■ Bleeding tendency may be caused by thrombocytopenia or circulating lupus anticoagulants.

Appropriate health care ■ Hospitalisation may be required for otherwise minor procedures, and postoperative discharge may be delayed ■ Bleeding tests should be performed before any surgical dental treatment is undertaken.

Pain and anxiety control **Local anaesthesia** Local anaesthesia is the preferred method. **Conscious sedation** Conscious sedation may be undertaken with routine precautions, although caution is advised when using sedative drugs if SLE is associated with significant pulmonary and/or renal disease. **General anaesthesia** In view of the multi-system effects of SLE, consultation with the specialist physician and a thorough preoperative assessment in conjunction with the anaesthetist is essential.

Treatment modification **Surgery** The responsible physician should be consulted and the results of recent investigations obtained to determine disease activity, and risk of bleeding and infection. Elective surgery should be postponed until lupus activity subsides. Local haemostatic measures and a careful aseptic technique are usually sufficient. **Conservative dentistry** Results of one study of lymphocyte reactivity in SLE indicated that *in vitro* reactivity to inorganic mercury, silver, organic mercury and lead decreased significantly after the replacement of dental amalgams, leading the authors to recommend replacement of amalgams. However, there is no *in vivo* evidence to support this.

Drug use ■ Tetracyclines may cause photosensitivity rashes
■ Sulphonamides or penicillins may cause deterioration in SLE
■ Patients may be on corticosteroid or other immunosuppressive therapy.

Further reading ● Gonzales T S, Coleman G C 1999 Periodontal manifestations of collagen vascular disorders. Periodontol 2000 21:94–105 ● Hughes C T, Downey M C, Winkley G P 1998 Systemic lupus erythematosus: a review for dental professionals. J Dent Hyg 72:35–40 ● Prochazkova J, Sterzl I, Kucerova H, Bartova J, Stejskal V D 2004 The beneficial effect of amalgam replacement on health in patients with autoimmunity. Neuro Endocrinol Lett 25:211–218 ● Rhodus N L, Little J W, Johnson D K 1990 Electrocardiographic examination of dental patients with systemic lupus erythematosus. Spec Care Dentist 10:46–50.

LYMPHOMAS

Definition ■ Lymphomas are solid neoplasms that arise in lymphoid cells and spread to distant lymphoid organs such as the lymph nodes, spleen, liver or bone marrow ■ Lymphomas include: ● *Hodgkin's lymphoma (HL)* – a lymphocyte malignancy in which there is proliferation of multinucleated reticulum cells sometimes with mirror-image nuclei (Reed–Sternberg cells) ● *Non-Hodgkin's lymphoma (NHL)* – a diverse group of about 15 different malignancies, arising from lymph nodes or mucosa-associated lymphoid tissue (MALT), and commonly of B-cell origin; Reed–Sternberg cells are not present ● *Infrequent forms* – Burkitt's lymphoma, mycosis fungoides and Sézary´s syndrome.

General aspects

Aetiopathogenesis ■ HL aetiology remains unclear, but an autoimmune response to a viral infection has been suggested ■ NHL may be due to Epstein–Barr virus; the incidence has increased dramatically with the advent of HIV/AIDS ■ NHL of the stomach found in MALT may be caused by *Helicobacter pylori* infection.

Clinical presentation ■ Lymphomas present mainly with painless swelling of lymph nodes and/or hepatosplenomegaly ■ Systemic complaints such as fever, sweats, or weight loss suggest advanced disease ■ In advanced lymphomas, symptoms may result from nerve root compression, or obstruction of lymphatic drainage or vascular supply ■ Features of HL and NHL are summarised in Table 3.105.

Classification ■ HL histological types include: ● lymphocyte predominant ● lymphocyte depletion ● mixed cellularity ● nodular sclerosis ■ NHL histological types include: ● lymphocytic ● mixed lymphocytic-histiocytic ● histiocytic ● undifferentiated ■ The degree of differentiation may be low, intermediate or high. The main histological types are nodular and diffuse.

Staging The Ann Arbor staging system is used to stage HL: ■ Stage I: single lymph node (LN) ± local extralymphatic spread ■ Stage II: two or

Table 3.105 **Clinical features of HL/NHL**

	HL	NHL
Incidence	2.4 per 100 000 annually	8.2 per 100 000; more common in individuals with AIDS
Age	2 peaks: early adulthood and again later in the elderly	Classically seen in the elderly More common in younger age groups since the advent of HIV/AIDS
Symptoms/signs	Lymphadenopathy – spread is contiguous – in early disease, the nodes may fluctuate in size – ± alcohol related pain Hepatosplenomegaly General malaise Severe itching *Herpes zoster* (marker of depression of cell-mediated immunity)	Lymphadenopathy – spread is not contiguous – often presents as disseminated disease – predilection for the GIT and CNS High grade disease results in fever, anorexia, weight loss Nodal pressure/extranodal disease may result in: – superior vena cava obstruction – abdominal obstruction – back pain – bone pain ± signs of autoimmune haemolysis

more LN on the same side of the diaphragm ■ Stage III: LN on both sides of diaphragm ■ Stage IV: diffuse/disseminated spread with involvement of one or more extra-lymphatic organs ■ Note: each stage is also divided into ● A: no systemic symptoms ● B: sustained fever (> 38°C), > 10% weight loss over 6 months, night sweats.

Diagnosis ■ Lymphoma diagnostic methods, also used to stage the disease, include: ● chest/abdomen CT/MRI ● ultrasonography ● lymph node biopsy ● bone marrow biopsy.

Treatment The treatment is dependent on the histological type and classification of HL/NHL: ■ HL ● early stages – radiotherapy ● later stages – chemotherapy ■ NHL ● low grade – radiotherapy ● high grade – radiotherapy/chemotherapy.

Prognosis ■ Over 90% of patients in early stage of HL will survive at least 5 years, but only 50% of those in advanced stages ■ Over 75% of patients with nodular NHL will survive 10 years; however, most patients with high-grade diffuse NHL will, after treatment, be free of disease for only 3–5 years.

Oral findings

■ Lymphomas most commonly develop in cervical lymph nodes ■ Lymphomas may present as swellings or ulcers in the gingiva, floor of the mouth and especially in the palate or fauces (often associated with AIDS) ■ Isolated tooth mobility and lip paraesthesia may also be present – histopathological examination of tissue from the extraction sockets of mobile teeth is mandatory where these features are present ■ Oral candidosis and herpes zoster infection (involving the trigeminal area) are not uncommon in advanced disease ■ Oral complications may also arise from radiotherapy and/or chemotherapy.

Dental management

Risk assessment Dental management may be complicated by: ■ bleeding tendencies ■ liability to infection ■ anaemia ■ corticosteroid therapy ■ impaired respiratory function (pulmonary fibrosis due to mediastinal irradiation) ■ cardiac disease (after mediastinal irradiation) ■ acute leukaemia (7% of treated patients).

Appropriate health care ■ During the acute phase, treatment is restricted to emergency dental care only ■ Investigation of bleeding tendency and consultation with the physician are mandatory before any invasive procedure ■ Antibiotic prophylaxis should be considered before invasive procedures in immunosuppressed patients ■ Complex treatment may be unwarranted in patients with a very poor prognosis.

Pain and anxiety control **Local anaesthesia** Local anaesthesia is the preferred method. **Conscious sedation** CS may be undertaken with the routine precautions, although caution is advised when using

Table 3.106 **Key considerations for dental management in lymphomas (see text)**

	Management modifications*	Comments/possible complications
Risk assessment	3	Anaemia; corticosteroid therapy; bleeding tendency; radiotherapy consequences; liability to infection
Appropriate dental care	3	Disease prognosis; avoid elective dental care during acute phase; bleeding tests; antibiotic prophylaxis; specialist advice before invasive procedures
Pain and anxiety control		
– Local anaesthesia	1	
– Conscious sedation	2	
– General anaesthesia	3/4	Irradiation may have damaged lung or heart function
Patient access and positioning		
– Access to dental office	0	
– Timing of treatment	0	
– Patient positioning	0	Upright position in patients with pulmonary fibrosis
Treatment modification		
– Oral surgery	3	
– Implantology	3	
– Conservative/Endodontics	1	
– Fixed prosthetics	1	
– Removable prosthetics	1	
– Non-surgical periodontology	3	
– Surgical periodontology	3	
Hazardous and contraindicated drugs	2	Some patients receive corticosteroids or immunosuppressives

*0 = No special considerations. 1 = Caution advised. 2 = Specialised medical advice recommended in some cases. 3 = Specialised medical advice mandatory. 4 = Only to be performed in hospital environment. 5 = Should be avoided.

sedative drugs if there is associated lung/heart damage due to irradiation.

General anaesthesia Consultation with the specialist physician and a thorough preoperative assessment in conjunction with the anaesthetist is essential. The risks of lung/heart damage due to irradiation must be assessed.

Patient access and positioning Consider placing the patient in an upright position if there is heart/lung damage due to mediastinal irradiation.

Further reading • Friedlander A H, Sung E C, Child J S 2003 Radiation-induced heart disease after Hodgkin's disease and breast cancer treatment: dental implications. J Am Dent Assoc 134:1615–1620 • Herrin H K 1999 The oral implications of Hodgkin's disease. Gen Dent 47:572–575

MALIGNANT HYPERTHERMIA

Definition ■ Malignant hyperthermia (malignant hyperpyrexia; MH; MHS; King–Denborough syndrome) is a rare, potentially lethal, inherited condition, characterised by a rapid rise in temperature when the patient takes one of the drugs that can trigger an attack ■ Although the incidence of genetic MH predisposition is 1:10000, clinical incidence is about 1:30000 – i.e. not every patient with a genetic predisposition to MH develops a MH crisis during exposure to triggering agents ■ Males are predominantly affected ■ 40% of reported cases have been in children under 14 years of age.

General aspects

Aetiopathogenesis ■ In some cases, an inherited dominant autosomal pattern has been described; others are found associated with rare disorders such as the autosomal recessive Schwartz–Jampel syndrome (chondrodystrophic myotonia) ■ The most common drug trigger is the combination of halogenated volatile GA agents (e.g. halothane), and muscle relaxants ■ Several non-anaesthetic triggers that have been described in susceptible persons include: • severe exercise in hot conditions • neuroleptic drugs • alcohol • infections ■ The syndrome is thought to be due to a reduction in the reuptake of calcium by the sarcoplasmic reticulum necessary for termination of muscle contraction ■ Consequently, muscle contraction is sustained, resulting in signs of hypermetabolism, including acidosis, tachycardia, hypercarbia, glycolysis, hypoxemia and heat production (hyperthermia) ■ The aetiology of the disturbed intracellular calcium homeostasis is not precisely known, although a general membrane defect has been proposed.

Clinical presentation ■ Poor muscular relaxation after induction of GA, or complete failure of the jaw to relax after suxamethonium has been administered ■ Rise in temperature with tachycardia or arrhythmias and hypotension ■ Late complications – pulmonary oedema, acute renal failure and disseminated intravascular coagulation.

Diagnosis ■ Serum creatine kinase level – raised ■ Serum pyrophosphate level – raised ■ Muscle biopsy – raised myophosphorylase A levels, and excessive *in vitro* response of muscle to halothane, suxamethonium or caffeine.

Treatment ■ Stop the trigger drug ■ Administer dantrolene sodium.

Prognosis The mortality rate may approach 80%.

Dental management

Risk assessment Oral infections should be treated quickly and effectively since they may precipitate attacks.

Pain and anxiety control **Local anaesthesia** ■ LA is safe in malignant hyperthermia; amide local anaesthetic agents, including lidocaine, articaine and prilocaine, were once thought to be weak triggers, but this has been discounted ■ Since the earliest signs of an MH reaction are rapid breathing and heart rate, along with increasing blood pressure, there may be confusion with a reaction to the LA, since epinephrine can cause similar signs ■ Since other agents are also effective to manage bleeding from the gingivae, the risk of using epinephrine in an unmonitored MH patient outweighs the benefit – prilocaine or mepivacaine epinephrine-free are recommended for LA. **Conscious sedation** Malignant hyperpyrexia has been reported after administration of nitrous oxide but this is extremely rare, and thus conscious sedation can usually be safely carried out using relative analgesia and close monitoring. **General anaesthesia** ■ Inquiry into the family history is essential before giving a GA as there are no absolutely reliable predictive tests; moreover, absence of reaction to a previous GA does not completely exclude the possibility of a reaction on the next occasion: the syndrome may develop after a single GA exposure or after several uneventful exposures ■ For major oral surgery, specialist GA care is needed ■ Thiopentone is usually used since intravenous agents are usually safe (Table 3.107) ■ In the event of hyperthermia, the drug and surgery must be stopped and the patient cooled. Oxygen and a bicarbonate intravenous infusion (2 mEq/kg), to counteract the metabolic acidosis, should also be given. Dantrolene sodium (1–2 mg/kg IV every 5–10 min to a total dose of 10 mg/kg) or procainamide are effective in controlling the disease. Dantrolene given preoperatively and postoperatively for about 3 days (4–7 mg/kg/day) may prevent hyperthermia.

Further reading
● Chen L W, Chang W K, Tsou M Y et al 1996 A child with suspected malignant hyperthermia during general anesthesia for dental surgery. Acta Anaesthesiol Sin 34:167–171 ● Monaghan A, Hindle I 1994 Malignant hyperpyrexia

Table 3.107 **Drugs contraindicated, and safer alternatives, in malignant hyperpyrexia in susceptible subjects**

	Contraindicated	Safer to use
General anaesthetics	Halothane Ether Cyclopropane Ketamine Enflurane	Nitrous oxide Thiopentone
Muscle relaxants	Suxamethonium Curare	Pancuronium
Antidepressants	Tricyclic antidepressants Monoamine oxidase inhibitors	

Table 3.108 **Key considerations for dental management in malignant hyperthermia (see text)**

	Management modifications*	Comments/possible complications
Risk assessment	2	Oral infections
Appropriate dental care	2	Select drugs; preoperative dantrolene
Pain and anxiety control		
– Local anaesthesia	2	Avoid epinephrine
– Conscious sedation	3/4	Monitor closely
– General anaesthesia	3/4	Avoid halothane
Patient access and positioning		
– Access to dental office	0	
– Timing of treatment	0	
– Patient positioning	0	
Treatment modification		
– Oral surgery	2	
– Implantology	2	
– Conservative/Endodontics	2	
– Fixed prosthetics	2	
– Removable prosthetics	2	
– Non-surgical periodontology	2	
– Surgical periodontology	2	
Hazardous and contraindicated drugs	2	Select drugs (see Table 3.107)

*0 = No special considerations. 1 = Caution advised. 2 = Specialised medical advice recommended in some cases. 3 = Specialised medical advice mandatory. 4 = Only to be performed in hospital environment. 5 = Should be avoided.

in oral surgery – case report and literature review. Br J Oral Maxillofac Surg 32:190–193

● Murray C, Sasaki S S, Berg D 1999 Local anesthesia and malignant hyperthermia: review of the literature and recommendations for the dermatologic surgeon. Dermatol Surg 25:626–630.

MANIA

Definition Mania is a syndrome of elation, 'butterfly' thinking, poor judgment, and extrovert social behaviour. It typically occurs as a symptom of *bipolar disorder* (a mood disorder characterised by both manic and depressive episodes).

General aspects

Aetiopathogenesis The aetiology appears to be related to increased brain norepinephrine and decreased serotonin (5-hydroxytryptamine) and dopamine. Down-regulation of the postsynaptic receptor systems has also been implicated.

Clinical presentation Mania is characterised by: ■ abnormal or excessive elation, 'high', overly good, euphoric mood ■ grandiose notions and unrealistic beliefs in one's abilities and powers ■ excessive talking ■ racing thoughts, jumping from one idea to another (butterfly mind) ■ distractibility ■ excessive sexual desire ■ greatly increased energy and provocative, intrusive, or aggressive behaviour ■ poor judgment ■ inappropriate social behaviour ■ spending sprees ■ abuse of drugs, particularly cocaine, alcohol and sleeping medications ■ denial that anything is wrong ■ less need for sleep.

Classification **Bipolar I disorder (mania with/without major depression)** This is classic mania, which usually involves recurrent episodes of depression. Sometimes, there are: ■ psychotic symptoms, commonly hallucinations (hearing, seeing, or otherwise sensing the presence of things not actually there) ■ delusions (false, strongly held beliefs not influenced by logical reasoning or explained by a person's usual cultural concepts). **Bipolar II disorder (hypomania with major depression)** This is a less severe disorder, with a lower level of mania (hypomania), which may feel good to the person who experiences it and may even be associated with good functioning and enhanced productivity.

Diagnosis Mania is diagnosed if the elevated mood comes with three or more of the other clinical features listed above, for most of the day, nearly every day, for 1 week or longer.

Treatment ■ Cognitive behavioural therapy (CBT) may be effective ■ Lithium and valproate are the most useful mood-stabilising drugs ■ Carbamazepine has also been successfully used.

Prognosis ■ Untreated patients with bipolar disorder will have a mean of 10 episodes (an episode lasts about 9 months) during their lives ■ They have a higher risk of hospitalisations and suicides than in unipolar psychosis (major depression).

Oral findings

■ Lithium can cause dehydration and a dry mouth or impaired taste; xerostomia results in higher rate of caries ■ Manic-depressive patients may also be treated with other antidepressant drugs with side effects such as xerostomia ■ Carbamazepine can depress bone marrow (agranulocytosis); mouth ulcers secondary to folic acid deficiency anaemia may be seen.

Dental management

Risk assessment Patients during an episode of acute mania should be treated in a hospital or other specialist centre setting. Elective dental treatment may be best deferred until they are controlled.

Pain and anxiety control **Local anaesthesia** LA may be used with caution, as the patient's level of cooperation should be assessed. **Conscious sedation** Diazepam should be avoided as it interacts with

Table 3.109 **Potential interactions with lithium**

Drug interacting with lithium	Consequences
Carbamazepine	Lithium toxicity
Diazepam	Hypothermia
Droperidol and other neuroleptics	Facial dyskinesias
Non-steroidal anti-inflammatory analgesics	Lithium toxicity
Metronidazole	Lithium toxicity
Phenytoin	Lithium toxicity
SSRIs	May produce the serotonin syndrome
Suxamethonium and other muscle relaxants	Prolonged muscle relaxation
Tetracyclines	Lithium toxicity

Table 3.110 **Key considerations for dental management in mania (see text)**

	Management modifications*	Comments/possible complications
Risk assessment	2/3	Inappropriate behaviour
Appropriate dental care	2–4	
Pain and anxiety control		
– Local anaesthesia	1	
– Conscious sedation	2	Avoid diazepam
– General anaesthesia	3/4	Avoid muscle relaxants; arrhythmias
Patient access and positioning		
– Access to dental office	1	
– Timing of treatment	1	
– Patient positioning	1	
Treatment modification		
– Oral surgery	2	
– Implantology	2	
– Conservative/Endodontics	2	
– Fixed prosthetics	2	
– Removable prosthetics	2	
– Non-surgical periodontology	2	
– Surgical periodontology	2	
Imaging	1	
Hazardous and contraindicated drugs	2	Avoid NSAIDs, metronidazole and tetracyclines

*0 = No special considerations. 1 = Caution advised. 2 = Specialised medical advice recommended in some cases. 3 = Specialised medical advice mandatory. 4 = Only to be performed in hospital environment. 5 = Should be avoided.

lithium. **General anaesthesia** Lithium treatment should be monitored by blood levels, since arrhythmias may arise, particularly during GA. Lithium can also interact with many drugs, and therefore it may be advisable to stop/replace lithium treatment 2–3 days before GA (Table 3.109).

Drug use ■ NSAIDs should be avoided since they can induce lithium toxicity; acetaminophen/paracetamol or codeine are safe to use in this regard ■ Antimicrobials (metronidazole and tetracyclines) should be avoided since they can also induce lithium toxicity.

Further reading ● Clark D B 2003 Dental care for the patient with bipolar disorder. J Can Dent Assoc 69:20–24 ● Friedlander A H, Birch N J 1990 Dental conditions in patients with bipolar disorder on long-term lithium maintenance therapy. Spec Care Dentist 10:148–151 ● Friedlander A H, Friedlander I K, Marder S R 2002 Bipolar I disorder: psychopathology, medical management and dental implications. J Am Dent Assoc 133:1209–1217 ● Reebye U N, Reebye P N, Cottrell D A, Misri N 2003 Mood disorders and dental implications. J Mass Dent Soc 52:38–42.

MARIJUANA ABUSE

General aspects

Background ■ Marijuana is the most commonly used illicit drug in the developed world ■ It is derived from a dry, shredded green/brown mix of flowers, stems, seeds, and leaves of the hemp plant *Cannabis sativa* or *Cannabis indica* ■ It usually is smoked as a cigarette (joint, nail), or in a pipe (bong) ■ It also is smoked in blunts, which are cigars that have been emptied of tobacco and refilled with marijuana, often in combination with another drug ■ Use also might include mixing marijuana in food or brewing it as a tea ■ As a more concentrated, resinous form it is called hashish which is chewed, and, as a sticky black liquid, hash oil ■ Recently, medicinal cannabis and cannabinoids have been suggested for the management of neurological disorders including multiple sclerosis and Alzheimer's disease.

Pathogenesis The main active chemical in marijuana is THC (delta-9-tetrahydrocannabinol). This binds to brain receptors, which are in high density in the parts of the brain that influence pleasure, memory, thought, concentration, sensory and time perception, and coordinated movement.

Clinical presentation ■ Findings that may indicate a drug addiction problem are as for amphetamine/LSD/MDMA abuse ■ The most significant risks from drug abuse are behavioural disturbances and psychoses ■ The clinical effect normally comes on within half an hour and lasts for 2–3 hours; when it is taken by mouth the onset is delayed sometimes up to 2–3 hours, and the effect may last twice as long ■ There are normally no characteristic physical effects, apart from redness of the eyes and the breath may smell of marijuana ■ When the drug is smoked there may be some initial rawness and burning in the throat, and tightness in the chest ■ When the subject is initially anxious, headache may result ■ There may be nausea and vomiting ■ Once the effect of the drug has worn off there may be an increase in appetite, even ravenous hunger ■ The effects of cannabis in moderate amounts are predominantly psychological: ● sense of excitement or tension ● sometimes apprehension or hilarity ● followed as a rule by a sense of heightened awareness: colours, sounds and social intercourse appear more intense and meaningful ● a sense of wellbeing is then usual ● after this, a phase of tranquillity and of passive enjoyment of the environment normally follows until, after a few hours, fatigue sets in and the subject sleeps. Although a 'hangover' may follow this is not common.

Adverse effects Adverse effects of marijuana can include: ■ depression, anxiety, and personality disturbances ■ impaired attention, memory, and learning ■ increased blood pressure and heart rate and lowered oxygen-carrying capacity of blood ■ a predisposition to respiratory illnesses such as infections, daily cough and sputum production, and obstructed airways ■ immune impairment ■ babies born to women who used marijuana during pregnancy have more behavioural problems and poorer performance on tasks of visual perception, language comprehension, sustained attention, and memory. **Severe adverse effects** ■ There have been isolated reports in which death has been attributed directly to marijuana, but these are very rare and their validity cannot be confirmed ■ However, smoking marijuana doubles or triples the risk of lung cancers, and it may be associated with some oral cancer.

Withdrawal and treatment No medications are currently available for treating marijuana misuse, but recent discoveries about the workings of THC receptors have raised the possibility of developing some.

Oral findings

There is a tendency to a dry mouth, and concern that cannabis use may predispose to oral cancer.

Dental management

Risk assessment There are no specific aspects of cannabis addiction that influence dental management in most patients, but recognition of individuals who may be abusing drugs is critical, as behavioural problems may interfere with dental treatment. Care should be taken with any patient who makes suspicious requests for medication (as detailed for amphetamine/LSD/MDMA abuse). Short-term memory loss may affect the validity of consent for subsequent appointment.

Pain and anxiety control **Local anaesthesia** LA should be given with caution due to the potentially uncooperative behaviour of the patient. **Conscious sedation** CS should be given with caution and the patient advised not to use marijuana concurrently. **General anaesthesia** GA should be given with caution and the patient advised not to use marijuana concurrently.

Table 3.111 **Key considerations for dental management in marijuana abuse (see text)**

	Management modifications*	Comments/possible complications
Risk assessment	2	Drug abuser recognition; abnormal behaviour; short term memory loss
Pain and anxiety control		
– Local anaesthesia	1	
– Conscious sedation	1	
– General anaesthesia	4	
Patient access and positioning		
– Access to dental office	0	
– Timing of treatment	1	
– Patient positioning	0	
Treatment modification		
– Oral surgery	1	
– Implantology	1	
– Conservative/Endodontics	1	
– Fixed prosthetics	1	
– Removable prosthetics	1	
– Non-surgical periodontology	1	
– Surgical periodontology	1	
Hazardous and contraindicated drugs	1	

*0 = No special considerations. 1 = Caution advised. 2 = Specialised medical advice recommended in some cases. 3 = Specialised medical advice mandatory. 4 = Only to be performed in hospital environment. 5 = Should be avoided.

Further reading ● van der Bijl P 2003 Substance abuse – concerns in dentistry: an overview. S Afr Dent J 58:382–385 ● Cornelius J R, Clark D B, Weyant R et al 2004 Dental abnormalities in children of fathers with substance use disorders. Addict Behav 29:979–982 ● Sandler N A 2001 Patients who abuse drugs. Oral Surg Oral Med Oral Pathol Oral Radiol Endod 91:12–14.

MITRAL VALVE DISEASE

MITRAL STENOSIS

Definition Mitral stenosis is a narrowing of the mitral valve that generates an increasing pressure in the left atrium of the heart.

General aspects

Aetiopathogenesis Caused by rheumatic fever, congenital defects and others.

Clinical presentation Features are related to increased pressure in the pulmonary veins: ■ dyspnoea and fatigue ■ chest pain ■ systemic emboli.

Diagnosis ■ Doppler echo ■ Echocardiography ■ ECG ■ Cardiac catheterisation.

Treatment ■ Diuretics ■ Digoxin ■ Anticoagulants (warfarin) ■ Surgery (balloon valvuloplasty, valvotomy or valve replacement).

Prognosis Prognosis is influenced by the severity of the stenosis, thrombotic episodes and development of pulmonary hypertension and/or infective endocarditis. Life expectancy of untreated symptomatic patients is about 5 years.

MITRAL REGURGITATION

Definition The blood propulsed to the left ventricle during systolic contraction returns into the left atrium during diastolic dilatation due to a valve closure defect.

General aspects

Aetiopathogenesis ■ Regurgitation because of left ventricular dilatation, valve calcification or damage (rheumatic carditis, infective endocarditis) ■ Valve prolapse ■ Damaged chordae tendinae or muscles ■ Drugs (fenfluramine, phentermine).

Clinical presentation Features include: ■ dyspnoea ■ fatigue ■ palpitations.

Diagnosis ■ Echocardiography ■ Doppler echo ■ Cardiac catheterisation ■ ECG.

Treatment ■ Digoxin ■ Surgery (valvotomy, grafts or prosthetic valves).

Prognosis Advanced regurgitation may lead to pulmonary hypertension and cardiac failure, and predisposes to infective endocarditis.

MITRAL PROLAPSE

Definition ■ Mitral prolapse is a protrusion of the valves into the left atrium during systole ■ It may exist in isolation but is sometimes associated with mitral regurgitation ■ Mitral valve prolapse may also be associated with: • atrial septal defect • patent ductus arteriosus.

General aspects

Aetiopathogenesis ■ Mitral valve prolapse (MVP) has a strong hereditary tendency ■ It is the most common cardiac defect, thought to affect about 3–4% of the general population, and to be more common in women ■ Although most cases are idiopathic, MVP is a characteristic feature of a range of other conditions (Ehlers–Danlos syndrome, Marfan syndrome, Down syndrome, Turner's syndrome, cardiomyopathies, pseudoxanthoma elasticum, muscular dystrophy, polycystic kidney disease, osteogenesis imperfecta, thyrotoxicosis, ischaemic heart disease, panic disorder and lupus erythematosus).

Clinical presentation ■ Mitral valve prolapse may cause no symptoms whatsoever ■ Some patients develop symptoms such as pain, irregular or racing pulse, or fatigue – but not before the early teenage years, when the adolescent growth spurt occurs ■ Most patients with mitral valve prolapse who exhibit symptoms are actually experiencing dysautonomia from panic disorder – up to 50% of patients with panic disorder are reported to have mitral valve prolapse.

Diagnosis ■ Echocardiography ■ ECG.

Treatment ■ Beta-blockers (propranolol) ■ Prosthetic valve replacement.

Prognosis Usually the prognosis of MVP is good, especially in cases of mild prolapse without regurgitation. Mitral valve prolapse with regurgitation predisposes to infective endocarditis.

Dental management of mitral valve disease

Risk assessment ■ Patients with mitral stenosis or regurgitation may be susceptible to infective endocarditis (see Endocarditis) ■ If the mitral valve has been replaced by a prosthetic valve, this is particularly susceptible to infective endocarditis ■ Some patients having heart surgery may still have a residual lesion postoperatively – this makes them a poor risk for general anaesthesia and a high risk for endocarditis; some are on anticoagulant treatment, immunosuppression or on other drugs.

Appropriate health care ■ For patients scheduled for cardiac surgery, a meticulous pre-surgery oral assessment is required and dental treatment undertaken with particular attention to establishing optimal oral hygiene and eradicating sources of potential infection; dental treatment should be completed before surgery ■ Generally speaking, teeth with a reasonable prognosis (shallow caries and periodontal pocketing) should be conserved but those with a poor pulpal or periodontal prognosis are best removed before cardiac surgery ■ Elective dental care should be avoided for the first 6 months after cardiac surgery – when there may be continued susceptibility to endocarditis.

Pain and anxiety control It is essential that oral health care should be provided with minimal stress and minimal pain. **Local anaesthesia** An aspirating syringe should be used to give LA. The use of epinephrine should be minimised. **Conscious sedation** Conscious sedation requires special sedation care, in hospital or other specialist centres. **General anaesthesia** GA requires special care, and close consultation with the patient's cardiologist.

Table 3.112 **Key considerations for dental management in mitral valve disease (see text)**

	Management modifications*	Comments/possible complications
Risk assessment	2	Infective endocarditis
Appropriate dental care	2	Ideally before any planned cardiac surgery; delay 6 months after surgery; antibiotic prophylaxis
Pain and anxiety control		
– Local anaesthesia	1	Aspirating syringe; minimise epinephrine use
– Conscious sedation	3/4	
– General anaesthesia	3/4	
Patient access and positioning		
– Access to dental office	0	
– Timing of treatment	0	
– Patient positioning	0	
Treatment modification		
– Oral surgery	1	
– Implantology	1	
– Conservative/Endodontics	0	
– Fixed prosthetics	0	
– Removable prosthetics	0	
– Non-surgical periodontology	1	
– Surgical periodontology	1	
Hazardous and contraindicated drugs	2	Some patients are treated with anticoagulants

*0 = No special considerations. 1 = Caution advised. 2 = Specialised medical advice recommended in some cases. 3 = Specialised medical advice mandatory. 4 = Only to be performed in hospital environment. 5 = Should be avoided.

Drug use Some drugs usually prescribed in dentistry can interact with anticoagulant therapy (see Warfarinisation).

Further reading
● Carmona I T, Diz Dios P, Seoane Leston J, Limeres Posse J 2001 Guidelines for antibiotic prophylaxis of bacterial endocarditis in patients undergoing dental therapy. Rev Clin Esp 201:21–24 ● Friedlander A H, Marder S R, Sung E C, Child J S 2004 Panic disorder: psychopathology, medical management and dental implications. J Am Dent Assoc 135:771–778 ● Martin M V, Gosney M A, Longman L P, Figures K H 2001 Murmurs, infective endocarditis and dentistry. Dent Update 28:76–82.

MOTOR NEURONE DISEASE

Definition Motor neurone diseases (MND) are a group of uncommon lethal degenerative diseases affecting especially males in old age and causing damage to motor neurones (especially anterior horn cells) with resultant muscular atrophy, weakness, and spasticity, but no sensory or intellectual abnormalities.

General aspects

Classification The clinical subtypes of MND are distinguished by the major site of degeneration of the motor neurones. They include: ■ *Progressive muscular atrophy* – affects the anterior horn below the foramen magnum, with lower motor neurone lesions causing wasting and weakness that starts in the hands and spreads proximally. It has the best prognosis. ■ *Progressive bulbar palsy* – affects anterior horn cells of the brainstem and thus cranial nerve motor neurones arising in the medulla (IX–XII inclusive). It is characterised by wasting, weakness and fasciculation of the muscles of the pharynx, tongue, palate, sternocleidomastoid and trapezius. It has the worst prognosis. ■ *Amyotrophic lateral sclerosis (ALS)* – affects the anterior horn and pyramidal tract, damaging upper and lower motor neurones and resulting in wasting and weakness of the hands and spasticity of the legs. This is the most common sub-type and has an intermediate prognosis.

Aetiopathogenesis The aetiology is unclear but may be viral (slow virus such as polio or polio-like virus). Premature aging, exposure to heavy metals, immunological abnormalities and biochemical deficiencies have also been implicated.

Clinical presentation Early signs and symptoms (Fig. 3.28) of ALS: ■ fatigue ■ muscle cramps and twitching in arms, shoulders and tongue, spreading to the trunk ■ slow loss of strength and coordination in one or more limbs ■ weakness in feet and ankles, resulting in a stiff and clumsy gait and in dragging feet ■ difficulty swallowing, speaking or breathing ■ the disease may affect bulbar functions such as chewing, swallowing, speaking and breathing ■ involvement of the brainstem leads to pseudobulbar palsy – bulbar palsy with emotional lability (involuntary weeping or laughing).

Diagnosis ■ Clinical findings – muscle fasciculation, weakness, wasting, spastic dysarthria and exaggerated reflexes ■ Nerve conduction studies ■ Electromyography (EMG).

Treatment ■ Riluzole may slow the progress of ALS ■ Also sometimes needed are: ● physical and occupational therapy ● speech therapy ● nutritional support ● breathing assistance.

Prognosis The disease is unremittingly progressive. Protection of the airway may be impaired and patients with this degree of disability are usually hospitalised. Morphine or pethidine are frequently needed for terminal care. Typically death occurs within 5 years, usually from respiratory paralysis. However, even in the late stages, sensory, bowel, bladder and cognitive functions are spared.

Oral findings

Clinical manifestations are consequence of weakness and fasciculations of oral musculature, and include: ■ dysarthria ■ dysphagia ■ drooling.

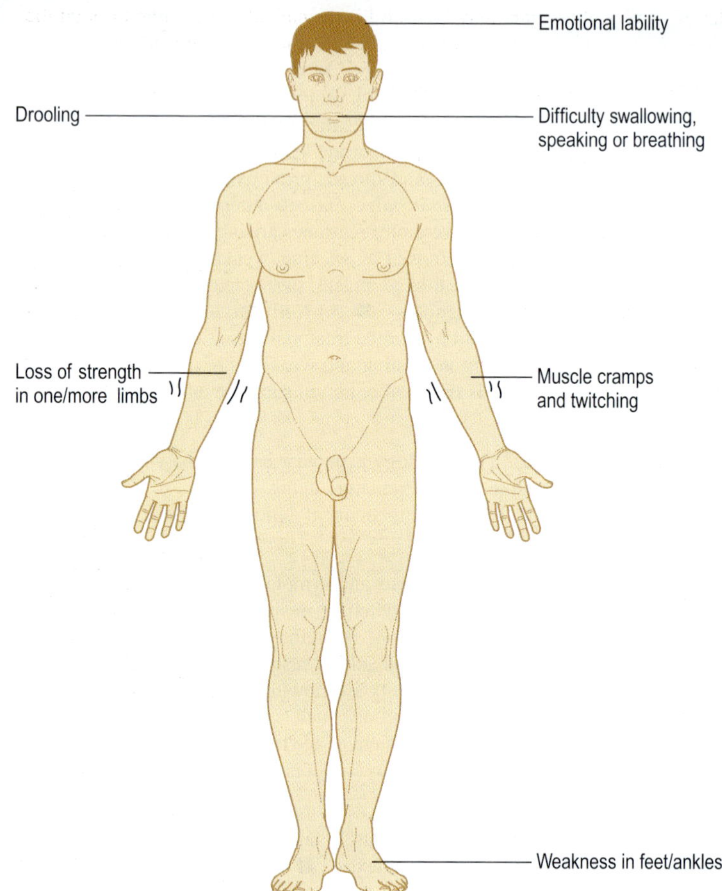

Figure 3.28 **Clinical presentation of motor neurone disease**

Dental management

Risk assessment ■ Weakness or paralysis of the neck and head and oral musculature can impede dental treatment ■ There is an increased risk of aspiration during dental treatment ■ These individuals develop severe respiratory problems due to the effect on the muscles that control breathing, and deficits in protective airway reflexes ■ Oral hygiene may be impaired.

Appropriate health care ■ Dental treatment is influenced by the prognosis and the ability of the patient to maintain good oral hygiene ■ Short appointments are desirable ■ Patients may have to be transferred from wheelchair to the dental chair ■ Domiciliary care may be required for patients with advanced disease ■ Rubber dam may be useful if the patient can breathe through the nose ■ Mouth props may help to facilitate most dental procedures.

Patient access and positioning The patient should be placed at 45 degrees (to protect the airway), not in a supine position.

Pain and anxiety management **Local anaesthesia** LA may be provided with routine precautions. **Conscious sedation** Specialist advice is mandatory before CS is provided, due to the risk of further compromising respiration. **General anaesthesia** Specialist advice is mandatory before GA is provided, due to the risks associated with hypoventilation and hypoxia.

Treatment modification **Removable prosthetics** Patients may have difficulty inserting and removing removable prostheses. Complete dentures should be avoided since oral muscle function will diminish. Mucous membrane supported prostheses tend to be unstable and although patients may request

Table 3.113 **Key considerations for dental management in motor neurone disease (see text)**

	Management modifications*	Comments/possible complications
Risk assessment	2	Difficult management due to head and neck paralysis; aspiration
Appropriate dental care	2/4	Short appointments; mouth props; rubber dam
Pain and anxiety control		
– Local anaesthesia	0	
– Conscious sedation	3	Breathing difficulty
– General anaesthesia	3/4	Breathing difficulty
Patient access and positioning		
– Access to dental office	1	Physical assistance required
– Timing of treatment	0	
– Patient positioning	1	Some are chairbound; otherwise place at 45 degrees
Treatment modification		
– Oral surgery	1	
– Implantology	1/5	
– Conservative/Endodontics	1/5	
– Fixed prosthetics	1/5	
– Removable prosthetics	1/5	Unstable prostheses
– Non-surgical periodontology	1	
– Surgical periodontology	1/5	
Hazardous and contraindicated drugs	0	

*0 = No special considerations. 1 = Caution advised. 2 = Specialised medical advice recommended in some cases. 3 = Specialised medical advice mandatory. 4 = Only to be performed in hospital environment. 5 = Should be avoided.

relines, the results may not be good, due to paralysis and fasciculation of the oral musculature. Indeed, an unstable denture may impede respiration and deglutition.

Further reading ● Asher R S, Alfred T 1993 Dental management of long-term amyotrophic lateral sclerosis: case report. Spec Care Dentist 13:241–244 ● Griffiths J 2002 Guidelines for oral health care for people with a physical disability. J Disability Oral Health 3:51–58 ● Talacko A A, Reade P C 1990 Progressive bulbar palsy: a case report of a type of motor neuron disease presenting with oral symptoms. Oral Surg Oral Med Oral Pathol 69:182–184 ● Targan B 1996 Differential diagnosis of facial paralysis and Bell's palsy identifiable for dental surgeons – a review of the literature. J NJ Dent Assoc 67:19–22 ● Walshe T 1988 Approach to patients with degenerative disorders of the nervous system. Gerodontics 4:156–157.

MULTIPLE SCLEROSIS (DISSEMINATED SCLEROSIS)

Definition Multiple sclerosis (MS) is a chronic relapsing demyelinating CNS disease affecting the corticospinal tract. It is the most common human demyelinating disease and causes a variety of sensory, motor and psychological symptoms.

General aspects

Background ■ MS is one of the commonest neurological conditions of young adults in the Western world, with an estimated 58 000–63 000 people with the disease in England and Wales ■ Pain and spasticity are two of the commonest symptoms ■ The importance of these symptoms is not simply their frequency, but also the impact they have on daily life ■ As the disease progresses, so does the spasticity, resulting in muscle spasms, immobility, disturbed sleep, pain and fatigue ■ Disability resulting from spasticity can lead to patients requiring extensive nursing care and support.

Aetiopathogenesis ■ The aetiology remains unclear, but autoimmune mechanisms triggered by a virus have been implicated ■ MS is a progressive disorder causing multifocal plaques of demyelination, leading to four important neurological disturbances: ● decreased conduction velocity ● differential rate of impulse transmission ● partial conduction blocking ● complete failure of impulse transmission.

Clinical presentation ■ MS affects mainly females, with a mean age of onset about 30 years ■ Manifestations vary over time and locations, but progressive disability is common and demyelination eventually causes paralysis ■ Some common initial presentations include: ● unilateral optic neuritis (rapid visual deterioration and pain on eye movement) ● limb paraesthesia/anaesthesia ● leg weakness ● cerebellar symptoms (diplopia/ataxia) ■ Psychological symptoms may include mood swings, depression and cognitive impairment.

Classification Based on the clinical course, MS has been classified as: relapsing–remitting, primary progressive, secondary progressive and progressive-relapsing (Table 3.114).

Table 3.114 **Multiple sclerosis subtypes**

Subtypes	Frequency	Features
Relapsing-remitting	80% of patients	Short acute attacks about once each year
Primary progressive	10%	Progressive deterioration from outset
Secondary progressive	40% of patients with relapsing-remitting MS	Progressive deterioration in patients with relapsing-remitting MS, after about 10 years
Progressive-relapsing	Rare	Relapses in patients with primary progressive MS

Diagnosis ■ Clinical findings during acute attack ■ Lumbar puncture – increased IgG in cerebrospinal fluid ■ Evoked potentials ■ MRI.

Treatment ■ Corticosteroids ■ Beta interferon ■ Glatiramer ■ Tizanidine.

Prognosis ■ Most patients survive at least 20–30 years ■ After 25 years more than 75% of patients are still alive ■ Remissions, complete and partial, are common ■ Occasionally there are fulminant cases.

Oral findings

■ There are no specific oral manifestations of MS but this diagnosis should always be considered in: ● a young patient presenting with trigeminal neuralgia, particularly if bilateral or if there have been other neurological disturbances, or if the pain lasts minutes or hours ● facial palsy not associated with retro-aural pain or with loss of taste sensation, such as may be seen in Bell's palsy ● abnormal perioral sensation, such as extreme hypersensitivity or facial anaesthesia ● facial myokymia (worm-like movements) or hemispasm ● abnormal speech ('scanning speech') ● cerebellar tremor ■ Atropinics used in the treatment of the bladder dysfunction may cause dry mouth, as may tizanidine ■ Glatiramer may cause facial oedema.

Dental management

Risk assessment and appropriate health care ■ Patients with chronic visual and motor complications of MS are considered ASA III ■ Dental care may need to be modified in light of: ● restricted mobility; patients may have to be transferred from wheelchair to dental chair ● psychological disorders ● involuntary mandibular movements ● some patients develop trigeminal neuralgia (tic douloureux), usually bilaterally ● difficulty localising orofacial pain; all diagnostic tools must be used before performing extractions or endodontic therapy ● communication difficulties – not uncommon in advanced MS ● respiratory problems, the effect on respiratory muscles, and deficits in protective airway reflexes compromise the airway.

Preventive dentistry ■ Regular preventive care is important since the ability to maintain good oral hygiene may be impaired ■ Oral health care plans must consider limitations of motor skills ■ The preventive dental programme may require involvement of family member, partner or care provider.

Pain and anxiety management **Local anaesthesia** LA may be provided with routine precautions. **Conscious sedation** Specialist advice is mandatory before CS is provided, due to the risk of further compromising respiration. Nitrous oxide is probably best avoided since it may theoretically cause further demyelination. **General anaesthesia** Specialist advice is mandatory before GA is provided, due to the risks associated with hypoventilation and hypoxia.

Patient access and positioning **Access to dental surgery** Physical assistance is often required to help the patient with MS get in

Table 3.115 **Key considerations for dental management in multiple sclerosis (see text)**

	Management modifications*	Comments/possible complications
Risk assessment	2	Uncontrollable movements; poor cooperation; communication difficulties
Appropriate dental care	2/4	Adapt to physical needs
Pain and anxiety control		
– Local anaesthesia	0	
– Conscious sedation	3	Avoid nitrous oxide
– General anaesthesia	3/4	
Patient access and positioning		
– Access to dental office	1	Physical assistance may be required
– Timing of treatment	1	In the morning
– Patient positioning	1	Some are chairbound; consider respiratory function
Treatment modification		
– Oral surgery	1	
– Implantology	1	
– Conservative/Endodontics	1	
– Fixed prosthetics	1	
– Removable prosthetics	1	
– Non-surgical periodontology	1	
– Surgical periodontology	1	
Hazardous and contraindicated drugs	1	Some patients are on corticosteroids

*0 = No special considerations. 1 = Caution advised. 2 = Specialised medical advice recommended in some cases. 3 = Specialised medical advice mandatory. 4 = Only to be performed in hospital environment. 5 = Should be avoided.

and out of the dental chair. **Timing of treatment** Short appointments in the morning are recommended. **Patient positioning** Patients with severe MS are best not treated fully supine, as respiration may be embarrassed.

Treatment modification **Fixed prosthetics and conservation** Rubber dam may be useful if the patient can breathe through the nose. Provision of complex dental prostheses will be influenced by the ability of the patient to maintain adequate oral hygiene.

Drug use Some patients are on corticosteroids, with their attendant complications.

Further reading ● Fiske J, Griffiths J, Thompson S 2002 Multiple sclerosis and oral care. Dent Update 29:273–283 ● Greenwood M, Meechan J G 2003 General medicine and surgery for dental practitioners Part 4: Neurological disorders. Br Dent J 195:19–25 ● Griffiths J 2002 Guidelines for oral health care for people with a physical disability. J Disability Oral Health 3:51–58 ● Hutchinson S, Clark S 2001 Multiple sclerosis presenting to the dental practitioner: a report of two cases. Dent Update 28:516–517.

MUSCULAR DYSTROPHIES

Definition ■ Muscular dystrophies (MD) are a group of uncommon genetically determined diseases, characterised by progressive painless skeletal muscle degeneration ■ They are the main crippling diseases of childhood.

General aspects

Aetiopathogenesis The aetiopathogenesis remains unclear, and may be related to neural, vascular, or biochemical dysfunction. Inheritance patterns differ with the type of dystrophy (Table 3.116).

Clinical presentation ■ The disease appears as the infant begins to walk, when there is a waddling gait and severe lumbar lordosis ■ The child has difficulty in standing ■ On attempting to stand the child begins with both hands and feet on the floor then moves the hands up the legs until in an upright posture (Gower's sign) ■ Weakness spreads to all other muscles but tends to spare those of the head, neck and hands ■ The affected muscles enlarge (pseudohypertrophy) ■ Typically the child becomes chairbound before puberty ■ Skeletal deformity in the head, neck and chest may occur ■ Cardiac disease (cardiomyopathy), respiratory impairment and intellectual deterioration may occur.

Classification Duchenne muscular dystrophy is the most common but other types are shown in Table 3.116.

Diagnosis ■ Serum creatine phosphokinase levels – raised ■ Serum aspartate transaminase (AST) levels – raised ■ Serum lactate dehydrogenase (LDH) levels – raised ■ Muscle biopsy.

Treatment ■ Physical therapy (possibly orthopaedic surgery) ■ Genetic counselling.

Table 3.116 Muscular dystrophies

Type	Inheritance*	Muscles affected	Pseudohypertrophy	Onset	Progress	Other features
Duchenne	X	All	Usual	Early childhood	Rapid	Cardiomyopathy Death in early adulthood
Becker	X	All	Usual	Late childhood	Variable	More benign than Duchenne type
Childhood	AR	All	Usual	Late childhood	Variable	More benign than Duchenne type
Limb girdle	AR	Pelvic and shoulder girdles	Occasional	Adolescence	Variable	Severely disabling May be cardiomyopathy
Facioscapulohumeral	AD	Starts in face and shoulder	Rare	Adolescence	Slow	Most benign type Normal life expectancy Pouting of lips with facial weakness
Scapuloperoneal	AD or X	Scapular Peroneal All	Occasional	Adolescence	Slow	Cardiac conduction defects Relatively benign
Congenital muscular	AR		Rare	Birth	Variable	–
Distal myopathy	AD	Distal	Rare	Any age	Slow	–
Oculopharyngeal	AD	Facial and sternomastoid	Rare	Adult	Slow	Dysphagia may be prominent Weakness of masticatory muscles and tongue

*AD = autosomal dominant, AR = autosomal recessive, X = x-linked.

Prognosis Muscular dystrophies are eventually fatal due to the onset of infectious and respiratory diseases, and pulmonary dysfunction. A respirator is necessary in later stages. Patients often fail to survive beyond their twenties.

Oral findings

The oral findings are variable. ■ In muscular dystrophies where there is facial myopathy (classically in the facioscapulohumeral type), there is lack of facial expression and, often, inability to whistle; electromyography shows involvement of the masseter muscles ■ A large tongue and malocclusions are often seen, especially expansion of the arches with posterior crossbite, and anterior open bite ■ Mouth breathing may be present ■ Tooth eruption may be delayed ■ Myotonic subjects differ from normal subjects in head length, head breadth, cephalic index, bizygomatic face width, nose breadth, maxillary arch widths, palatal depth, anterior and posterior face heights, cranial base lengths, cranial base angles, and other cephalometric measures ■ Weakness of facial and neck muscles causes decreased protective reflexes, and a decrease in the ability to swallow secretions ■ Poor oral hygiene may be present due to an inability to provide self care.

Dental management

Risk assessment Cardiomyopathy and respiratory muscle weakness are the major complications.

Appropriate health care ■ The patient's disease stage and prognosis and motor skills must be assessed when treatment planning ■ The preventive dental programme may require involvement of a family member, partner or care provider ■ Frequent recall appointments, topical fluoride, and antiplaque agents are required.

Pain and anxiety control **Local anaesthesia** LA may be provided with routine precautions. **Conscious sedation** Opioids and benzodiazepines are best avoided due to the risk of respiratory depression. **General anaesthesia** ■ Cardiomyopathies and respiratory disease are contraindications to GA ■ Endotracheal intubation may be difficult due to skeletal deformity in the head and neck ■ Volatile anaesthetics can produce severe respiratory depression ■ There is a risk of post-intubation regurgitation and aspiration ■ There may be a risk of malignant hyperthermia.

Patient access and positioning ■ The patient may have to be transferred from wheelchair to dental chair and a hoist or physical assistance to get in and out of the dental chair is often required ■ Domiciliary care may be more appropriate in advanced stages of MD ■ Some patients use orthopaedic devices ■ Patients with severe MD require short appointments ■ Patients with severe MD can develop severe respiratory problems – they should be placed at 45 degrees, not in a supine position (to protect airway) and rubber dam may be helpful if the patient can breathe through the nose.

Further reading ● Eckardt L, Harzer W 1996 Facial structure and functional findings in patients with progressive muscular dystrophy (Duchenne). Am J Orthod

Table 3.117 **Key considerations for dental management in muscular dystrophies (see text)**

	Management modifications*	Comments/possible complications
Risk assessment	2	Cardiac and respiratory complications
Appropriate dental care	2/4	Disease stage and prognosis
Pain and anxiety control		
– Local anaesthesia	0	
– Conscious sedation	2	Avoid benzodiazepines and opioids
– General anaesthesia	3–5	Difficult endotracheal intubation; avoid volatile anaesthetics; aspiration; malignant hyperthermia
Patient access and positioning		
– Access to dental office	1	Physical assistance required
– Timing of treatment	0	
– Patient positioning	1	Orthopaedic devices; some are chairbound; otherwise position at 45 degrees
Treatment modification		
– Oral surgery	1	
– Implantology	1	
– Conservative/Endodontics	1	
– Fixed prosthetics	1	
– Removable prosthetics	1	
– Non-surgical periodontology	1	
– Surgical periodontology	1	
Hazardous and contraindicated drugs	0	

*0 = No special considerations. 1 = Caution advised. 2 = Specialised medical advice recommended in some cases. 3 = Specialised medical advice mandatory. 4 = Only to be performed in hospital environment. 5 = Should be avoided.

Dentofacial Orthop 110:185–190 ● Erturk N, Dogan S 1991 The effect of neuromuscular diseases on the development of dental and occlusal characteristics. Quintessence Int 22:317–321 ● Guler A U, Ceylan G, Ozkoc O, Aydiin M, Cengiz N 2003 Prosthetic treatment of a patient with facioscapulohumeral muscular dystrophy: a clinical report. J Prosthet Dent 90:321–324 ● Kiliaridis S, Katsaros C 1998 The effects of myotonic dystrophy and Duchenne muscular dystrophy on the orofacial muscles and dentofacial morphology. Acta Odontol Scand 56:369–374 ● Shimizu H, Takizawa Y, Pulkkinen L et al 1999 Epidermolysis bullosa simplex associated with muscular dystrophy: phenotype-genotype correlations and review of the literature. J Am Acad Dermatol 41:950–956 ● Staley R N, Bishara S E, Hanson J W, Nowak A J 1992 Craniofacial development in myotonic dystrophy. Cleft Palate Craniofac J 29:456–462 ● Suda N, Matsuda A, Yoda S et al 2004 Orthodontic treatment of a case of Becker muscular dystrophy. Orthod Craniofac Res 7:55–62 ● Symons A L, Townsend G C, Hughes T E 2002 Dental characteristics of patients with Duchenne muscular dystrophy. ASDC J Dent Child 69:234,277–283.

MYASTHENIA GRAVIS

Definition Myasthenia gravis (MG) is an autoimmune disorder characterised by muscular weakness, which affects mainly adult females.

General aspects

Aetiopathogenesis Antibodies to acetylcholine receptors result in the progressive loss of receptors, and in poor neuromuscular transmission.

Clinical presentation Symptoms (Fig. 3.29) vary according to the amount of activity undergone, the onset of infection, or stress of any kind. An individual with MG may appear perfectly normal one moment, and a few hours, or even minutes later, is droopy and listless. Features include: ■ Muscle weakness: ● initially extraocular ● bulbar ● facial (jaw drop) ● neck ● limbs ● quiet speech ■ Aggravated by: ● pregnancy ● emotion ● some antimicrobials (gentamicin, tetracyclines) ● beta-blockers ■ MG is sometimes associated with a connective tissue disease, hyperthyroidism or thymic tumour.

Classification Based on the main muscular groups involved, myasthenia gravis is classified as bulbar or ocular, and generalised.

Diagnosis ■ Edrophonium test ■ Acetylcholine receptor antibodies ■ Neurophysiology ■ CT mediastinum (for thymus enlargement).

Treatment ■ Anticholinesterase (e.g. pyridostigmine) ■ Corticosteroids ■ Thymectomy.

Prognosis There may be minimal restriction of activity in many cases. In generalised MG, there is an increased risk of aspiration and ventilatory problems.

Oral findings

■ Masticatory muscle fatigue is often conspicuous ■ Dysphagia, dysphonia and dysarthria are common ■ Occasionally there is also furrowing, atrophy or paresis of the tongue, or uvula palsy ■ Salivation is increased if an anticholinesterase, alone, is being taken ■ Occasionally, Sjögren's syndrome or other autoimmune disorders, particularly pemphigus, may be associated ■ If there is a thymoma, there may be chronic mucocutaneous candidosis.

Dental management

Risk assessment ■ Stress and oral infections may trigger a myasthenic crisis ■ There is an increased risk of aspiration during dental procedures.

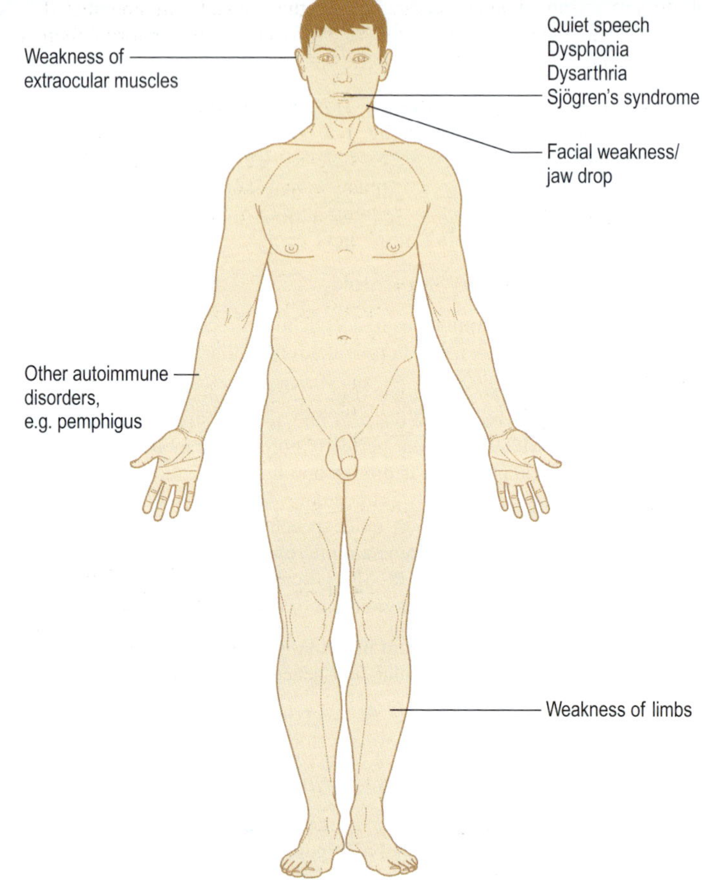

Figure 3.29 **Clinical presentation of myasthenia gravis**

Appropriate health care ■ Dental treatment is best carried out during a period of remission ■ Dental treatment of patients with severe MG should be performed in a hospital or other specialist centre setting.

Pain and anxiety control **Local anaesthesia** ■ LA is preferred, but minimal doses should be given ■ Lidocaine, prilocaine, articaine or mepivacaine can safely be used ■ The older ester types of LA (such as procaine) are contraindicated. **Conscious sedation** ■ A small dose of a benzodiazepine may be given if the patient is anxious ■ Intravenous sedation must not be given in the general dental surgery since bulbar or respiratory involvement impairs respiration – hospital care is preferred. **General anaesthesia** ■ Many drugs used in GA, such as opioids, barbiturates, suxamethonium, curare or anaesthetic agents, are potentiated by or aggravate the myasthenic state ■ Postoperative respiratory infection can result and may also cause MG to worsen.

Patient access and positioning **Timing of treatment** Treatment is best carried out early in the day, within 1–2 hours of routine medication with anticholinesterases, since weakness increases during the day and fatigue or emotional stress may precipitate a myasthenic crisis. **Patient positioning** The patient should be seated upright or at most at 45 degrees, in order to prevent respiratory compromise.

Treatment modification **Implantology** Dental implants may help to stabilise removable prostheses. **Removable prosthetics** Mucous membrane-supported prostheses may be unstable due to muscular weakness.

Drug use ■ Drugs to be avoided, since they increase weakness, include tetracyclines, clindamycin, lincomycin, quinolones, sulphonamides and aminoglycosides ■ Penicillin or erythromycin can safely be used

Table 3.118 **Key considerations for dental management in myasthenia gravis (see text)**

	Management modifications*	Comments/possible complications
Risk assessment	2	Myasthenic crisis; aspiration
Appropriate dental care	2/4	During a remission
Pain and anxiety control		
– Local anaesthesia	2	Minimal doses; avoid ester type
– Conscious sedation	2/4	Avoid intravenous sedation
– General anaesthesia	3/4	Avoid drugs that aggravate MG
Patient access and positioning		
– Access to dental office	0	
– Timing of treatment	1	Early morning; 1–2 h after medication intake
– Patient positioning	1	Upright position
Treatment modification		
– Oral surgery	1	
– Implantology	1	
– Conservative/Endodontics	1	
– Fixed prosthetics	1	
– Removable prosthetics	1/5	Unstable prostheses
– Non-surgical periodontology	1	
– Surgical periodontology	1	
Hazardous and contraindicated drugs	2	Avoid aspirin, clindamycin and tetracyclines

*0 = No special considerations. 1 = Caution advised. 2 = Specialised medical advice recommended in some cases. 3 = Specialised medical advice mandatory. 4 = Only to be performed in hospital environment. 5 = Should be avoided.

■ Occasionally, aspirin has produced a cholinergic crisis in those on anticholinesterases; acetaminophen/paracetamol and codeine do not have this potential disadvantage ■ Corticosteroids and other immunosuppressants may also complicate dental treatment.

Further reading ● Lotia S, Randall C, Dawson L J, Longman L P 2004 Dental management of the myasthenic patient. Dent Update 31:237–242 ● Patton L L, Howard J F Jr 1997 Myasthenia gravis: dental treatment considerations. Spec Care Dentist 17:25–32 ● Weijnen F G, van der Bilt A, Kuks J B, van der Glas H W, Oudenaarde I, Bosman F 2002 Masticatory performance in patients with myasthenia gravis. Arch Oral Biol 47:393–398.

NEUTROPENIA AND NEUTROPHIL DEFECTS

Definition ■ *Leucopenia* is defined as low levels of circulating functional leucocytes, either in absolute numbers or as functionally effective cells ■ *Neutropenia* is defined as a low level of circulating functional neutrophils, either in absolute numbers ($< 2000 \times 10^6$/L) or as functionally effective phagocytes ■ *Agranulocytosis* is the term given to the clinical syndrome characterised by marked decrease in the number of granulocytes and by lesions of the throat and other mucous membranes, of the gastrointestinal tract and of the skin. It is also called granulocytopenia or Schutz's disease.

General aspects

Aetiopathogenesis Neutropenia may be congenital or acquired (Box 3.20). It can develop in isolation or be associated with other effects of depressed marrow function, notably anaemia and bleeding tendencies, as in acute leukaemia and aplastic anaemia.

Box 3.20 Causes of neutropenia

Intrinsic (congenital) neutropenia
● Congenital severe neutropenia (Kostmann's syndrome) ● Congenital benign neutropenia ● Reticular dysgenesis ● Cyclic neutropenia ● Schwachman–Diamond syndrome ● Severe chronic neutropenias, related to: immunoglobulinopathies, phenotypic abnormalities, metabolic alterations

Acquired neutropenia
● Caused by drugs: predictable – cytostatics and immunodepressants; idiosyncratic – penicillins, aminopyridine, NSAIDs, quinidine, sulphonamides, procainamide, phenothiazine ● Post-infection ● Bone marrow transplantation ● Radiotherapy ● Nutritional deficiencies: vitamin B_{12}, folate, copper

Classification **Reduced number of neutrophils** Based on the absolute neutrophil count in peripheral blood, neutropenia is classified as: ■ Mild: 1000–2000 neutrophils × 10^6/L ■ Moderate: 500–1000 neutrophils × 10^6/L ■ Severe: < 500 neutrophils × 10^6/L. **Neutrophil defects** Neutrophils may be present in normal numbers but malfunction due to: ■ leucocyte adhesion defects (LAD) ■ alteration in chemotaxis ■ opsonisation defects ■ phagocytosis defects ■ killing defects (granule alterations, oxidative activity deficiency).

Clinical presentation The clinical presentation of neutropenias is the same as that of neutrophil defects: ■ fever, weakness or prostration and sore throat ■ recurrent infections ■ Gram-positive oral microorganisms such as Viridans streptococci, mainly *S. mitis* and *S. sanguis,* may cause septicaemias, with serious morbidity and mortality. Predisposing factors appear to be the presence of mucositis, the use of high doses of chemotherapy such as cytosine arabinoside, and the failure to use intravenous antibiotics at the time of the bacteraemia.

Diagnosis ■ Full blood picture ■ Bone marrow biopsy.

Treatment ■ Treatment depends on the underlying cause ■ Granulocyte colony stimulating factors (G-CSF) are now available and may be of benefit ■ Control infections: ● Viridans streptococci are usually sensitive to penicillin, beta-lactams, vancomycin, roxithromycin, rifampicin, macrolides, teicoplanin, lincosamides and aminoglycosides; co-trimoxazole is not effective and there is increasing resistance to penicillin after prolonged exposure to it ● Gram-negative infections should be treated with ticarcillin, mecillinam or a third generation cephalosporin such as ceftazidime or cefotaxime ● if fever develops, samples of blood, urine, sputum and faeces should be taken for culture to exclude septicaemia; the patient should be started on empirical systemic antibiotics, usually initially piperacillin/tazobactam plus gentamicin or, if penicillin-allergic, ceftazidime.

Prognosis Complications of septicaemia include adult respiratory distress syndrome, pneumonia, shock or endocarditis. Mortality rates are as high as 30%. Patients should therefore be nursed in laminar-airflow rooms, and surgical procedures must be carried out under antibiotic cover.

Oral findings

Infections and ulcers are the main oral manifestations. ■ Apparently minor oral infections in severe neutropenia may result in gangrenous stomatitis and are a potential source of sometimes fatal metastatic infections or septicaemia ■ Oral infections can be caused by a variety of organisms but can usually be controlled with topical or systemic antibiotic therapy, or occasionally with antiseptics such as chlorhexidine ■ Mixed infections can often be controlled by a broad-spectrum antimicrobial such as tetracycline, but this should be given together with an antifungal drug because of the risk of superinfection ■ Failure to respond to such treatment indicates that the causative bacteria are not sensitive; bacteriological investigation is mandatory ■ Ulcers may resolve after G-CSF treatment ■ Periodontal disease may be accelerated and results in premature tooth loss ■ Enamel hypoplasia, caries, delayed tooth eruption and pre-pubertal periodontitis have been described in patients with primary neutrophil dysfunction.

Dental management

Risk assessment ■ Infection risk: surgical procedures should be covered with antibiotics ■ Thrombocytopenia with haemorrhagic tendencies may be present in association with cytotoxic drugs ■ Risks associated with corticosteroid treatment.

Appropriate health care Dental treatment of patients with severe neutropenia should be carried out in a hospital or other specialist centre.

Preventive dentistry Rigorous preventive measures, including dietary advice, oral health promotion, topical fluorides and fissure sealants, are particularly important.

Pain and anxiety control **Local anaesthesia** LA is the method of choice. Use of a preoperative rinse with chlorhexidine mouthwash is advisable. **Conscious sedation** CS may be undertaken but consideration should be given to any underlying disease, particularly in acquired neutropenia. **General anaesthesia** GA may be undertaken but consideration should be given to any underlying disease, particularly in acquired neutropenia. A bleeding tendency, which may compromise the airway, should also be identified.

Patient access and positioning **Timing of treatment** Two days after the last G-CSF dose there initially is a significant decrease in the circulating neutrophil count (up to 50%) – it takes up to 7 days to reach normal levels again. Although the most appropriate time to undertaken dental treatment is therefore one week after the last dose of G-CSF, the physician should be consulted.

Treatment modification **Surgery** Prophylactic measures to minimise the risk of bacteraemia related to oral procedures include: ■ chlorhexidine mouth rinse ■ antibiotic administration before and after surgery ■ primary closure of the surgical wound ■ in patients with mild and moderate neutropenia able to undergo surgical dental treatment – subcutaneous or intravenous administration of G-CSF 0.5×10^6 units/kg/day over 3–5 days has been recommended. **Implantology** Implantology has been successfully carried out in patients on G-CSF treatment. **Periodontology** The regular removal of plaque and calculus, as well as the use of chlorhexidine and periodontal treatment in patients with neutropenia, help to maintain periodontal health. G-CSF may be indicated before scaling.

Further reading

● Chin E A 1998 A brief overview of the oral complications in pediatric oncology patients and suggested management strategies. ASDC J Dent Child 65:468–473 ● Diz-Dios P, Ocampo-Hermida A, Fernandez-Feijoo J 2002 Quantitative and functional neutrophil deficiencies. Med Oral 7:206–221 ● Graber C J, de Almeida K N, Atkinson J C et al 2001 Dental health and viridans streptococcal bacteremia in allogeneic hematopoietic stem cell transplant recipients. Bone Marrow Transplant 27:537–542.

Table 3.119 **Key considerations for dental management in neutropenia (see text)**

	Management modifications*	Comments/possible complications
Risk assessment	2	Infection; bleeding tendency
Appropriate dental care	2/4	Antibiotic cover; full blood picture; bleeding tests
Pain and anxiety control		
– Local anaesthesia	1	Chlorhexidine rinse
– Conscious sedation	2	Consider underlying disease
– General anaesthesia	2	Consider underlying disease
Patient access and positioning		
– Access to dental office	0	
– Timing of treatment	2	Avoid 2–7 days after G-CSF intake
– Patient positioning	0	
Treatment modification		
– Oral surgery	2	Chlorhexidine; antibiotic cover; primary closure of surgical wound; possibly G-CSF
– Implantology	2	See oral surgery
– Conservative/Endodontics	1	
– Fixed prosthetics	1	
– Removable prosthetics	1	
– Non-surgical periodontology	2	See oral surgery
– Surgical periodontology	2	See oral surgery
Hazardous and contraindicated drugs	0	Some patients are on corticosteroids

*0 = No special considerations. 1 = Caution advised. 2 = Specialised medical advice recommended in some cases. 3 = Specialised medical advice mandatory. 4 = Only to be performed in hospital environment. 5 = Should be avoided.

NICOTINE ABUSE

Definition ■ Nicotine ($C_{10}H_{14}N_2$) is a naturally occurring liquid alkaloid ■ It is absorbed readily from tobacco smoke in the lungs, and represents one of the most heavily used addictive drugs ■ It is both a stimulant and a sedative to the CNS ■ In addition to nicotine, which normally makes up about 5% of a tobacco plant, cigarette smoke is primarily composed of a dozen gases (mainly carbon monoxide) and tar, but also about 4000 other compounds, including nitrosamines and aromatic amines, which are known carcinogens.

General aspects

Pathogenesis ■ Nicotine binds to a CNS receptor and, like cocaine, heroin and marijuana, raises the level of dopamine as well as opioids and glucose, and activates the nucleus accumbens ■ Nicotine also causes a discharge of epinephrine from the adrenals and other endocrine glands, which stimulates the CNS.

Clinical presentation ■ Common signs of nicotine use are: ● breath may smell of tobacco ● nicotine on fingers ■ Drug-associated diseases include: ● oral and head and neck cancer ● lung cancer ● atherosclerotic heart disease ● chronic obstructive pulmonary disease ■ Pregnant women who smoke cigarettes run a greater risk of having stillborn or premature infants or infants with low birth weight – children of women who smoked while pregnant have a raised risk for developing conduct disorders ■ Many smokers also drink alcohol, in some cases excessively.

Severe adverse effects ■ Tobacco use is the major cause of cancer of the lung, oesophagus, mouth and bladder, stroke, ischaemic heart disease, hypertension and a leading cause of death ■ Passive smoking also causes lung cancer in adults and greatly increases the risk of respiratory illnesses in children and sudden infant death.

Withdrawal and treatment ■ Addiction to nicotine results in withdrawal symptoms when a person tries to stop smoking, with excessive anger, hostility and aggression ■ Pharmacological treatment combined with psychological treatment results in some of the highest long-term abstinence rates, and includes: ● nicotine chewing gum ● nicotine transdermal patch ● bupropion.

Oral findings

■ Smoking may cause mucosal keratinisation and pigmentary incompetence and is linked to oral cancer ■ Oral snuff dipping and chewing tobacco predispose to leukoplakia and oral cancer ■ Smoking also predisposes to periodontal disease (particularly necrotising gingivitis), dry socket, candidosis, halitosis and xerostomia ■ Cigarette smoking is the most common cause of extrinsic staining of teeth ■ Stopping smoking reduces the risk of oral cancer so that by 5 years it is down to that of a non-smoker ■ However, stopping smoking is not merely difficult but may bring other problems: ● aggravation or the onset of recurrent aphthae ● increased consumption of sweets as a substitute for smoking, leading to caries and/or weight gain ● use of nicotine-containing chewing gum may reduce the risk of aphthae but may produce hypersalivation.

Dental management

Risk assessment ■ Patients with a smoking history may have hyperactive airways, which predispose them to laryngospasm, diminished oxygen saturation, coughing and copious secretions ■ In addition smokers may be resistant to sedative drugs ■ Difficulties in dental management of smokers may be related to associated disorders such as: ● chronic obstructive airway disease ● ischaemic heart disease ● alcoholism ● peptic ulcer ■ Smokers have delayed healing after surgery; scarring is more frequent.

Pain and anxiety control **Local anaesthesia** LA may be given safely with routine precautions. **Conscious sedation** ■ Patients with a smoking history of greater than 30 pack-years are particularly prone to arterial oxygen desaturation during CS; close monitoring is required ■ Smoking may increase the requirement for sedative drugs. **General anaesthesia** ■ GA should be undertaken with caution as: ● some constituents of tobacco smoke cause cardiovascular problems, increasing the blood pressure, heart rate, and the systemic vascular resistance ● some cause respiratory problems, interfering with oxygen uptake, transport, and delivery ● others interfere with respiratory function both during and after anaesthesia ● drug metabolism may be altered ● various effects on muscle relaxants have been

Table 3.120 **Key considerations for dental management in nicotine abuse (see text)**

	Management modifications*	Comments/possible complications
Risk assessment	1	Associated disorders; resistance to sedation; hyperacute airways; delayed healing
Pain and anxiety control		
– Local anaesthesia	0	
– Conscious sedation	1	Lung disease; resistance
– General anaesthesia	1	Lung disease; deep vein thrombosis; resistance to GA
Patient access and positioning		
– Access to dental office	0	
– Timing of treatment	0	
– Patient positioning	0	
Treatment modification		
– Oral surgery	1	Heavy smokers – poor healing
– Implantology	1/5	See oral surgery
– Conservative/Endodontics	1	
– Fixed prosthetics	1/5	Heavy smokers; staining
– Removable prosthetics	1	
– Non-surgical periodontology	1	Periodontitis
– Surgical periodontology	1/5	See oral surgery
Hazardous and contraindicated drugs	1	Avoid opioids

*0 = No special considerations. 1 = Caution advised. 2 = Specialised medical advice recommended in some cases. 3 = Specialised medical advice mandatory. 4 = Only to be performed in hospital environment. 5 = Should be avoided.

reported ● smoking may be a risk factor for the development of deep venous thrombosis, particularly when compounded by prolonged bed rest; compression stockings may be indicated ■ It is advisable to ask the patient to stop smoking for at least 1 week prior to surgery, or, if not achievable, at least for 24 hours before surgery ■ Avoid opioids as smokers have a greater tendency to develop hypoxia postoperatively.

Further reading ● van der Bijl P 2003 Substance abuse – concerns in dentistry: an overview. S Afr Dent J 58:382–385 ● Christen A G 2001 Tobacco cessation, the dental profession, and the role of dental education. J Dent Educ 65:368–374 ● Cornelius J R, Clark D B, Weyant R et al 2004 Dental abnormalities in children of fathers with substance use disorders. Addict Behav 29:979–982 ● Johnson G K, Hill M 2004 Cigarette smoking and the periodontal patient. J Periodontol 75:196–209 ● Sandler N A 2001 Patients who abuse drugs. Oral Surg Oral Med Oral Pathol Oral Radiol Endod 91:12–14.

OSTEOARTHRITIS

Definition Osteoarthritis (osteoarthrosis) is a common joint disease, caused by degeneration of the articular cartilage, especially prevalent in females over 50 years.

General aspects

Aetiopathogenesis ■ Primary osteoarthritis is not related to any obvious predisposing factor ■ Secondary osteoarthritis usually follows trauma, but may also be seen in joint instability or certain metabolic diseases ■ Pathogenesis includes: ● release of degradative enzymes from leucocytes ● dysfunction of proteoglycans ● degradation of cartilage surface ● bone metabolism alteration ● bone sclerosis and osteophyte production (compensatory bone thickening).

Clinical presentation ■ Osteoarthritis (Fig. 3.30) causes: ● pain ● stiffness ● loss of function mainly in weight-bearing joints on movement ● Heberden's nodes (osteophytes of the distal interphalangeal joint of the fingers) – may be seen but are not normally painful ■ Although it typically involves the hips and distal intercarpophalangeal joints, it may also affect other joints: ● first metacarpophalangeal ● first metatarsophalangeal ● cervical spine ● lumbar spine ● knees.

Diagnosis ■ Full blood picture – normal ■ Erythrocyte sedimentation rate – normal ■ Rheumatoid factor – normal ■ Radiology – loss of joint space, subchondral sclerosis, marginal osteophytes.

Treatment ■ Drugs (acetaminophen/paracetamol or NSAIDs) ■ Weight reduction ■ Walking aids ■ Joint replacement.

Oral findings

Osteoarthritis may affect the temporomandibular joints (TMJ) in some elderly patients, with osteophytes demonstrable. However, those with osteoarthritis

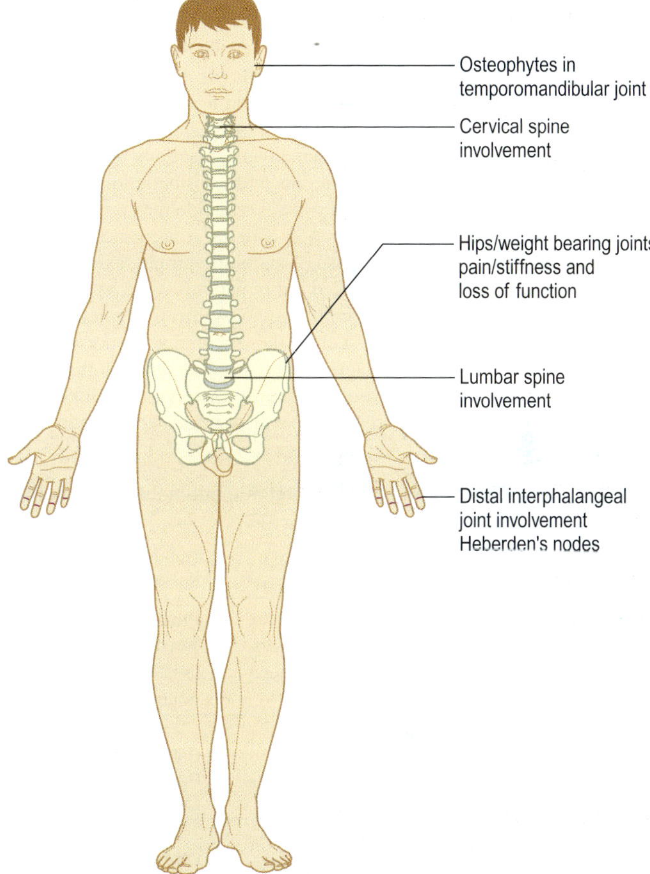

Figure 3.30 **Clinical presentation of osteoarthritis**

of other joints do not appear to have significantly more involvement of the temporomandibular joints than controls. Furthermore, the radiographic severity of TMJ osteoarthritis does not correlate with symptoms. TMJ osteoarthritis is rarely of clinical significance, so patients should not be made unnecessarily anxious.

Dental management

Risk assessment ■ Most infections of prosthetic joints have been due to non-oral microorganisms such as staphylococci ■ Only occasional infections of prosthetic joints have been with oral organisms such as *Streptococcus sanguis* ■ The prevalence of prosthetic joint infections of oral origin in patients who have undergone total joint arthroplasties is estimated at about 5–10% of all cases.

Appropriate dental care ■ There is no reliable evidence of a need for antibiotic prophylaxis before most dental treatment in most patients with prosthetic joints, and the British Society for Antimicrobial Chemotherapy does not recommend it ■ The risks from adverse reactions to antibiotics, were they to be given routinely to all patients with prosthetic joints, would probably exceed any benefit ■ However, guidelines issued by the American Dental Association in conjunction with the American Association of Orthopedic Surgeons advocate the use of antibiotic prophylaxis where dental at-risk procedures are to be carried out in patients who have recent new joints (within 2 years), where the joint has previously been infected, or where the patient is immunocompromised, such as those with diabetes or rheumatoid disease ■ Although these do not agree with current practice in the UK, some UK orthopaedic surgeons nevertheless insist upon it – careful negotiation is required in these cases, and the risk to the patient evaluated on an individual

Table 3.121 **Key considerations for dental management in osteoarthritis (see text)**

	Management modifications*	Comments/possible complications
Risk assessment	1	Prosthetic joint infection; bleeding tendency for patients on aspirin
Appropriate dental care	1	Antibiotic prophylaxis
Pain and anxiety control		
– Local anaesthesia	1	Patient positioning
– Conscious sedation	1	Patient positioning
– General anaesthesia	1	Cervical spine stiffness
Patient access and positioning		
– Access to dental office	1	Difficulties due to age and immobility
– Timing of treatment	1	Late morning or afternoon
– Patient positioning	1	Neck and leg supports
Treatment modification		
– Oral surgery	1	Patient positioning; bleeding
– Implantology	1	
– Conservative/Endodontics	0	
– Fixed prosthetics	0	
– Removable prosthetics	0	
– Non-surgical periodontology	1	
– Surgical periodontology	1	
Hazardous and contraindicated drugs	1	Some patients are on aspirin or corticosteroids

*0 = No special considerations. 1 = Caution advised. 2 = Specialised medical advice recommended in some cases. 3 = Specialised medical advice mandatory. 4 = Only to be performed in hospital environment. 5 = Should be avoided.

basis ■ Dental management may be complicated by a bleeding tendency if the patient is anticoagulated occasionally (after arthroplasty) or takes high doses of aspirin.

Preventive dentistry Manual dexterity and the ability to maintain good oral hygiene may be limited. Modified toothbrush handles and electric toothbrushes may be useful.

Pain and anxiety management **Local anaesthesia** LA may be given safely with routine precautions, but care should be taken with regard to patient positioning. **Conscious sedation** CS may be given safely with routine precautions, but care should be taken with regard to patient positioning. **General anaesthesia** Care should be taken with regard to patient positioning, particularly when there is significant cervical spine stiffness.

Patient access and positioning **Access to dental surgery** Age and immobility may influence access to dental care. Escorts, transport and/or domiciliary care may also need to be considered.
Timing of treatment Stiffness usually improves during the day: short appointments in the late morning or in the afternoon are recommended.
Patient positioning Supine positioning may be uncomfortable, and neck and leg supports may be needed.

Drug use Some patients are on aspirin or corticosteroids.

Further reading
● Gidarakou I K, Tallents R H, Kyrkanides S, Stein S, Moss M 2003 Comparison of skeletal and dental morphology in asymptomatic volunteers and symptomatic patients with bilateral degenerative joint disease. Angle Orthod 73:71–78 ● Nilner M 2003 Musculoskeletal disorders and the occlusal interface: II. Int J Prosthodont 16(Suppl):85–87 ● Seymour R A, Whitworth J M, Martin M 2003 Antibiotic prophylaxis for patients with joint prostheses – still a dilemma for dental practitioners. Br Dent J 194:649–653

OSTEOPOROSIS

Definition Osteoporosis is a loss of bone mineral density characterised by reduced mineralised bone mass, especially common in older women.

General aspects

Aetiopathogenesis ■ This metabolic bone disease results from an imbalance in osteoblastic and osteoclastic activities ■ Primary osteoporosis is caused by androgen–oestrogen deficiency, lack of vitamin D and lack of exercise ■ Secondary osteoporosis is caused by corticosteroid use, hyperparathyroidism, diabetes, chronic liver disease, malabsorption or hyperthyroidism.

Clinical presentation ■ Osteoporosis is usually asymptomatic ■ However, increased bone fragility may lead to vertebral crush fractures or femoral neck fractures ■ Osteoporosis may also cause persistent lower back pain, kyphosis and loss of height.

Diagnosis ■ Radiography ■ Bone densitometry – reduced ■ Serum calcium – normal ■ Serum phosphorus – normal or low ■ Serum alkaline phosphatase – normal or low.

Treatment ■ Prevention – exercise, calcium supplementation, hormone replacement therapy (HRT), avoiding risk factors ■ Treatment – bisphosphonates, HRT or vitamin D.

Prognosis The rate of death in osteoporotic patients who fracture their hip reaches 20% within one year.

Oral findings

■ Jaw osteoporosis is particularly a problem in women; systemic treatment of osteoporosis may improve the jaw osteoporosis ■ There is a correlation of osteoporosis with excessive alveolar bone loss in the elderly and pathological fracture ■ There may be an association with periodontitis.

Dental management

Risk assessment There is an increased risk of bone fracture with surgery. ■ Bisphosphonates such as Pamidronate (Aredia) and Zoledronate (Zometal), in particular can lead to painful refractory bone exposures in the jaws (sometimes termed osteochemonecrosis or osteonecrosis of the jaws; ONJ), typically following oral surgical procedures (see Cancer).

Pain and anxiety control **Local anaesthesia** LA may be used with routine precautions. **Conscious sedation** CS may be used with routine precautions. **General anaesthesia** Patients with osteoporosis may be at risk during GA if there is associated vertebral collapse and chest deformity. Furthermore, they may have any of the additional problems of the elderly.

Patient access and positioning Care must be taken to provide adequate neck support. Patients with advanced osteoporosis may have reduced mobility and require assistance/an escort.

Treatment modification **Surgery** Delayed alveolar bone healing is not uncommon following dental extractions and there is an increased risk of jaw fracture. **Implantology** Although there is no evidence that osteoporosis is a contraindication to implants, such patients may not be a good risk group for sinus lifts. **Removable prosthetics** Resorption of the alveolar ridge makes dental prostheses unstable, and patients often request soft-relining of their prosthesis.

Imaging The jaws are thinned and granular. The lamina dura appears thinned. The maxillary sinus may extend between the roots of molars. Panoramic radiography may demonstrate spinal osteoporosis.

Drug use Calcium inactivates tetracycline. Bisphosphonates occasionally cause osteochemonecrosis, affecting the jaws.

Table 3.122 **Key considerations for dental management in osteoporosis (see text)**

	Management modifications*	Comments/possible complications
Risk assessment	1	Jaw fracture Osteochemonecrosis due to bisphosphonates
Appropriate dental care	1	
Pain and anxiety control		
– Local anaesthesia	0	
– Conscious sedation	0	
– General anaesthesia	1	Neck and chest deformities
Patient access and positioning		
– Access to dental office	1	Assistance/escort
– Timing of treatment	0	
– Patient positioning	1	Neck support; mobility reduced
Treatment modification		
– Oral surgery	1	Jaw fracture; delayed alveolar bone healing Osteochemonecrosis due to bisphosphonates
– Implantology	1	Avoid sinus lifts
– Conservative/Endodontics	0	
– Fixed prosthetics	0	
– Removable prosthetics	1	Unstable prosthesis; soft-relining required
– Non-surgical periodontology	0	
– Surgical periodontology	1	Impaired bone remodelling
Imaging	1	Typical radiological features
Hazardous and contraindicated drugs	1	Avoid tetracyclines

*0 = No special considerations. 1 = Caution advised. 2 = Specialised medical advice recommended in some cases. 3 = Specialised medical advice mandatory. 4 = Only to be performed in hospital environment. 5 = Should be avoided.

Further reading ● Keller J C, Stewart M, Roehm M, Schneider G B 2004 Osteoporosis-like bone conditions affect osseointegration of implants. Int J Oral Maxillofac Implants 19:687–694 ● Maupome G, Gullion C M, White B A, Wyatt C C, Williams P M 2003 Oral disorders and chronic systemic diseases in very old adults living in institutions. Spec Care Dentist 23:199–208 ● Taguchi A, Suei Y, Sanada M et al 2004 Validation of dental panoramic radiography measures for identifying postmenopausal women with spinal osteoporosis. AJR Am J Roentgenol 183:1755–1760.

PAGET'S DISEASE

Definition ■ Paget's disease is a disorder characterised by excessive bone turnover ■ It causes remodelling and enlargement of skull, pelvis and long bones ■ The highest incidence of Paget's disease is in the UK (mainly in older 'Anglo-Saxons') and is lower in other European countries ■ Worldwide the incidence appears to be decreasing.

General aspects

Aetiopathogenesis ■ The aetiology remains unknown: ● evidence of a genetic susceptibility to Paget's disease is accumulating, with chromosomes 6 (the HLA locus) and 18q emerging as strong candidates ● possible role of viruses (paramyxovirus, measles, canine distemper virus) ● endocrinopathies ■ There are osteolytic phases where bone resorption predominates, and osteosclerotic phases where there is appositional bone growth ■ Familial Paget's disease is associated with more severe disease.

Clinical presentation ■ May be asymptomatic ■ Can cause bone pain and swelling ■ Leg deformities, kyphosis and loss of height, enlarged skull with headache, deafness or visual impairment may also be seen (Fig. 3.31) ■ Increased bone vascularity with arteriovenous shunting can result in high output cardiac failure ■ Quality of life may be reduced and psychological problems are often present.

Diagnosis ■ Radiography ■ Bone scintigraphy ■ Serum alkaline phosphatase level – raised ■ Plasma calcium and phosphorus levels – normal ■ Urinary hydroxyproline level – raised.

Treatment ■ Analgesia ■ Bisphosphonates ■ Calcitonin.

Prognosis About 1% of patients develop an osteosarcoma.

Oral findings

■ Typically, enlargement of the maxilla causes symmetrical bulging in the malar region (leontiasis ossea) ■ The intraoral features are gross symmetrical widening of the alveolar ridges, sometimes loss of lamina dura, root resorption and hypercementosis – often forming enormous craggy masses that may become fused to the surrounding bone ■ Pulp calcification may be seen ■ Benign giant cell tumours may be seen ■ Osteosarcoma is particularly rare in the jaws, where no fully authenticated case appears to have been reported ■ Alendronate may induce mouth ulcers or osteochemonecrosis.

Dental management

Risk assessment ■ In the early stages of Paget's disease, the highly vascular bone may bleed freely; later, the poor blood supply to the bone makes it susceptible to chronic suppurative osteomyelitis as a result of such trauma ■ Patients with Paget's disease involving facial or maxillo-mandibular parts

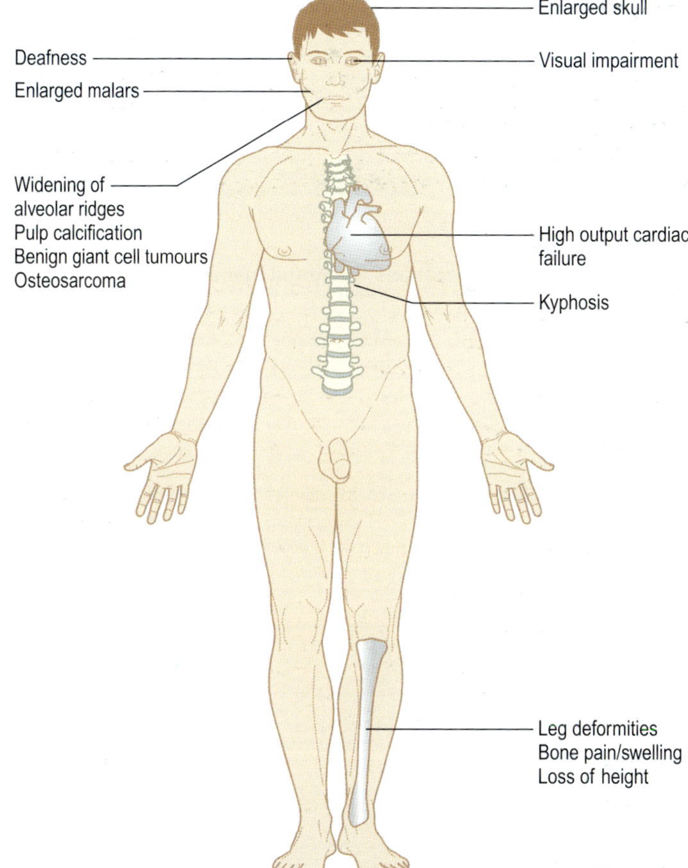

Figure 3.31 **Clinical presentation of Paget's disease**

of the skeleton have a higher prevalence of heart disease and of deteriorating senses of hearing, sight and smell ■ Psychosocial problems may be present ■ Bisphosphonates such as Pamidronate (Aredia) and Zoledronate (Zometal), in particular, can lead to painful refractory bone exposures in the jaws (sometimes termed osteochemonecrosis or osteonecrosis of the jaws; ONJ), typically following oral surgical procedures (see Cancer).

Appropriate dental care ■ Local haemostatic measures (e.g. sutures, packs) are recommended after oral surgery, particularly in early stages of the disease ■ Prophylactic administration of an antibiotic such as penicillin (immediately before and for 3–4 days after the operation) may help prevent postoperative infection.

Pain and anxiety control **Local anaesthesia** LA may be used with routine precautions. **Conscious sedation** CS may be used with routine precautions. **General anaesthesia** If the patient is in heart failure, the usual precautions have to be taken but, since GA may be needed for dental extractions, the risk of excessive bleeding or infection needs to be kept in mind. Chest deformity may also complicate GA.

Treatment modification **Surgery** ■ Serious complications may follow efforts to extract severely hypercementosed teeth. Attempts using forceps may

Table 3.123 **Key considerations for dental management in Paget's disease (see text)**

	Management modifications*	Comments/possible complications
Risk assessment	2	Increased heart disease; impaired sight and hearing; bleeding tendency; osteomyelitis Osteochemonecrosis due to bisphosphonates
Appropriate dental care	2	Penicillin prophylaxis; haemostatic measures
Pain and anxiety control		
– Local anaesthesia	0	
– Conscious sedation	0	
– General anaesthesia	3/4	Heart disease; chest deformity; bleeding; infection
Patient access and positioning		
– Access to dental office	0	
– Timing of treatment	0	
– Patient positioning	1	Kyphosis
Treatment modification		
– Oral surgery	2/4	Hypercementosis; bleeding Osteochemonecrosis due to bisphosphonates
– Implantology	2/4	Hypercementosis; bleeding
– Conservative/Endodontics	1	Pulp calcification
– Fixed prosthetics	1	
– Removable prosthetics	1/2	Prosthesis replacement
– Non-surgical periodontology	1	Bleeding tendency
– Surgical periodontology	2	Bleeding tendency
Imaging	1	Typical radiological features
Hazardous and contraindicated drugs	0	

*0 = No special considerations. 1 = Caution advised. 2 = Specialised medical advice recommended in some cases. 3 = Specialised medical advice mandatory. 4 = Only to be performed in hospital environment. 5 = Should be avoided.

fail to move the tooth, or cause fracture of the alveolar bone. Alternatively, the tooth may be mobilised but retained as if in a ball-and-socket joint. ■ If hypercementosis is severe, a surgical approach with adequate exposure should be used for extractions. **Removable prosthetics** Dentures may have to be replaced more frequently as the alveolar ridge enlarges.

Imaging **Radiology** When the skull is affected, a typical early feature is a large irregular area of relative radiolucency (osteoporosis circumscripta). Later, there is increased radio-opacity with loss of the normal landmarks and an irregular cotton-wool appearance. Basilar invagination may be seen. The maxilla is occasionally and the mandible rarely involved.

Further reading ● Bender I B 2003 Paget's disease. J Endod 29:720–723 ● Seed R, Nixon P P 2004 Generalised hypercementosis: a case report. Prim Dent Care 11:119–122 ● Wheeler T T, Alberts M A, Dolan T A, McGorray S P 1995 Dental, visual, auditory and olfactory complications in Paget's disease of bone. J Am Geriatr Soc 43:1384–1391.

PANCREATIC TRANSPLANTATION

Definition ■ Pancreas transplantation is the surgical replacement of a diseased pancreas with a healthy one, used to ameliorate type I diabetes and produce complete insulin independence ■ The pancreas usually comes from a cadaveric organ donor, however, select cases of living donor pancreas transplants have been performed ■ About 85% of pancreatic transplants are performed with a kidney transplant (both organs from the same donor) in diabetic patients with renal failure – this is referred to as a simultaneous pancreas–kidney (SPK) transplant ■ About 10% of cases are performed after a previously successful kidney transplant – this is referred to as a pancreas-after-kidney transplant ■ An alternative new therapy that also may ameliorate diabetes is islet transplantation – experimental and not yet as efficient as pancreatic transplantation.

General aspects

Treatment All transplant recipients require life-long immunosuppression to prevent a T-cell, alloimmune rejection response, using: ■ *muromonab-CD3* – a mouse antihuman monospecific antibody against CD3 antigen on T lymphocytes ■ *daclizumab* – a humanised monoclonal antibody that blocks the interleukin-2 (IL-2) receptor on activated T cells ■ *basiliximab* – a chimeric monoclonal antibody that also blocks the IL-2 receptor.

Prognosis The 1-year survival after pancreas transplantation is around 70%.

Oral findings

- Diabetic patients may show oral manifestations of diabetes
- Immunosuppression-related oral infections may develop.

Dental management

Risk assessment ■ The risks associated with diabetes and bacteraemia should be considered.

Appropriate health care ■ A meticulous pre-surgery oral assessment is required and dental treatment undertaken with particular attention to establishing optimal oral hygiene and eradicating sources of potential infection ■ Dental treatment should be completed before surgery ■ If surgical treatment is needed, antibiotic prophylaxis is warranted for 6 months post-transplantation ■ Elective dental care is best deferred until 6 months post-transplantation.

Pain and anxiety control Local anaesthesia LA may be used safely with the usual routine precautions. A preoperative rinse with chlorhexidine mouthwash is advisable. Conscious sedation CS may be used safely with the usual routine precautions. General anaesthesia Close

Table 3.124 **Key considerations for dental management in pancreatic transplantation (see text)**

	Management modifications*	Comments/possible complications
Risk assessment	3	Diabetes; bacteraemia
Appropriate dental care	2	Assess before surgery; antibiotic prophylaxis; delay elective dental care until 6 months post-surgery
Pain and anxiety control		
– Local anaesthesia	1	Chlorhexidine rinse
– Conscious sedation	0	
– General anaesthesia	3/4	Dehydration
Patient access and positioning		
– Access to dental office	0	
– Timing of treatment	0	
– Patient positioning	0	
Treatment modification		
– Oral surgery	2	
– Implantology	2	
– Conservative/Endodontics	1	
– Fixed prosthetics	1	
– Removable prosthetics	0	
– Non-surgical periodontology	1	
– Surgical periodontology	2	
Hazardous and contraindicated drugs	2	see Renal transplantation section

*0 = No special considerations. 1 = Caution advised. 2 = Specialised medical advice recommended in some cases. 3 = Specialised medical advice mandatory. 4 = Only to be performed in hospital environment. 5 = Should be avoided.

consultation with the physician and a thorough preoperative assessment with the anaesthetist are required. The risk of dehydration increases during GA. Monitoring liquid intake and excretion (bladder catheter) is then mandatory.

Further reading ● Elkhammas E A, Henry M L, Ferguson R M et al 2004 Simultaneous pancreas–kidney transplantation: overview of the Ohio State experience. Yonsei Med J 45:1095–1100 ● Larsen J L 2004 Pancreas transplantation: indications and consequences. Endocr Rev 25:919–946.

PARALYSES (HEAD AND NECK)

BULBAR PALSY

Definition Bulbar palsy is a lower motor neurone paralysis affecting tongue, muscles of chewing/swallowing and face.

General aspects

Aetiopathogenesis This disorder is due to brainstem nuclei dysfunction, caused by: ■ motor neurone disease ■ Guillain–Barré syndrome ■ poliomyelitis ■ syringobulbia ■ tumours.

Clinical features/oral findings

■ Oral manifestations are the consequence of weakness and fasciculations of oral musculature, and include: ● tongue – flaccid and fasciculating ● jaw jerk (may be absent) ● speech – altered (quiet, nasal or hoarse) ● drooling ■ It is possible to determine that the lesion is a lower motor type, as the forehead muscles are spared because of crossover innervation at a higher level (i.e. frowning is not possible in upper motor neurone disorders).

Dental management

Risk assessment Involuntary movements can be hazardous during dental treatment.

Appropriate health care ■ Oral hygiene may be impaired as in other disabilities ■ Mouth props and rubber dam are strongly recommended ■ The airways should be protected.

Pain and anxiety control Local anaesthesia LA may be used safely with the usual routine precautions, taking care to avoid injury due to the patient's involuntary movements. Conscious sedation CS may be used safely with the usual routine precautions, taking care to avoid injury due to the patient's involuntary movements. General anaesthesia Close consultation with the physician and a thorough preoperative assessment with the anaesthetist, particularly in view of potential problems with intubation.

Table 3.125 **Key considerations for dental management in bulbar palsy (see text)**

	Management modifications*	Comments/possible complications
Risk assessment	2	Involuntary movements
Appropriate dental care	2	Impaired oral hygiene; mouth props; rubber dam
Pain and anxiety control		
– Local anaesthesia	1	
– Conscious sedation	1	
– General anaesthesia	3/4	
Patient access and positioning		
– Access to dental office	0	
– Timing of treatment	0	
– Patient positioning	0	
Treatment modification		
– Oral surgery	1	
– Implantology	1	
– Conservative/Endodontics	1	
– Fixed prosthetics	1	
– Removable prosthetics	1/5	Unstable prostheses
– Non-surgical periodontology	1	
– Surgical periodontology	1	
Hazardous and contraindicated drugs	0	

*0 = No special considerations. 1 = Caution advised. 2 = Specialised medical advice recommended in some cases. 3 = Specialised medical advice mandatory. 4 = Only to be performed in hospital environment. 5 = Should be avoided.

Treatment modification **Implantology** Dental implants may be needed to help to stabilise the prosthesis. **Removable prosthetics** Mucous membrane supported prostheses may become unstable due to muscular weakness. Results of relining are poor.

PSEUDOBULBAR PALSY

Definition Pseudobulbar palsy is an upper motor neurone paralysis affecting the tongue, muscles of chewing/swallowing and face.

General aspects

Aetiopathogenesis This disorder is due to lesion above mid-pons, caused by: ■ strokes ■ multiple sclerosis ■ motor neurone disease.

Oral findings

Oral manifestations are the consequence of muscular involvement, and include: ■ tongue – spastic ■ jaw jerk – exaggerated ■ speech – slurred, 'Donald Duck'-like.

Dental management

See Bulbar palsy (above).

BELL'S AND OTHER FACIAL PALSIES

Definition Bell's palsy is a lower motor neurone neuropathy affecting the facial (VIIth cranial) nerve alone. It is usually transitory and self-limiting.

General aspects

Aetiopathogenesis ■ In Bell's palsy there is facial nerve inflammation with demyelination and oedema, further hazarding the blood supply to the nerve ■ Most cases are linked to herpes simplex virus infection ■ Other causes of VII nerve palsy include: ● other infections (other herpesviruses, HIV, polio, TB, Lyme disease, leprosy) ● cerebral tumours ● stroke ● multiple sclerosis ● diabetes ● sarcoidosis ● Guillain–Barré syndrome ● Melkersson–Rosenthal syndrome/Crohn's disease ● tumours or trauma affecting pons, skull base, middle ear or parotid ● iatrogenic injection of local anaesthesia.

Clinical presentation Symptoms ■ Acute onset of typically unilateral upper and lower facial paralysis (over a 48-h period) ■ Posterior auricular pain ■ Decreased tearing ■ Hyperacusis ■ Taste disturbances. Signs ■ Initial inspection of the patient demonstrates flattening of the forehead and nasolabial fold on the side affected with the palsy ■ When the patient is asked to raise the eyebrows, the side of the forehead with the palsy will remain flat ■ When the patient is asked to smile, the face becomes distorted and lateralises to the side opposite the palsy ■ The patient is not able to close the eye completely on the affected side. On attempted eye closure, the eye rolls upward and inward on the affected side – this is known as Bell phenomenon and is considered a normal response to eye closure.

Diagnosis Clinical findings and neurological examination.

Treatment ■ Corticosteroids (prednisone or prednisolone) ■ Aciclovir ■ Eye pad and ophthalmological consultation.

Prognosis ■ Hyperacusis, severe taste impairment and diminished salivation or lacrimation are signs of a poor prognosis ■ In about 5% of patients, palsy remains after 9 months.

Oral findings

■ Lips are unresponsive to motor commands ■ Loss of taste in some (due to chorda tympani involvement) ■ Anomalous lacrimation during eating, retraction of the labial commissure when the eye is closed, and hemifacial spasm, suggest anomalous nerve regeneration.

Dental management

Appropriate health care If a patient develops Bell's palsy during dental treatment due to iatrogenic injection of local anaesthesia (an inferior alveolar LA block injection may be misplaced and LA enter the parotid gland, diffusing through to affect the facial nerve): ■ stop dental treatment ■ reassure the patient ■ give no drugs ■ reassess after 24 hours.

Further reading ● Bsoul S A, Terezhalmy G T, Moore W S 2004 Bell's palsy. Quintessence Int 35:506–507 ● Dawidjan B 2001 Idiopathic facial paralysis: a review and case study. J Dent Hyg 75:316–321 ● Luker J, Scully C 1990 The lateral medullary syndrome. Oral Surg Oral Med Oral Pathol Oral Radiol Endod 69:322–324 ● Rover B C, Morgano S M 1988 Prevention of self-inflicted trauma: dental intervention to prevent chronic lip chewing by a patient with a diagnosis of progressive bulbar palsy. Spec Care Dentist 8:37–39 ● Talacko A A, Reade P C 1990 Progressive bulbar palsy: a case report of a type of motor neuron disease presenting with oral symptoms. Oral Surg Oral Med Oral Pathol Oral Radiol Endod 69:182–184.

PARKINSONISM

Definition Parkinson's disease is a progressive neurological disorder characterised by tremor, rigidity, and a short shuffling gait, which usually presents after the age of 50.

General aspects

Aetiopathogenesis ■ Although the cause remains unclear, Parkinson's disease is characterised by: ● a degeneration of dopamine neurones in brain basal ganglia substantia nigra (primary and much secondary Parkinson's disease) ● or by drugs, such as phenothiazines, which block dopamine (Parkinsonism); this is always reversible ■ Secondary Parkinson's disease may also follow exposure to: ● recurrent head trauma (e.g. boxing) ● toxins (such as the illicit drug MPTP) ● encephalitis ● cerebrovascular disease ● pesticides.

Clinical presentation Symptoms (Fig. 3.32) include: ■ tremor – pill-rolling of thumb over fingers, worst at rest ■ difficulty starting/stopping walking ■ slowness (bradykinesia) – and slow monotonous speech ■ rigidity – throughout movements ('lead pipe') ■ mask-like face ■ depression (50–60%).

Diagnosis Diagnosis is made based on clinical findings.

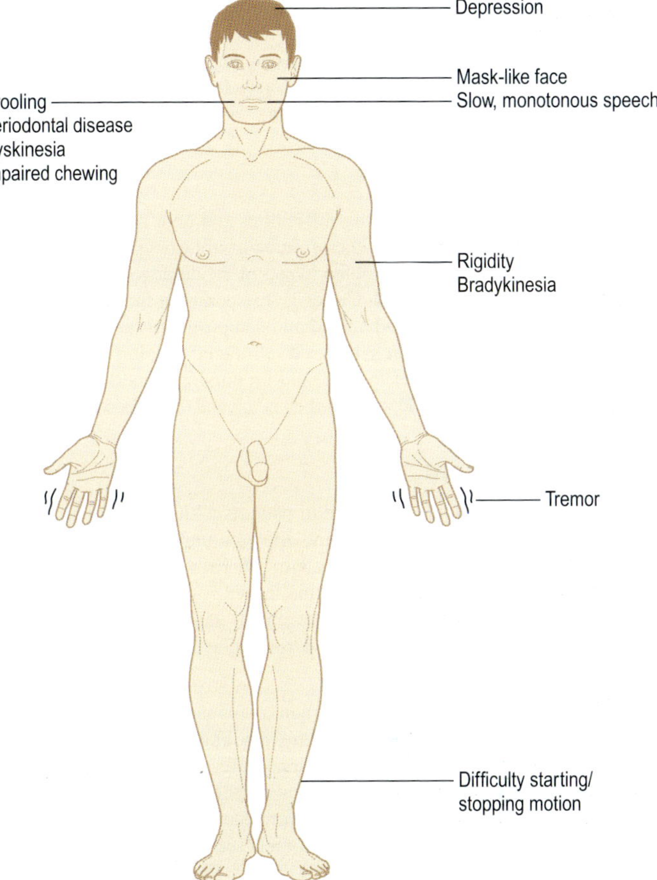

Figure 3.32 **Clinical presentation of Parkinsonism**

Treatment ■ Dopaminergic drugs: ● levodopa (dopamine precursor) ● carbidopa or benserazide (dopa-decarboxylase inhibitors) ● dopamine agonists (apomorphine, ropinirole, pramipexole), including those derived from ergot (pergolide, lisuride, bromocriptine, cabergoline) – the latter can cause pulmonary, pericardial or retroperitoneal fibrosis ● entacapone and tolcapone (catechol o-methyl transferase [COMT] inhibitors) ■ Antimuscarinic drugs (benzatropine, orphenadrine, procyclidine, trihexylphenidyl [benzhexol]) ■ Selegeline, a monoamine oxidase inhibitor, differs from other MAOIs in that it should not cause the acute hypertensive episodes found with most drugs ■ Stereotactic surgery – improves the tremor.

Prognosis ■ There is a slow progression over many years and Parkinson's disease is not generally fatal ■ However, about one-third of patients also develop a gradual dementia later in the disease, manifesting with confusion, paranoia, and visual hallucinations ■ The psychosocial impact of the condition on the patient, family and carers may be profound.

Oral findings

■ The patient may have swallowing difficulties and poor control of oral secretions; drooling of saliva may therefore be troublesome ■ Conversely, medications routinely used to control the effects of the disease (i.e. antimuscarinic drugs) may cause xerostomia ■ Caries is less common than in controls ■ Periodontal disease may be advanced and can progress due to xerostomia ■ Levodopa may cause reddish saliva ■ Orofacial involuntary movements (dyskinesia) such as 'flycatcher tongue' and lip pursing are side effects of levodopa and bromocriptine ■ Impaired chewing and slow speech are common.

Dental management

Risk assessment ■ It is essential in patients with Parkinson's disease not to let the blankness of expression and apparent unresponsiveness be mistaken for lack of reaction or intelligence ■ However, dementia in not uncommon in advanced Parkinsonism; this makes communication and consent problematic ■ Involuntary movements can make the use of sharp and rotating instruments hazardous ■ Drooling and head position may compromise access.

Appropriate health care ■ Treatment plans must consider limitations of tremor and motor skills ■ Sympathetic handling is particularly important, since anxiety increases the tremor, which may affect the tongue and/or lips ■ Questions should require a simple yes/no response as the patient may take time to answer verbally or with head/eye movement ■ The regular use of mouth prop and (if the patient can control their secretions) rubber dam, are recommended.

Preventive dentistry ■ Oral hygiene may be compromised by physical limitations; assistance and education of carers and/or family may be required ■ Dietary advice, topical fluoride and salivary substitutes may be useful in patients with hyposalivation ■ Antiseptics such as chlorhexidine will reduce infectious complications.

Pain and anxiety control **Local anaesthesia** COMT inhibitors may interact with epinephrine to cause tachycardia, arrhythmias and hypertension. **Conscious sedation** Nitrous oxide may be useful. **General anaesthesia** GA may be required for patients with severe uncontrollable movements.

Patient access and positioning **Access to dental surgery** Some patients will need assistance to get into and out of the dental chair. **Timing of treatment** Short appointments are recommended. **Patient positioning** ■ The patient should be seated upright or at most at

Table 3.126 **Key considerations for dental management in Parkinsonism (see text)**

	Management modifications*	Comments/possible complications
Risk assessment	2	Difficult communication; involuntary movements
Appropriate dental care	2/4	Sympathetic handling; mouth prop; rubber dam
Pain and anxiety control		
– Local anaesthesia	1	Avoid epinephrine
– Conscious sedation	1	
– General anaesthesia	3/4	For severe disease
Patient access and positioning		
– Access to dental office	1	Assistance required
– Timing of treatment	1	Short appointments
– Patient positioning	1	Semi-reclined; orthostatic hypotension; possibly physical restriction
Treatment modification		
– Oral surgery	1	
– Implantology	1	Implant supported prosthesis
– Conservative/Endodontics	1	
– Fixed prosthetics	1	
– Removable prosthetics	1	Soft mouth guard
– Non-surgical periodontology	1	
– Surgical periodontology	1	
Hazardous and contraindicated drugs	1	Avoid macrolides

*0 = No special considerations. 1 = Caution advised. 2 = Specialised medical advice recommended in some cases. 3 = Specialised medical advice mandatory. 4 = Only to be performed in hospital environment. 5 = Should be avoided.

45 degrees, in order to prevent respiratory compromise ■ L-dopa and some other agents may cause hypotension – patients should be raised upright only cautiously and carefully assisted out of the dental chair ■ Some degree of physical restraint may be required for patients with uncontrollable movements, but consent should be sought.

Treatment modification **Implantology** Implant-supported prostheses may help to reduce oral dyskinesia in some patients. **Fixed prosthetics and conservation** Orofacial involuntary movements (dyskinesia) may make the use of rotating dental instruments hazardous. **Removable prosthetics** A soft mouth guard may be useful in patients with oral dyskinesia to prevent soft tissue damage. **Periodontology** Frequent periodical recalls are necessary in patients with xerostomia and/or impaired oral hygiene.

Drug use Erythromycin and other macrolides may increase bromocriptine or cabergoline levels.

Further reading ● Dirks S J, Paunovich E D, Terezhalmy G T, Chiodo L K 2003 The patient with Parkinson's disease. Quintessence Int 34:379–393 ● Nakayama Y, Washio M, Mori M 2004 Oral health conditions in patients with Parkinson's disease. J Epidemiol 14:143–150 ● Scully C, Shotts R 2001 The mouth in neurological disorders. Practitioner 245:539–549 ● Wächter R, Diz Dios P, Fabinger A, Kartun D, Krekeler G, Schilli W 1998 Implantes dentales en pacientes con enfermedad de Parkinson. Avances en Perioncia e Implantología Oral 10:31–35.

PHOBIAS

Definitions There are four main types of phobia: ■ *Claustrophobia* – fear of closed spaces, is probably the most common phobic disorder ■ *Agoraphobia* – fear of being in public places from which escape might be difficult or help unavailable ■ *Social phobia* – overwhelming anxiety and excessive self-consciousness in normal social situations ■ *Simple, or specific phobias (phobic neurosis)* – a morbid irrational fear, or anxiety out of all proportion to the threat: ● phobic neuroses differ from anxiety neuroses in that the phobic anxiety arises only in specific circumstances, whereas patients with anxiety neuroses are generally anxious ● common specific phobias are centred on heights, tunnels, driving, water, flying, insects, dogs, injuries involving blood, and dental procedures ● dental 'phobia' is more extreme than straightforward anxiety and is characterised by avoidance behaviour – previous frightening dental experiences are often the major factor in its development.

General aspects

Clinical presentation ■ Blushing ■ Profuse sweating ■ Trembling ■ Nausea ■ Difficulty in talking ■ Muscle tension ■ Increased pulse rate ■ Accelerated breathing ■ Sweating ■ Stomach cramps.

Treatment ■ Supportive or intensive psychotherapy ■ Behaviour therapy aims at desensitisation by slow and gradual exposure to the frightening situation ■ Implosion is a technique where patients are asked to imagine a persistently frightening situation for 1 or 2 hours ■ Anxiolytic drugs have a limited role: ● buspirone is particularly useful since it lacks the psychomotor impairment, dependency and some other features of benzodiazepines ● benzodiazepines such as diazepam, lorazepam, oxazepam or alprazolam can be used but are habituating ● antidepressants, especially tricyclics, are used if there is a significant depressive component.

Prognosis ■ When phobias are centred on threats such as flying, anaesthetics or dental treatment, normal life is possible if such threats can be avoided ■ Phobias may also be a minor part of an anxiety state, personality disorder or a more severe disorder such as depression, obsessive neurosis, or schizophrenia.

Oral findings in dental phobia

Neglected dental disease is not uncommon due to fear of dental treatment and avoidance behaviour. Antidepressant medication may result in xerostomia, increasing the caries risk.

Dental management

Risk assessment Phobic patients: ■ are often not just dentally anxious but may show a range of other complaints ■ report poorer perceived dental health, a longer interval since their last dental appointment, a higher frequency of past fear behaviours, more physical symptoms during the last dental injection, and a higher percentage of symptoms of anxiety and depression ■ may genuinely want dental care but can be unable to cooperate, may be unaware of their response to their anxiety and, as a consequence, may be hostile in their responses or behaviour ■ may chat incessantly, have a

Table 3.127 **Key considerations for dental management in phobia (see text)**

	Management modifications*	Comments/possible complications
Risk assessment	2	Associated disorders
Pain and anxiety control		
– Local anaesthesia	1	Avoid sight of needle; topical LA
– Conscious sedation	0	
– General anaesthesia	0/4	
Patient access and positioning		
– Access to dental office	0	
– Timing of treatment	1	Early morning
– Patient positioning	0	
Treatment modification		
– Oral surgery	0	
– Implantology	2	Not recommended
– Conservative/Endodontics	0	
– Fixed prosthetics	2	Not recommended
– Removable prosthetics	0	
– Non-surgical periodontology	0	
– Surgical periodontology	0	
Imaging	1	Avoid CT and MRI
Hazardous and contraindicated drugs	1	Some patients receive psychoactive drugs/ antidepressant therapy

*0 = No special considerations. 1 = Caution advised. 2 = Specialised medical advice recommended in some cases. 3 = Specialised medical advice mandatory. 4 = Only to be performed in hospital environment. 5 = Should be avoided.

history of failed appointments, and appear tense and agitated ('white knuckle syndrome') ■ may have difficulties resulting from: alcoholism, drug dependence, or drug treatment with major tranquillisers, MAOIs or tricyclics.

Appropriate health care ■ Patients with dental phobia often fear: ● the noise and vibration of the drill ● the sight of the injection needle ● sitting in the dental chair ■ A true dental phobic is not common, but when seen demands great patience and time ■ The main aids are: ● confident reassurance ● patience ● careful painlessly performed dental procedures ● desensitisation ■ Complex oral rehabilitation requiring multiple appointments, such as fixed prostheses, are not recommended in the early stages.

Pain and anxiety control **Local anaesthesia** Although LA may be used with routine precautions, care must be taken to ensure the patient avoids the sight of the needle. Topical LA is very useful and distraction techniques (e.g. asking the patient to raise their legs, wriggle their toes) help to facilitate the use of LA. **Conscious sedation** Anxiolytics such as oral buspirone or diazepam, supplemented if necessary with inhalational or intravenous sedation, may help. **General anaesthesia** General anaesthesia may be indicated in some patients.

Patient access and positioning **Timing of treatment.** Early morning appointments, with premedication, and no waiting, can help.

Imaging ■ Some people find it impossible to undergo MRI, CT or radiation therapy because of their claustrophobia.

Drug use Some patients are on antidepressant therapy/psychoactive drugs.

Further reading ● Little J W 2003 Anxiety disorders: dental implications. Gen Dent 2003;51:562–568 ● Lundgren J, Berggren U, Carlsson S G 2004 Psychophysiological reactions in dental phobic patients with direct vs. indirect fear acquisition. J Behav Ther Exp Psychiatry 35:3–12 ● Moore R, Brodsgaard I, Rosenberg N 2004 The contribution of embarrassment to phobic dental anxiety: a qualitative research study. BMC Psychiatry 4:10.

PORPHYRIAS

Definition Porphyrias are rare genetic errors in haem biosynthesis, which result in the accumulation of toxic precursors (porphobilinogen and aminolaevulinic acid) (Table 3.128).

General aspects

Aetiopathogenesis An extraordinarily wide array of factors can cause exacerbations of porphyria, including: ■ drugs (e.g. benzodiazepines, oral contraceptives, phenytoin, rifampicin and sulphonamides) ■ alcohol (in some cases the disease may be controlled by withdrawal of alcohol) ■ fasting ■ infections ■ pregnancy.

Table 3.128 **Main types and characteristics of porphyrias**

	Type	Alternative name	Particular features
Acute	Variegate porphyria*	South African (Afrikaans) genetic porphyria	Acute, severe abdominal pain; cardiovascular disturbances; neuropsychiatric disturbance; autonomic dysfunction; rashes
	Acute intermittent porphyria*	Swedish porphyria	Acute, severe abdominal pain; cardiovascular disturbances; neuropsychiatric disturbance; autonomic dysfunction
	Hereditary coproporphyria*	Coproporphyria	Acute, severe abdominal pain; cardiovascular disturbances; neuropsychiatric disturbance; autonomic dysfunction
Non-acute	Porphyria cutanea tarda	Cutaneous hepatic porphyria	Photosensitivity and iron overload. Drugs do not precipitate acute attacks but the condition is aggravated by alcohol, oestrogens, iron and polychlorinated aromatic compounds
	Congenital porphyria**	Erythropoietic porphyria, Gunther's disease	Red teeth; hypertrichosis; severe mutilating photosensitivity rashes; haemolytic anaemia

*Clinically significant.
**Erythropoietic.

Clinical presentation Acute exacerbations may be associated with: ■ Neuropsychiatric disturbances: ● typically a peripheral sensory and motor neuropathy ● sometimes agitation, mania, depression, hallucinations, and schizophrenic-like behaviour ■ Cardiovascular disturbances: ● tachycardia and hypertension in the majority sometimes followed by postural hypotension ■ Occasionally also: ● respiratory embarrassment ● major convulsions ● gastrointestinal disturbances ● autonomic dysfunction ● severe hyponatraemia ● cutaneous photosensitivity.

Classification The forms are clinically significant, since acute illness is precipitated by drugs. They are: ■ *Variegate porphyria* – the commonest form, found mainly in South Africans of Afrikaans descent ■ *Acute intermittent porphyria* – less common but found in all population groups ■ *Hereditary coproporphyria* – rare.

Diagnosis Diagnosis is confirmed by demonstrating 5-aminolaevulinic acid (ALA) and porphobilinogen in the urine.

Box 3.21 Drugs considered unsafe for use in porphyria

Local anaesthetics
- Articaine • Lidocaine (may be used with caution) • Mepivacaine • Prilocaine (may be used with caution)

General anaesthetics
- Barbiturates • Enflurane • Halothane

Analgesics
- Dextropropoxyphene • Diclofenac • Mefenamic acid • Indometacin • Pentazocine • Opioids

Antibiotics
- Doxycycline • Erythromycin • Flucloxacillin • Sulphonamides

Antifungals
- Fluconazole • Itraconazole • Ketoconazole • Miconazole • Griseofulvin

Psychoactive drugs
- Barbiturates • Carbamazepine • Chlordiazepoxide • Diazepam • Dichloralphenazone • Meprobamate • Monoamine oxidase inhibitors • Phenytoin • Tricyclics

Endocrine active drugs
- Androgens • Chlorpropamide • Contraceptive pill • Oestrogens • Progestogens

Others
- Ethanol (alcohol) • Clonidine • Danazol • Pentoxifylline

Treatment ■ Reduction of hepatic iron overload through phlebotomy ■ Treatment of attacks is to stop the triggering drug and to give haem arginate, fluids, electrolytes and glucose.

Prognosis Patients with porphyrias may develop acute attacks that are potentially fatal but, between attacks, patients may appear normal – apart from severe photosensitivity rashes.

Oral findings

Erythropoietic porphyria is characterised by red/brown discoloration of the teeth (which fluoresce in ultraviolet light). Fewer than 100 cases have probably ever been reported, but it has been suggested that this disease might have been the source of the werewolf legend because of the red teeth (thought to be dripping with blood), the hairy distorted facial features and avoidance of daylight.

Dental management

Risk assessment ■ Dental treatment should be avoided during porphyria attacks ■ Liver function and blood tests may be performed before dental operative procedures.

Box 3.22 Drugs considered probably safe for use in porphyria

Antiemetics
● Cyclizine ● Domperidone ● Meclozine ● Prochlorperazine ● Promazine

Antihistamines
● Chlorpheninamine ● Diphenhydramine ● Ketotifen ● Loratadine ● Mequitazine ● Promethazine ● Trimeprazine

Antibacterial agents
● Aminoglycosides ● Ciprofloxacin ● Co-amoxiclav ● Ethambutol ● Minocycline ● Pentamidine ● Sodium fusidate ● Streptomycin ● Vancomycin

Local anaesthetics
● Amethocaine ● Bupivacaine ● Procaine ● Tetracaine ● Epinephrine

Immunisations
● Immunoglobulins ● Vaccines

Antidepressants
● Amitriptyline ● Fluoxetine ● Lofepramine ● Mianserin

Antipsychotics
● Chlorpromazine ● Fluphenazine ● Haloperidol ● Pipothiazine ● Trifluoperazine

Antivirals/antifungals
● Aciclovir ● Amphotericin ● Famciclovir ● Flucytosine ● Ganciclovir ● Valaciclovir ● Zalcitabine

Anticonvulsants
● Clobazam ● Clonazepam ● Gabapentin ● Sodium valproate

Drugs used in anaesthesia
● Atropine ● Cyclopropane ● Ether ● Isoflurane ● Neostigmine ● Nitrous oxide ● Pancuronium ● Propofol ● Suxamethonium

Analgesics
● Alfentanil ● Aspirin ● Buprenorphine ● Co-codamol ● Co-dydramol ● Codeine phosphate ● Dextromethorphan ● Dextromoramide ● Diamorphine ● Diflunisal ● Dihydrocodeine ● Fenbufen ● Fentanyl ● Flurbiprofen ● Ibuprofen ● Ketoprofen ● Methadone ● Morphine ● Nalbuphine ● Paracetamol/acetaminophen ● Pethidine ● Sulindac ● Tiaprofenic acid

Others
● Corticosteroids ● Midazolam ● Sucralfate ● Temazepam ● Tranexamic acid ● Vitamins

http://www.uq.edu.au/porphyria
http://www.cs.nsw.gov.au/csls/RPAH/porphyria/druglist1.htm

Pain and anxiety control **Analgesia** Aspirin, acetaminophen and codeine can be safely used. **Local anaesthesia** ■ Bupivacaine is considered safe ■ Articaine, lidocaine, prilocaine and mepivacaine are probably contraindicated. **Conscious sedation** ■ Many benzodiazepines,

Table 3.129 **Key considerations for dental management in porphyria (see text)**

	Management modifications*	Comments/possible complications
Risk assessment	1	Liver function, blood test
Pain and anxiety control		
– Local anaesthesia	1	Avoid some local anaesthetics
– Conscious sedation	1	Avoid some benzodiazepines
– General anaesthesia	4	Avoid some general anaesthetics
Patient access and positioning		
– Access to dental office	0	
– Timing of treatment	1	Evening
– Patient positioning	0	
Treatment modification		
– Oral surgery	0	Avoid some drugs
– Implantology	0	
– Conservative/Endodontics	1	Avoid light-cured fillings
– Fixed prosthetics	0	
– Removable prosthetics	0	
– Non-surgical periodontology	0	
– Surgical periodontology	0	
Hazardous and contraindicated drugs	2	Many drugs are contraindicated

*0 = No special considerations. 1 = Caution advised. 2 = Specialised medical advice recommended in some cases. 3 = Specialised medical advice mandatory. 4 = Only to be performed in hospital environment. 5 = Should be avoided.

including diazepam, are absolutely contraindicated ■ Midazolam and flumazenil, however, are considered probably safe ■ Nitrous oxide is safe. **General anaesthesia** Barbiturates (including the intravenous barbiturates), enflurane, and halothane are absolutely contraindicated.

Patient access and positioning **Timing of treatment** Evening or early morning appointments will reduce sunlight exposure during the journey to the dental office.

Treatment modification **Fixed prosthetics and conservation** Light-cured fillings are better avoided, although there is no evidence that the light used produces skin or mucosal lesions.

Drug use Drugs that are liable to precipitate attacks are absolutely contraindicated (Box 3.21), and include: ■ some anaesthetics ■ antifungals ■ benzodiazepines ■ antibiotics (cephalosporins, erythromycin, flucloxacillin, sulphonamides, trimethoprim, tetracyclines) ■ analgesics (mefenamic acid, pentazocine).

Drugs considered safe for use in porphyria are shown in Box 3.22. Assessing the safety of drugs in porphyria is an inexact science, and for many drugs no information is available. For some others, the data are of doubtful validity and often conflicting.

Further reading ● Brown G J, Welbury R R 2002 The management of porphyria in dental practice. Br Dent J 193:145–146 ● Moore A W 3rd, Coke J M 2000 Acute porphyric disorders. Oral Surg Oral Med Oral Pathol Oral Radiol Endod 90:257–262.

PREGNANCY

Definition Pregnancy is a major event in any woman's life and is associated with physiological changes affecting especially the endocrine, cardiovascular and haematological systems – and often attitude, mood or behaviour.

General aspects

The fetus

■ Any woman of childbearing age is a potential candidate for pregnancy but may not be aware of pregnancy for 2 or more months when, unfortunately, the fetus is most vulnerable to damage from drugs, radiation and infections.

■ Fetal development during the first 3 months of pregnancy is a complex process of organogenesis – the fetus is then especially at risk from developmental defects. About 10–20% of all pregnancies abort at this time, often because of fetal defects.

■ The most critical period is the 3rd to 8th week, when differentiation is occurring. Precautions to avoid fetal damage and developmental defects should therefore be adequate if carried out from the time of the first missed menstruation.

■ Most developmental defects are of unknown aetiology – there may be hereditary influences, but drugs (including alcohol and tobacco), infections and radiation can be implicated in some cases.

■ Alcohol can cause serious fetal damage; even a single exposure to high alcohol levels can cause significant brain damage and most will suffer effects, ranging from mild learning disabilities to major physical, mental and intellectual impairment.

■ Tobacco smoking during or after pregnancy can seriously damage the fetus or child. Smoking increases the risk of stillbirth, diminishes the infant's birth weight, and impairs the child's subsequent mental and physical development. Smoking by either parent after the child's birth increases the child's risk of respiratory tract infection, severe asthma, and sudden death.

■ Infections early in pregnancy may damage the fetus; this applies especially to those that cause the TORCH syndrome (Toxoplasmosis, Rubella, Cytomegalovirus, Herpesviruses). Consequences vary, depending on the fetal age and infecting agent, but range from hearing damage to learning disability, cardiac anomalies, or death.

■ In contrast, it is now recognised that folic acid supplements are an important way of minimising the risk of neural tube defects such as spina bifida, and of facial clefts.

Clinical presentation Many hormones increase in pregnancy, especially sex hormones, prolactin and thyroid hormones, but levels of luteinising hormone (LH) and follicle stimulating hormone (FSH) fall. Sequelae may include: ■ nausea ■ vomiting ■ deepened pigmentation, particularly of the nipples and sometimes the face (chloasma) ■ glycosuria, impaired glucose tolerance, and sometimes diabetes ■ tachycardia, and initially often a slight fall in blood pressure with the possibility of syncope or postural hypotension. In later pregnancy, when the mother is supine the fetus may press on and occlude the venous return to the heart via the vena cava, causing the 'supine hypotensive syndrome'.

Prognosis Medical complications in pregnancy can include: ■ *Hypertension* – a dangerous complication; this leads to increased morbidity and mortality in both fetus and mother. Hypertension may be asymptomatic but, when associated with oedema and proteinuria (pre-eclampsia), may culminate in eclampsia (hypertension, oedema, proteinuria and convulsions) that may be fatal. The fetus is also at risk. ■ *Blood hypercoagulability* – can lead to venous thrombosis, particularly postoperatively, or occasionally disseminated intravascular coagulopathy ■ *Anaemia* – expansion of the blood volume may cause an apparent anaemia but, in about 20%, true anaemia also develops, mainly because of fetal demands for iron and folate. Most patients are given both of these haematinics. Pregnancy may worsen pre-existing anaemias, especially sickle cell anaemia. ■ *Supine hypotension syndrome* – up to 10% of patients may be affected.

Oral findings

■ In some pregnant women, gingivitis is aggravated (pregnancy gingivitis) or may even (in about 1%) result in a pyogenic granuloma at the gingival margin (pregnancy epulis) – these conditions typically arise after the second month, and resolve on parturition ■ Chronic periodontal disease in the mother has been linked with low birth weight babies ■ In a few women subject to recurrent aphthae, ulcers may stop (or occasionally become more severe) during pregnancy ■ Some pregnant women have a hypersensitive gag reflex ■ Halitosis and enamel erosion are not uncommon, due to hypersensitive gag reflex and acid regurgitation from the stomach.

Dental management

Risk assessment ■ Drugs may be teratogenic ■ Very low-dose radiation exposure of the maternal head/neck region during pregnancy is associated with an increased risk of having a low birth weight infant ■ *Hazards to pregnant dental staff* may include exposure to: ● infections by some viruses, such as cytomegalovirus or rubella ● radiation ● inhalational anaesthetic or sedation agents – nitrous oxide scavenging must always be used ● mercury vapour. Experimental and clinical data do not suggest that there should be any restriction on use of amalgams or work restriction of dental personnel, provided that work practices are up to accepted standards. Concern has been expressed, particularly in Sweden, about the risk of placental transfer of mercury as a result of exposure to the metal during pregnancy. However, measurements taken at the Department of Odontological Toxicology at the Karolinska Institute on female dental personnel and their newborn babies and non-exposed controls have shown no significant differences in the plasma mercury levels or in the fetal/maternal ratios of mercury levels.

Appropriate health care ■ Because of the risk of coincidental mishaps, it is wise to try to avoid giving any drugs or using radiation, and best to postpone as much active treatment as possible until after parturition – particularly in those with a history of abortions and those who have at last achieved pregnancy after years of failure ■ Dental health education is usefully given ■ During the first trimester the only safe course of action is to protect the patient as far as possible from infections and to avoid the use of radiography and drugs, particularly general anaesthetics ■ In the second and third trimesters the fetus is growing and maturing but can still be affected by infections, drugs such as tetracyclines, and possibly other factors ■ Dental treatment, if required, is best carried out during the second trimester; advanced restorative procedures are probably best postponed until the periodontal state improves after parturition and prolonged sessions of treatment are better tolerated ■ In the third trimester the supine hypotension syndrome may result if the patient is laid flat – if this occurs, the patient should be placed on one side to allow venous return to recover ■ In the last month of pregnancy, elective dental care is best avoided as it is uncomfortable for the patient. Moreover, premature labour or even abortion may also be ascribed, without justification, to dental treatment.

Preventive dentistry ■ Pregnancy is the ideal opportunity to begin a preventive dental education programme ■ The mother's teeth do not, of course, lose calcium as a result of fetal demands and there is no reason to expect caries to become more active unless the mother develops a capricious desire for sweets ■ Prenatal fluorides are not indicated as there is little evidence of benefit to the fetus ■ Advice on any need for fluoride administration to the infant can be given.

Pain and anxiety control **Local anaesthesia** Dental treatment of pregnant women under local anaesthesia is safe but drugs and procedures should be avoided unless absolutely necessary, until the second trimester. There is some evidence to suggest that prilocaine and procaine should be avoided. **Conscious sedation** ■ Sedation with diazepam or midazolam are particular hazards and must be avoided in the first trimester and in the last month of the third trimester ■ Nitrous oxide is able to interfere with vitamin B_{12} and folate metabolism, but does not appear to be teratogenic. However, it is should be avoided where possible. If it is indicated, it is advisable to: ● restrict nitrous oxide to the second or third trimester when unavoidable ● limit the duration of exposure to less than 30 minutes ● use 50% oxygen ● avoid repeated exposures ● use scavenging in the dental surgery to minimise staff exposure ● it may be a sensible precaution for pregnant staff to avoid areas where nitrous oxide is in use.

General anaesthesia ■ General anaesthesia is best avoided unless essential – there is scanty evidence of teratogenic effects in humans from exposure to general anaesthetic agents, but (apart from the above comments concerning nitrous oxide), it is possible that barbiturates and benzodiazepines

Table 3.130 **Drugs to avoid in pregnant mothers***

Drug	Potential effects on fetus
Aciclovir (systemic)	Teratogenicity?
Alcohol	Fetal alcohol syndrome
Aspirin	Premature closure of ductus arteriosus Persistent pulmonary hypertension Bleeding tendency
Carbamazepine	Neural tube defects Vitamin K impairment and bleeding tendency
Carbimazole	Goitre
Cocaine	Ankyloglossia
Codeine	Respiratory depression
Corticosteroids	Adrenal suppression Growth retardation
Co-trimoxazole	Haemolysis Teratogenicity Methaemoglobinaemia
Diazepam	Cleft lip/palate
Felypressin	Oxytocic
Fluconazole	Congenital anomalies
Gentamicin	Deafness
Lithium	Cardiac abnormalities
Nitrous oxide (repeated large doses)	Congenital anomalies
NSAIDs	Premature closure of ductus arteriosus Persistent pulmonary hypertension Bleeding tendency
Pentazocine	Fetal addiction and withdrawal symptoms
Phenytoin	Fetal phenytoin syndrome
Prilocaine	Methaemoglobinaemia
Retinoids	Neural tube defects
Tetracyclines	Discoloured teeth and bones
Thalidomide	Phocomelia
Valproate	Neural tube defects
Vancomycin	Toxicity (monitor levels)
Warfarin	Long bone and cartilage abnormalities Bleeding tendency

*Drugs of abuse may cause neonatal addiction.

Table 3.131 **Known risks to fetus of some drugs used systemically in dentistry**

Category[a]	B	C	D and X
	Either safe to fetus in animal models without human data, or risk in animal models but safe in human studies	Risk to fetus in animal models but no human studies available, or no human studies support safety	Definitive human data demonstrating risk to fetus
Use in dentistry	Where necessary	Only if really essential and after consulting physician	*Do not use*
Local anaesthetics	Lidocaine	Articaine[b]	
	Prilocaine[c]	Bupivacaine	
		Mepivacaine	
Sedative agents	Promethazine		Benzodiazepines
			Nitrous oxide[d]
Analgesics	Meperidine	Codeine	Aspirin
	Paracetamol/acetaminophen	Diflunisal	NSAIDs[e]
Antimicrobials	Azithromycin	Aciclovir	Doxycycline
	Cefadroxil	Ciprofloxacin	Minocycline
	Cefuroxime	Clarithromycin	Tetracyclines
	Cephalexin	Fluconazole	Co-trimoxazole[f]
	Clindamycin		

Table 3.131 **Known risks to fetus of some drugs used systemically in dentistry—cont'd**

Category[a]	B	C	D and X
Antimicrobials	Erythromycin		
	Loracarbef		
	Metronidazole		
	Penciclovir (cream)		
	Penicillins		
Others		Corticosteroids (even topical)	Antidepressants
			Carbamazepine
			Colchicine
			Danazol
			Phenytoin
			Povidone-iodine applications
			Retinoids
			Thalidomide
			Warfarin

[a]US Federal Drug Agency (FDA) pregnancy categories; category A has not been included as this represents drugs with no risk to the fetus.
[b]Sometimes categorised as B.
[c]Prilocaine, at least in theory, can cause methaemoglobinaemia.
[d]Nitrous oxide, though able to interfere with vitamin B_{12} and folate metabolism, does not appear to be teratogenic in normal use though it is advisable to restrict use to the second or third trimester.
[e]May be safer in first and second trimesters.
[f]Co-trimoxazole may cause neonatal haemolysis.

are teratogenic ■ When a general anaesthetic is given but there is a mishap to the fetus, the mother may blame the anaesthetist, even though this may be quite unjustifiable ■ Another hazard is an increased tendency to vomit during GA induction in the third trimester ■ The greater risk is late in pregnancy when GA may induce respiratory depression in the fetus.

Patient access and positioning **Timing of treatment** Appointments are preferable in the afternoon, because the tendency to vomit is usually greater in the morning. **Patient positioning** Avoid laying the mother flat, in order to prevent supine hypotension syndrome, particularly in the third trimester. Lateral left side position is recommended. **Treatment modification** As has been previously stated, complex dental procedures are best postponed until after parturition.

Table 3.132 **Key considerations for dental management in pregnancy (see text)**

	Management modifications*	Comments/possible complications
Risk assessment	1	Drugs; irradiation; infection
Appropriate dental care	1/5	Postpone elective dental care
Pain and anxiety control		
– Local anaesthesia	1	Avoid some local anaesthetics
– Conscious sedation	5	
– General anaesthesia	5	
Patient access and positioning		
– Access to dental office	0	
– Timing of treatment	1	Afternoon
– Patient positioning	1	Avoid supine position
Treatment modification		
– Oral surgery	1	Only simple procedures
– Implantology	5	Postpone until after parturition
– Conservative/Endodontics	1	Only simple procedures
– Fixed prosthetics	5	Postpone until after parturition
– Removable prosthetics	1	Only simple procedures
– Non-surgical periodontology	1	Only simple procedures
– Surgical periodontology	5	Postpone until after parturition
Imaging	5	Postpone until after parturition
Hazardous and contraindicated drugs	1/2	Many drugs are contraindicated

*0 = No special considerations. 1 = Caution advised. 2 = Specialised medical advice recommended in some cases. 3 = Specialised medical advice mandatory. 4 = Only to be performed in hospital environment. 5 = Should be avoided.

Imaging ■ Radiography should be avoided in pregnancy, especially in the first trimester, even though dental radiography is unlikely to be a significant risk except if the beam is directed at the fetus such as in vertex-occlusal radiography ■ If radiography is essential, patients must wear a lead apron and exposure must be minimal. When an apron is used in dental radiography, gonadal and fetal exposure is negligible; a full mouth dental radiographic survey of 18 intraoral films using a lead apron gives an absorbed exposure of only 0.00001 cGy. It has been estimated that two periapical dental X-rays give an exposure 700 times less than that due to natural radiation for one day. ■ MRI is best avoided during the first trimester.

Drug use ■ Drugs may be teratogenic and should therefore be avoided where possible, especially in the first trimester (Tables 3.130, 3.131) ■ Penicillin is the drug of choice to treat oral infections ■ Aspirin and other NSAIDs may cause closure of the ductus arteriosus in utero, and fetal pulmonary hypertension, as well as delaying or prolonging labour, and therefore are contraindicated in the third trimester ■ Aspirin and other NSAIDs, in addition, cause a platelet defect and are best avoided throughout pregnancy ■ Therefore the use of analgesics should be minimised during the first trimester; if necessary, paracetamol/acetaminophen is recommended ■ Corticosteroids can suppress the fetal adrenals, and, if given, steroid cover is then needed for labour.

Further reading ● Franca C M, Mugayar L R 2004 Intrauterine infections: a literature review. Spec Care Dentist 24:250–253 ● Gajendra S, Kumar J V 2004 Oral health and pregnancy: a review. NY State Dent J 70:40–44 ● Hujoel P P, Bollen A M, Noonan C J, Del Aguila M A 2004 Antepartum dental radiography and infant low birth weight. Obstet Gynecol Surv 59:809–811 ● Suresh L, Radfar L 2004 Pregnancy and lactation. Oral Surg Oral Med Oral Pathol Oral Radiol Endod 97:672–682.

RADIOTHERAPY PATIENTS

General aspects

■ Radiotherapy is the treatment of disease with ionising radiation ■ Radiation dose or exposure is measured in units of absorbed radiation per unit of tissue. The Gray (Gy) represents 1 J/kg of tissue. Older literature uses the rad, which is equivalent to 0.01 Gy. The exposure and dose rate of radiation decrease according to an inverse square law, such that the exposure decreases by 4 when the distance increases by times 2. ■ External beam radiotherapy (RTP or DXR) is often used to treat head and neck, and oral cancer (Table 3.133) ■ External beam therapy is now commonly delivered via a medical linear accelerator or Cobalt-60 unit. These units deposit the maximum dose beneath the surface, therefore reducing the dose to the skin.

Oral findings

■ Several oral complications can follow radiotherapy involving the oral cavity and salivary glands (Box 3.23) ■ The most common complication is mucositis, which is inevitable though relatively transient ■ Some

Table 3.133 **Types of external beam radiotherapy used to treat cancer in the head and neck**

Type	Source	Used for
Electron beam	Electrical	Superficial lesions
Low voltage	X-ray	Superficial lesions
Orthovoltage	X-ray	Skin lesions
Supervoltage	^{60}Cobalt	Deeper lesions
Megavoltage	Linear accelerator or betatron	Larger lesions

Box 3.23 Oral complications of radiotherapy involving the mouth and salivary glands

- **Week 1** – nausea, vomiting
- **Week 2+** – mucositis, taste changes
- **Week 3+** – dry mouth
- **Later** – infections, caries, pulp pain and necrosis, tooth hypersensitivity, trismus, osteoradionecrosis, craniofacial defects

complications, such as xerostomia, may be inevitable but permanent ■ With improved radiation techniques, the application of lower radiation doses or use of shielding, use of amifostine and improved oral hygiene, these and other complications can often be reduced.

Mucositis ■ Mucositis is characterised by mucosal erythema, discomfort and sometimes ulceration ■ It is almost inevitable during radiotherapy, where the field involves the oral mucosa, and is particularly severe after chemoradiotherapy ■ Dysphagia and oral soreness become maximal 2–4 weeks after radiotherapy but usually subside within 2–3 weeks of completion ■ Radiation-induced mucositis is a function of cumulative tissue dose and typically begins at doses of about 15–20 Gy of standard fractionated radiation therapy; profound ulcerative mucositis is usually noted at doses of 30 Gy ■ The degree of mucositis is also determined by the radiation field size and fractionation schedules prescribed for individual patients, and appears modified by saliva volume, total epidermal growth factor (EGF) level, and the concentration of EGF in the oral environment ■ Mucositis healing is impaired by high-dose radiotherapy, hyperfractionated radiation therapy, chemo-radiotherapy and tobacco smoking ■ Mucositis can be reduced by: ● modifying the radiation treatment ● protecting the mucosa with midline mucosa-sparing blocks ● using amifostine ● other methods, including the use of: warm normal saline mouthwashes, benzydamine oral rinse, lidocaine viscous 2%, coumarin/ troxerutine ● some suggest: sucralfate, proteolytic enzymes, topical prostaglandin E2, growth factors, cytokines.

Xerostomia ■ Radiotherapy of tumours of the mouth, nasopharynx and oropharynx is especially liable to damage the salivary glands ■ It depresses salivary secretion and results in saliva of a higher viscosity but lower pH

■ Salivary secretion diminishes within a week of radiotherapy in virtually all patients ■ Some salivary function may return after many months ■ Both acute and long-term xerostomia can be reduced by: ● sparing at least one parotid gland during irradiation of patients with head and neck cancer ● giving amifostine, which is cytoprotective of acinar cells and also reduces the risk of infection associated with neutropenia, but it may cause severe nausea and vomiting ● possibly by stimulating salivation pre-radiotherapy, with pilocarpine or cevimeline ■ A saliva substitute such as carboxymethylcellulose may provide some symptomatic relief from xerostomia, as may salivary stimulants.

Infections Infections predisposed to by xerostomia include caries, oral candidosis and acute ascending sialadenitis.

Radiation caries ■ Radiation caries (Fig. 3.33) and dental hypersensitivity may follow radiotherapy, as a consequence of xerostomia and a softer, more cariogenic diet ■ Rampant dental caries may include areas such as incisal edges and cervical margins, which are normally free from caries ■ Caries begins at any time between 2 and 10 months after radiotherapy, and may possibly result in the crown breaking off from the root; a complete dentition may be destroyed within a year of irradiation ■ Caries may be reduced by: ● protecting salivary function as above ● control of dietary carbohydrates ● fluoride applications.

Loss of taste ■ Loss of taste (hypoguesia) may follow radiation damage to the taste buds, although they are relatively resistant to such injury ■ Xerostomia alone can disturb taste sensation ■ If more than 60 Gy have been given, loss of taste is usually permanent ■ In others, taste may start to recover within 2–4 months ■ Zinc supplements may help.

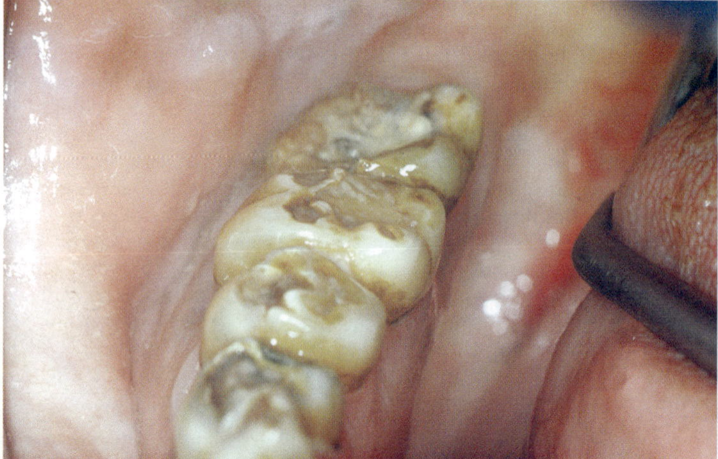

Figure 3.33 **Rampant radiation caries**

Trismus ■ It is important to exclude posterior invasion of carcinoma into pterygomasseteric muscles as a cause ■ Trismus may result from replacement fibrosis of the masticatory muscles following progressive endarteritis of affected tissues, with reduction in their blood supply after radiotherapy, but must be differentiated from recurrence of the tumour, and from osteoradionecrosis ■ The fibrosis becomes apparent 3–6 months after radiotherapy and can cause permanent limitation of jaw opening ■ Trismus may be improved by jaw-opening exercises with tongue spatulas or wedges, or use of a jaw motion rehabilitation system, such as Therabite®, three or more times a day.

Osteoradionecrosis ■ Osteoradionecrosis (ORN) is a potentially serious complication of radiotherapy (DXR) involving the jaws ■ Osteoradionecrosis appears to develop mainly in patients receiving more than 50–55 Gy; it is, however, a less frequent problem now, as megavoltage radiotherapy has less effect on bone than did orthovoltage therapy ■ ORN is particularly likely when internal radiotherapy (brachytherapy), e.g. iridium 192, is used ■ Skull bones are liable in decreasing order of frequency: ● frontal bone > zygoma > maxilla > mandible > temporal ■ The risk of ORN is increased by: ● duration elapsed after DXR ● any trauma ● oral infections involving bone, e.g. periodontal, and any additional immune or nutritional defect may also predispose ● chemotherapy ● malnutrition ● tobacco use ● alcohol use ■ ORN typically results from dental extractions carried out in the mandible after radiotherapy because of reduced bone vascularity following irradiation endarteritis ■ ORN may follow months or years after radiotherapy but about 30% of cases develop within 6 months ■ ORN is heralded by pain and swelling – the area of involved bone is often small (less than 2 cm diameter) ■ In severe cases the whole of the body of the mandible may become infected, both the overlying mucosa and skin may be destroyed and the bone may become exposed internally and externally ■ ORN may be prevented by avoiding operations such as dental extractions in patients who have irradiated jaw bones with endarteritis obliterans. This is best achieved by leaving only saveable teeth and removing any of dubious prognosis at least 10 days to 2 weeks before starting radiotherapy. Hyperbaric oxygen (HBO) may help prevent ORN. ■ ORN is managed with prophylactic antibiotics; typically the signs and symptoms of inflammation clear within a few weeks ■ Complete resolution can, however, take 2 or more years despite intensive antimicrobial treatment. Hyperbaric oxygen and possibly surgical bone decortication may be required.

Craniofacial defects ■ Craniofacial defects, tooth hypoplasia and retarded eruption can follow irradiation of developing teeth and growth centres in children ■ Children treated for neuroblastoma are at particularly high risk for abnormal dental development.

Dental management

Appropriate health care Dental care should be modified and adapted in three different stages: before, during and after radiotherapy.

Preventive dentistry ■ Before radiotherapy, meticulous oral hygiene should be implemented and preventive oral health care instituted ■ During radiotherapy, mucosal and salivary gland protection is critical: ● amifostine can minimise mucositis and xerostomia ● chlorhexidine mouthwash, 0.2%, helps maintain oral hygiene ● antifungal drugs such as nystatin suspension, 100 000 units/mL, as a mouthwash or pastilles used four times daily, may be required ■ After radiotherapy: ● oral hygiene and preventive dental care should be continued ● radiation caries and dental hypersensitivity can be controlled with a non-cariogenic diet, and daily topical fluoride applications (sodium fluoride mouthwash, stannous fluoride gel or acidulated fluoride phosphate gel); this may include daily application of fluoride by means of custom-fabricated carriers ● salivary substitutes and sialogogues are usually required.

Patient education ■ Smoking and alcohol should be discouraged during and after radiotherapy ■ A soft diet avoiding spices and acidic fruits should be recommended.

Pain and anxiety control **Local anaesthesia** Local anaesthetics without epinephrine are recommended. Intraligamentary technique may increase the ORN risk. **Conscious sedation** Conscious sedation may be provided with routine precautions. **General anaesthesia** General anaesthesia may be compromised by trismus.

Treatment modification **Surgery before radiotherapy** ■ Teeth of a dubious prognosis (e.g. grossly carious teeth with periodontal pockets over 7 mm) and unsaveable teeth in the radiation path should be extracted *before* radiotherapy ■ An interval of at least 10 days to 2 weeks between extracting the teeth and starting radiotherapy is ideal. The time interval permitted between extractions and radiotherapy is invariably a compromise because of the need to start radiotherapy as soon as possible. No bone should be left exposed in the mouth when radiotherapy begins since, once the blood supply is damaged by radiotherapy, wound healing is jeopardised. ■ Preprosthetic surgery should be performed at least 6 weeks before radiotherapy. **Surgery after radiotherapy** If extractions become unavoidable: ■ trauma should be kept to a minimum, raising the periosteum as little as possible, ensuring that sharp bone edges are removed, and suturing carefully ■ prophylactic antibiotics in adequate doses from 24–48 hours preoperatively are indicated and continued for at least 4 weeks; clindamycin 300 mg qds is an appropriate antibiotic since it penetrates bone well ■ Hyperbaric oxygen may be indicated. **Implantology** Osseointegrated implant insertion should be delayed no longer than 6 months, and insertion in directly irradiated bone should be avoided. Hyperbaric oxygen may be useful to help avoid ORN at other sites. **Fixed prosthetics and conservation** Restorative procedures should be carried out, when possible, before radiotherapy. After radiotherapy, dental restorations should be kept simple, ensuring the maintenance of acceptable aesthetics and function, using a restorative material with fluoride release where appropriate. **Removable prostheses** If dentures are required, they should

Table 3.134 **Key considerations for dental management in radiotherapy (RTP or DXR) patients (see text)**

	Management modifications*	Comments/possible complications
Appropriate dental care	1	Before, during and after RTP
Pain and anxiety control		
– Local anaesthesia	1	Avoid intraligamentary technique and epinephrine after RTP
– Conscious sedation	0	
– General anaesthesia	1	Trismus
Patient access and positioning		
– Access to dental office	0	
– Timing of treatment	0	
– Patient positioning	0	
Treatment modification		
– Oral surgery	2	2 weeks before RTP
– Implantology	1	Postpone 6 months after RTP
– Conservative/Endodontics	1	Poor prognosis after RTP
– Fixed prosthetics	1	Poor prognosis after RTP
– Removable prosthetics	1	Postpone 4–6 weeks after RTP
– Non-surgical periodontology	1	2 weeks before or 6 weeks after RTP
– Surgical periodontology	1	2 weeks before RTP
Hazardous and contraindicated drugs	0	

*0 = No special considerations. 1 = Caution advised. 2 = Specialised medical advice recommended in some cases. 3 = Specialised medical advice mandatory. 4 = Only to be performed in hospital environment. 5 = Should be avoided.

be fitted at least 4–6 weeks after radiotherapy, when initial mucositis subsides and there is only early fibrosis. **Endodontics** Spontaneous dental pulp necrosis and pulp chamber obliteration after radiotherapy have been described. However, endodontic treatment is preferred after radiotherapy, to avoid tooth extraction and the risks of ORN. **Periodontology** Periodontal surgery, if unavoidable, should be performed at least 2 weeks before radiotherapy. **Orthodontics** Orthodontic treatment is better avoided after radiotherapy.

Further reading ● Metges J P, Eschwege F, de Crevoisier R, Lusinchi A, Bourhis J, Wibault P 2000 Radiotherapy in head and neck cancer in the elderly: a challenge. Crit Rev Oncol Hematol 34:195–203 ● Shaw M J, Kumar N D, Duggal M et al 2000 Oral management of patients following oncology treatment: literature review. Br J Oral Maxillofac Surg 38:519–524 ● http://www.rcseng.ac.uk/dental/fds/pdf/oncolradio.doc

RENAL DISEASE (CHRONIC RENAL FAILURE; CRF)

Definition Chronic renal failure (CRF) is defined as an irreversible long-standing loss of renal function with deterioration of nephrons, which results in diminished glomerular filtration rate (GFR) and increased urea levels, leading to end-stage renal disease (ESRD) and ultimately to death.

General aspects

Aetiopathogenesis Common causes include: ■ glomerulonephritis ■ pyelonephritis ■ interstitial nephritis ■ diabetes ■ hypertension ■ drugs (e.g. acetaminophen rarely) ■ calculi ■ polycystic kidney ■ systemic lupus erythematosus.

Clinical presentation Features related to renal failure (Fig. 3.34) include: ■ weakness, fatigue ■ dyspnoea ■ depression, lethargy ■ anorexia, nausea, vomiting, peptic ulcer, diarrhoea ■ bone pain ■ bruising ■ hypertension.

Classification ■ CRF is classified according to the severity of failure as determined by the GFR (Box 3.24) ■ The GFR is the volume of fluid filtered by the kidney per minute and is normally 20 mL/min; it is measured by creatinine clearance.

Diagnosis ■ Urine 24-h protein ■ Creatinine clearance ■ Blood urea nitrogen (BUN) or urea levels ■ Renal ultrasound ■ Intravenous urogram ■ Diethylene-triamine-pentacetic acid (DTPA) scan.

Treatment ■ Psychosocial support ■ Nutritional advice ■ Counselling ■ Social work advice ■ Pharmacy support ■ Dialysis (haemodialysis or peritoneal dialysis) ■ Kidney transplantation.

Prognosis The prognosis is influenced by the age of the patient and the severity of the underlying disease. Infections and cardiovascular disease are the most common life-threatening complications. The annual mortality rate in patients on haemodialysis is around 10%.

Oral findings

■ Osseous lesions include: ● loss of the lamina dura ● osteoporosis and osteolytic areas (renal osteodystrophy) ● the TMJ is occasionally involved ● secondary hyperparathyroidism may lead to giant cell lesions ■ Common complaints are: ● dry mouth ● halitosis (uraemic fetor) ● metallic taste ■ Less common complaints are: ● insidious oral bleeding ● purpura can also be conspicuous ● the salivary glands may swell, salivary flow is reduced and there are protein and electrolyte changes ● accelerated calculus accumulation ■ A variety of mucosal lesions may be seen: ● the oral mucosa may be pale because of anaemia or orange stained due to carotene-like deposition ● oedema involving the soft palate and the ventral tongue is not uncommon ● there may be oral ulceration

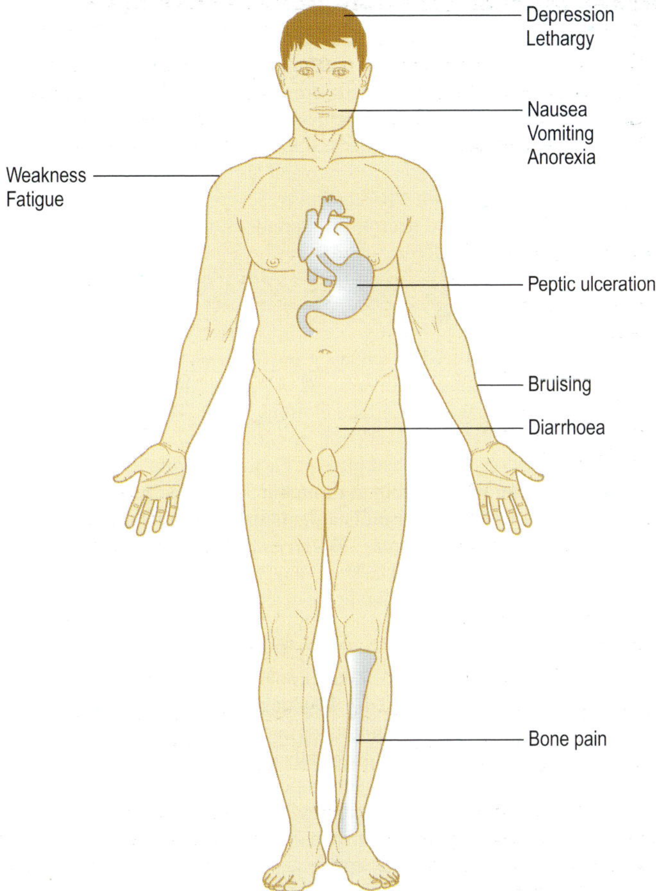

Figure 3.34 **Clinical presentation of renal failure**

Box 3.24 Classification of chronic renal failure (CRF)

• Mild CRF	GFR* 30–50 mL/min
• Moderate CRF	GFR 10–29 mL/min
• Severe CRF	GFR 5–9 mL/min
• End-stage RF (ESRD)	GFR <5 mL/min

*GFR = glomerular filtration rate.

covered with a grey pseudomembrane (uraemic stomatitis); healing of these lesions takes at least 3 weeks after blood urea levels return to normal ■ Paraesthesia of the tongue or lips may appear in patients with severe uraemia ■ In children with CRF, jaw growth is usually retarded and tooth eruption may be delayed; there may be malocclusion and enamel hypoplasia with brownish discoloration, but tetracycline staining of the teeth should no longer be seen ■ A lower caries rate and less periodontal disease have been reported in children with CRF; however, severe periodontal disease is not uncommon in adults, and necrotising periodontitis has been described in seriously ill patients with CRF.

Dental management

Risk assessment A bleeding tendency and infections are the most common complications during dental treatment: ■ *Bleeding*: the bleeding time is often prolonged but there is no defined clotting defect. The bleeding tendency is mainly because of platelet dysfunction, resulting from: ● abnormal platelet production ● diminished platelet Factor 3 (thromboxane) – which impairs conversion of prothrombin to thrombin ● raised prostacyclin (prostaglandin I) – leading to vasodilatation and poor platelet aggregation ● defective Von Willebrand factor. ■ *Infections*: infections are poorly controlled by the patient with CRF. They may spread locally as well as giving rise to septicaemia, and also accelerate tissue catabolism causing clinical deterioration. The increased risk of infection is related to: ● defective phagocyte function, which results from impaired interleukin-2 (IL-2), but increases in other cytokines (IL-1, IL-6, tumour necrosis factor) ● some patients are also immunosuppressed. ■ Consideration must also be given to the effect on dental management of underlying diseases, such as hypertension, diabetes, systemic lupus erythematosus, polyarteritis nodosa, myelomatosis and amyloidosis, or complications such as peptic ulceration ■ Major surgical procedures may be complicated by hyperkalaemia as a result of tissue damage, acidaemia and blood transfusion. Hyperkalaemia predisposes to arrhythmias and may cause cardiac arrest.

Appropriate health care The patient with CRF is often fatigued and may seem uncooperative at times. This is because of the immense psychosocial implications of their disease as well as the associated medical problems. The patient may appear depressed and poorly motivated. A sympathetic approach is essential. Medical advice is mandatory to ascertain the severity of the CRF, the degree of metabolic control and any associated risks. The main management problems in patients in CRF include:

Bleeding tendencies ■ The renal physician/haematologist should first be consulted ■ Although dialysis overall improves platelet function, the patient is often heparinised to facilitate it – hence treatment should not be undertaken on the same day as dialysis ■ Careful haemostasis should be ensured if surgical procedures are necessary ■ Should bleeding be prolonged, desmopressin (DDAVP) may achieve haemostasis for up to 4 hours. If this fails, cryoprecipitate may be effective, has a peak effect at

4–12 hours and lasts up to 36 hours. Conjugated oestrogens may aid haemostasis: the effect takes 2–5 days to develop but persists for 30 days. **Infections** ■ Infections can be difficult to recognise as signs of inflammation are masked ■ Odontogenic infections should be treated vigorously ■ Haemodialysis predisposes to blood-borne viral infections such as hepatitis virus infections ■ Tuberculosis is also more frequent, but is usually extrapulmonary and therefore does not constitute a risk to dental staff. **Prophylaxis of infections** ■ Patients with polycystic kidneys (who may have mitral valve prolapse), those receiving peritoneal dialysis, some on haemodialysis and those with transplants should be considered for antimicrobial prophylaxis before dental treatment that induces bleeding ■ Bacteraemia can result in peritonitis in those on continuous ambulatory peritoneal dialysis (CAPD) or continuous cycling peritonal dialysis (CCPD) ■ Patients with arteriovenous fistulas are not usually considered at risk from infection during dental treatment. Although vascular access infections caused by oral microorganisms have been reported in patients on haemodialysis, most are caused by skin organisms such as *Staphylococcus aureus* ■ Patients with prosthetic bridge grafts of polytetrafluorethylene or tunnelled cuffed catheters may need to be managed with precautions similar to those at risk from infective endocarditis; an alternative is to give 400 mg teicoplanin IV during dialysis, which gives cover for at least a day. **Impaired drug excretion** ■ Drugs that are directly nephrotoxic must be avoided (Table 3.135) ■ Drugs excreted mainly by the kidney may have undesirably enhanced or prolonged activity if doses are not reduced in renal failure – except in emergency, such drugs should be prescribed only after consultation with the renal physician ■ Drug therapy may need to be adjusted, depending on the degree of renal failure, the patient's dialysis schedule, or the presence of a transplant ■ Hypertension – many renal patients are on antihypertensive therapy, digoxin and diuretics, which may also complicate management.

Preventive dentistry Instructions on dietary control, oral hygiene and topical fluoride applications are strongly recommended.

Pain and anxiety control **Local anaesthesia** Local anaesthesia is safe unless there is a severe bleeding tendency. Lidocaine with epinephrine can be used at standard dosage. **Conscious sedation** Relative analgesia may be used. If it is necessary to give intravenous diazepam or midazolam, or take blood pressure, veins such as those at or above the elbow should be used because of the risk of consequent fistula infection or thrombophlebitis. If an A–V fistula is in place, this arm should not be used. The veins of the forearms and the saphenous veins are lifelines for patients on regular haemodialysis. **General anaesthesia** Light general anaesthesia with nitrous oxide is generally the technique of choice. CRF is invariably complicated by anaemia, which is a contraindication to general anaesthesia if the haemoglobin is below 10 g/dL. Some of the other difficulties with general anaesthesia are: ■ patients with CRF are highly sensitive to the myocardial depressant effects of halothane or cyclopropane, and this may result in hypotension at moderate levels of anaesthesia ■ myocardial depression and cardiac arrhythmias are

Table 3.135 **Dental drugs that may be used or contraindicated in patients with chronic renal failure[a]**

Safe (No dosage change usually required)	Fairly safe (Dosage change only in severe renal failure[b])	Less safe (Dosage reduction indicated[b] even in mild renal failure)	Avoid (Best avoided in any patient with renal failure)
Azithromycin	Ampicillin	Aciclovir[c]	Aminoglycosides
Cloxacillin	Amoxicillin	Cephalosporins[d]	Cephaloridine
Doxycycline	Benzylpenicillin	Ciprofloxacin	Cephalothin
Flucloxacillin	Clindamycin	Etafloxacin	Sulphonamides
Fucidin	Co-trimoxazole	Fluconazole	Tetracyclines[e]
Minocycline	Erythromycin	Levofloxacin	
Metronidazole	Ketoconazole	Ofloxacin	
Rifampicin	Lincomycin	Vancomycin	
	Phenoxymethyl penicillin		
Lidocaine			
Paracetamol/ acetaminophen	Codeine	NSAIDs and aspirin	Pethidine and opioids
Diazepam			
Midazolam			

[a]Many other drugs unlikely to be used in dentistry may be contraindicated: check the formulary.
[b]Severe renal failure – GFR < 10 mL/min; moderately severe renal failure – GFR < 30mL/min; mild renal failure – GFR < 50 mL/min.
[c]Systemic aciclovir.
[d]Except cephaloridine and cephalothin, which are contraindicated.
[e]Except doxycycline and minocycline.

especially likely in those with poorly controlled metabolic acidosis and hyperkalaemia ■ enflurane is metabolised to potentially nephrotoxic organic fluoride ions and therefore should only be used with caution if other nephrotoxic agents are used concurrently; isoflurane and sevoflurane are probably safer.

Patient access and positioning **Timing of treatment** Dental treatment is best carried out on the day after dialysis, when there has been maximal benefit from the dialysis and the effect of the heparin has worn off. In a dental emergency, heparin can be reversed by intravenous protamine sulphate but medical advice is mandatory. **Patient positioning** Patients on continuous ambulatory peritoneal dialysis may require adjustment in dental chair position.

Treatment modification **Surgery** There may be abnormal bone repair after extractions, with socket sclerosis. Some have recommended prophylactic antimicrobials for prevention of endovascular infections in ESRD. **Implantology** Patients with renal disease should be screened for bone disease before implant placement. Implants are not recommended in immunosuppressed patients and those on haemodialysis.
Fixed prosthetics and conservation Complex dental procedures and

Table 3.136 **Key considerations for dental management in dental treatment in chronic renal failure (see text)**

	Management modifications*	Comments/possible complications
Risk assessment	3	Bleeding; infections; impaired drug excretion; underlying disease; hyperkalaemia
Appropriate health care	3	Consult physician; psychosocial support; haemostatic support; consider antibiotic prophylaxis
Pain and anxiety control		
– Local anaesthesia	1	Bleeding tendency
– Conscious sedation	1	Preserve veins
– General anaesthesia	1/4	Anaemia; drug sensitivity
Patient access and positioning		
– Access to dental office	0	
– Timing of treatment	1	The day after dialysis
– Patient positioning	1	Adjust in CAPD patients
Treatment modification		
– Oral surgery	3	Delayed healing, bleeding
– Implantology	3	Avoid in some cases
– Conservative/Endodontics	1	Only single procedures
– Fixed prosthetics	1	Only single procedures
– Removable prosthetics	0	
– Non-surgical periodontology	3	Bleeding
– Surgical periodontology	3	Bleeding; tooth extraction recommended in some cases
Hazardous and contraindicated drugs	3	Many drugs are contraindicated

*0 = No special considerations. 1 = Caution advised. 2 = Specialised medical advice recommended in some cases. 3 = Specialised medical advice mandatory. 4 = Only to be performed in hospital environment. 5 = Should be avoided.
CAPD, continuous ambulatory peritoneal dialysis.

extensive prosthetic rehabilitation are not recommended.

Periodontology Frequent periodontal scaling is mandatory. Teeth with periodontal pockets deeper than 7 mm should be extracted.

Drug use Antimicrobial considerations include: ■ azithromycin, metronidazole, cloxacillin and fucidin and can be given in standard dosage ■ penicillins (other than phenoxymethyl penicillin and flucloxacillin), clindamycin and cephaloridine should be given in lower doses, since very high serum levels can be toxic to the central nervous system; benzylpenicillin has a significant potassium content and may also be neurotoxic and may therefore be contraindicated ■ Tetracyclines can worsen nitrogen retention and acidosis in CRF – most should be avoided, but doxycycline and minocycline can be safely given ■ Aspirin and other NSAIDs should be avoided since they aggravate gastrointestinal irritation and bleeding associated with CRF, their excretion may be delayed, and they may be nephrotoxic – especially in the elderly or where there is renal damage or cardiac failure. Some patients have peptic ulceration, which is a further contraindication to aspirin. COX-2 inhibitors may be nephrotoxic and are best avoided. ■ Fluorides can usually safely be given topically for caries prophylaxis but systemic fluorides should not be given, because of doubt about fluoride excretion by damaged kidneys.

Further reading ● Ganibegovic M 2000 Dental radiographic changes in chronic renal disease. Med Arh 54:115–118 ● Gudapati A, Ahmed P, Rada R 2002 Dental management of patients with renal failure. Gen Dent 50:508–510 ● Werner C W, Saad T F 1999 Prophylactic antibiotic therapy prior to dental treatment for patients with end-stage renal disease. Spec Care Dentist 19:106–111 ● Ziccardi V B, Saini J, Demas P N, Braun T W 1992 Management of the oral and maxillofacial surgery patient with end-stage renal disease. J Oral Maxillofac Surg 50:1207–1212.

RENAL TRANSPLANTATION

Definition ■ Renal (kidney) transplantation is the surgical replacement of a diseased kidney with a healthy one, now considered for most patients with end-stage renal disease (ESRD) who are medically suitable ■ A successful kidney transplant offers enhanced quality and duration of life and is more effective (medically and economically) than chronic dialysis therapy ■ The kidney can be from cadaveric or living donors.

General aspects

Treatment ■ All transplant recipients require life-long immunosuppression to prevent a T-cell, alloimmune rejection response ■ Induction immunosuppression consists of a short course of intensive treatment with intravenous antilymphocyte antibody (including daclizumab and basiliximab) ■ After transplantation, patients are immunosuppressed to prevent graft rejection, usually with a corticosteroid plus a steroid-sparing drug such as azathioprine or now, more commonly, ciclosporin or tacrolimus or sirolimus, or mycophenolate mofetil ■ After renal transplant, patients are thus susceptible to infections, including a liability to virally-induced neoplasia.

Prognosis Renal transplantation graft survival can be as high as 90% at one year, with an overall mortality of less than 5%, and about 70% survival at 5 years.

Oral findings

■ Patients waiting for a kidney transplant may show the typical oral findings associated with chronic renal failure ■ In immunosuppressed patients after transplantation: ● oral candidosis and recurrent herpes simplex infection are common • ciclosporin often induces gingival swelling • there is an increased prevalence of oral tumours (lymphoma, lip carcinoma and Kaposi's sarcoma) • dental pulp narrowing has been noted – apparently a corticosteroid effect.

Dental management

Risk assessment ■ Bacterial sepsis is a common complication occurring during the early postoperative months, when antibiotic cover is thus mandatory before any invasive procedure ■ Renal transplant patients also have an increased prevalence of infection with viral hepatitis B and C ■ Haematologic abnormalities, such as platelet-haemostatic dysfunction causing a bleeding tendency, may influence dental care ■ Cardiovascular disorders such as hypertension, atherosclerotic heart disease with myocardial infarction, congestive heart failure, and left ventricular hypertrophy are common and may also influence dental care ■ Gastrointestinal abnormalities, such as gastritis and peptic ulcer disease, are not uncommon, and may restrict drug use (e.g. NSAIDs).

Appropriate health care **Before transplantation** ■ A meticulous pre-transplant oral assessment is required and dental treatment undertaken with particular attention to establishing optimal oral hygiene and eradicating sources of potential infection ■ A full preventive oral health care programme should be then instituted. **After transplantation** ■ Elective dental care is best deferred until after 6 months post-transplantation ■ Invasive dental treatment should only be carried out after medical consultation and bearing in mind the bleeding tendency and infectious risk.

Preventive dentistry A meticulous oral hygiene programme is mandatory, because sepsis is the main post-transplantation complication.

Pain and anxiety control **Local anaesthesia** LA may be used safely with the usual routine precautions. A preoperative rinse with chlorhexidine mouthwash is advisable. **Conscious sedation** CS may be used safely with the usual routine precautions. **General anaesthesia** Close consultation with the physician and a thorough preoperative assessment with the anaesthetist are required.

Treatment modification **Surgery** ■ Teeth with poor prognosis should be extracted before transplantation ■ Antibiotic cover within the first 6 months after transplantation is mandatory to prevent bacteraemia and to avoid postoperative infection ■ Delayed wound healing and alveolar socket remodelling following dentoalveolar surgery have been described. **Implantology** Altered bone metabolism could influence implant osseointegration. Implants should be deferred for at least 6 months post-transplantation. **Fixed prosthetics and conservation** Complex tooth reconstruction and prosthetic rehabilitation should be postponed until after 6 months post-transplantation.

Drug use ■ A degree of renal dysfunction persists after transplantation – thus nephrotoxic drugs or drugs which are excreted by the kidneys should be avoided (Table 3.135) ■ Some patients may be on anticoagulants or platelet

Table 3.137 **Key considerations for dental management in renal transplantation (see text)**

	Management modifications*	Comments/possible complications
Risk assessment	2	Bleeding, infections, impaired drug excretion, hypertension
Appropriate dental care	1	Pre-transplant assessment; consider need for antibiotic prophylaxis ± steroid cover; postpone elective dental care for 6 months post transplantation
Pain and anxiety control		
– Local anaesthesia	1	Chlorhexidine rinse
– Conscious sedation	0	
– General anaesthesia	3/4	
Patient access and positioning		
– Access to dental office	0	
– Timing of treatment	0	
– Patient positioning	0	
Treatment modification		
– Oral surgery	2	Antibiotic prophylaxis; steroid cover; delayed healing, bleeding
– Implantology	2	Postpone 6 months
– Conservative/Endodontics	1	Postpone complex procedures
– Fixed prosthetics	1	Postpone complex procedures
– Removable prosthetics	0	
– Non-surgical periodontology	2	Bleeding
– Surgical periodontology	2	Delayed healing, bleeding
Hazardous and contraindicated drugs	2	Some drugs are contraindicated

*0 = No special considerations. 1 = Caution advised. 2 = Specialised medical advice recommended in some cases. 3 = Specialised medical advice mandatory. 4 = Only to be performed in hospital environment. 5 = Should be avoided.

antiaggregants ■ Patients receiving steroid therapy may require supplementation before dental treatment.

Further reading ● Al Nowaiser A, Lucas V S, Wilson M, Roberts G J, Trompeter R S 2004 Oral health and caries related microflora in children during the first three months following renal transplantation. Int J Paediatr Dent 14:118–126 ● Cohen D, Galbraith C 2001 General health management and long-term care of the renal transplant recipient. Am J Kidney Dis 38:S10–24 ● Fernandez de Preliasco M V, Viera M J, Sebelli P, Rodriguez Rilo L, Sanchez G A 2002 Compliance with medical and dental treatments in children and adolescent renal transplant patients. Acta Odontol Latinoam 15:21–27.

RHEUMATIC FEVER

Definition Rheumatic fever (RF) is an acute systemic inflammatory condition characterised by fever and arthritis 2–4 weeks after pharyngitis. It is caused by certain strains of beta-haemolytic streptococci.

General aspects

Aetiopathogenesis ■ Some patients develop antibodies to the streptococcal cell wall and in consequence it has been suggested that RF is an autoimmune–inflammatory disease ■ These antibodies cause vasculitis and inflammatory lesions of the joints, skin, and nervous system, and sometimes the heart (rheumatic carditis).

Clinical presentation Major features ■ Polyarthritis – involving large joints (ankles, knees) ■ Carditis – tachycardia, murmurs; the mitral valve is often affected ■ Skin – subcutaneous nodules or erythema marginatum ■ Sydenham's chorea (St Vitus' dance) – involuntary movements. Minor features ■ Previous rheumatic fever ■ Fever ■ Arthralgia ■ Increased erythrocyte sedimentation rate, C-reactive protein, leukocytosis, antistreptolysin O ■ ECG alterations (prolonged PR).

Diagnosis Diagnosis is made by: ■ evidence of streptococcal infection (throat swab, raised antistreptolysin O titre, raised DNase B titre) ■ presence of two major manifestations, or one major and two minor features.

Treatment ■ Benzylpenicillin ■ NSAIDs and possibly corticosteroids ■ Bed rest.

Prognosis ■ The acute phase lasts 6–12 weeks, but a definitive cure may take up to 6 months ■ RF recurrence rate is high – estimated as around 50% during the first 5 years; thus prophylactic therapy with penicillin (e.g. benzylpenicillin IM once a month) is required, sometimes prolonged until the age of 20 years ■ The mortality rate is about 0.5 per 100000.

Oral findings

Some patients have scarlet fever (as a first step of rheumatic fever), which produces: ■ facial rash (without circumoral involvement) ■ throat oedema ■ prominent fungiform papillae on the dorsum of the tongue (strawberry tongue).

Dental management

Risk assessment ■ Patients are rarely seen during an attack of acute rheumatic fever but emergency dental treatment may be necessary. No special precautions should be needed as there appears to be little risk of infective endocarditis at this stage. Treatment can be done under local anaesthesia in consultation with the physician. ■ Chronic rheumatic heart disease predisposes to infective endocarditis. All rheumatic heart lesions are at risk from infective endocarditis but the level of risk is not related to the severity of the defect. Asymptomatic cardiac lesions are often a greater risk for endocarditis than those that are severely disabling. Evaluation of a history of rheumatic fever and whether carditis or valve damage has occurred is difficult. The only way to be certain is to refer the patient to a cardiologist to decide whether there has been any carditis and valve damage. The simpler alternative is to give antibiotic cover on the assumption that the history is valid – but this means that at least 70% of such patients would receive the antibiotic unnecessarily, with the possibility of adverse effects.

Appropriate health care ■ Elective dental care should be postponed for 6 months after an episode of rheumatic fever ■ Referral to a cardiologist to assess possible cardiac damage is desirable.

Table 3.138 **Key considerations for dental management in rheumatic fever (see text)**

	Management modifications*	Comments/possible complications
Risk assessment	3	During acute attack – only emergency dental care
Appropriate dental care	2	Postpone elective dental care 6 months; referral to a cardiologist; antibiotic prophylaxis against endocarditis
Pain and anxiety control		
– Local anaesthesia	1	Use epinephrine with caution
– Conscious sedation	4/5	
– General anaesthesia	5	
Patient access and positioning		
– Access to dental office	0	
– Timing of treatment	0	
– Patient positioning	0	
Treatment modification		
– Oral surgery	0	
– Implantology	0	
– Conservative/Endodontics	0	
– Fixed prosthetics	0	
– Removable prosthetics	0	
– Non-surgical periodontology	0	
– Surgical periodontology	0	
Hazardous and contraindicated drugs	1	Many are given anticoagulants; possibly antibiotic resistance

*0 = No special considerations. 1 = Caution advised. 2 = Specialised medical advice recommended in some cases. 3 = Specialised medical advice mandatory. 4 = Only to be performed in hospital environment. 5 = Should be avoided.

Preventive dentistry Neglected oral health and some oral manipulations may produce a bacteraemia, which is a potential cause of bacterial endocarditis. In consequence, preventive measures to avoid caries and periodontal disease are mandatory.

Pain and anxiety control Local anaesthesia ■ An aspirating syringe should be used to give a local anaesthetic, since epinephrine in the anaesthetic given intravenously may (theoretically) increase hypertension and precipitate arrhythmias ■ Blood pressure tends to rise during oral surgery under local anaesthesia, and epinephrine theoretically can contribute to this – but this is usually of little practical importance. Conscious sedation Conscious sedation should be avoided in acute rheumatic fever. In those patients with subsequent rheumatic heart disease, CS requires special care, usually in a hospital or other specialist centre environment. General anaesthesia General anaesthesia should be avoided in acute rheumatic fever, because of the possibility of myocarditis.

Drug use ■ The risk of allergy and drug resistance emerging in patients with rheumatic fever on long-term penicillin prophylaxis is controversial. In consequence, some authors recommend using an antibiotic prophylactic regimen for penicillin-allergic patients before dental manipulations. ■ Many patients are anticoagulated.

Further reading ● Aboul Dahab O M, Darhous M S, Abdel Rahman R 1993 The incidence of *Streptococcus pyogenes* in throat and plaque cultures in cases with acute throat infections. Egypt Dent J 39:527–532 ● Guggenheimer J, Orchard T J, Moore P A, Myers D E, Rossie K M 1998 Reliability of self-reported heart murmur history: possible impact on antibiotic use in dentistry. J Am Dent Assoc 129:861–866 ● Strom B L, Abrutyn E, Berlin J A et al 1998 Dental and cardiac risk factors for infective endocarditis. A population-based, case-control study. Ann Intern Med 129:761–769.

RHEUMATOID ARTHRITIS

Definition Rheumatoid arthritis (RA) is a chronic systemic disease, characterised by persistent, symmetrical, deforming peripheral arthropathy, which typically affects mainly females between 30 and 50 years of age.

General aspects

Aetiopathogenesis ■ RA is considered an autoimmune disease related to antigen–antibody complexes, probably triggered by endogenous or infectious agents ■ It results in a recurrent synovial inflammation and articular cartilage destruction ■ The autoantibody is IgG directed against IgM ■ A genetic background involving the HLA system and DR4 antigen has also been suggested to play a role.

Clinical presentation ■ Mainly swollen, painful, stiff hands and feet on rising in the mornings (Fig. 3.35) ■ Metacarpo-phalangeal and proximal

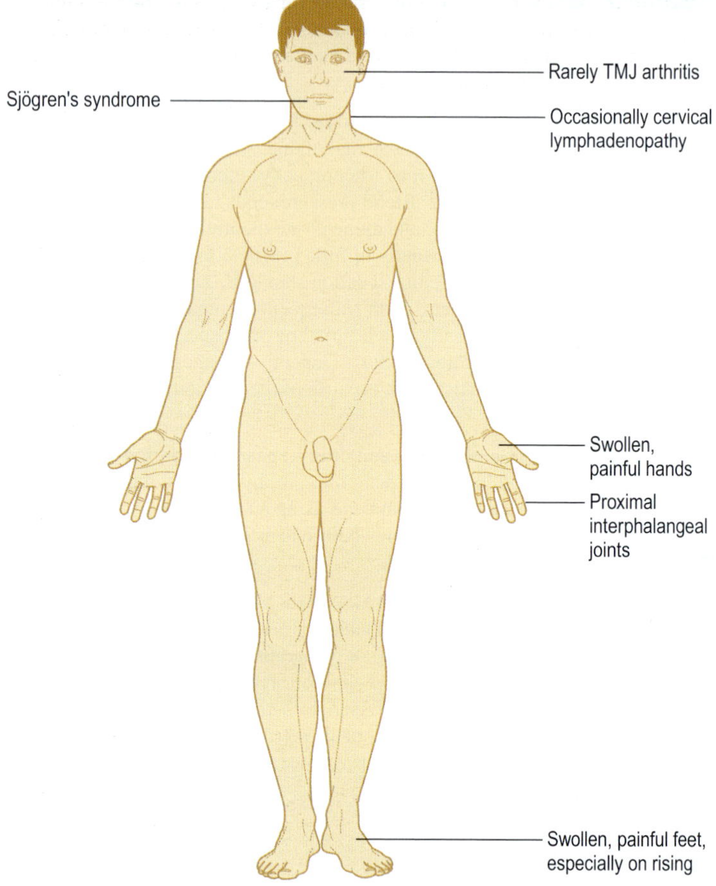

Figure 3.35 **Clinical presentation of rheumatoid arthritis**

interphalangeal joint swelling ■ Occasional cervical lymphadenopathy ■ Rheumatoid nodules (fibrinoid nodules over subcutaneous pressure points but occasionally involving lungs, heart or intestine) ■ Sjögren's syndrome ■ Rarely, TMJ arthritis ■ The psychosocial implications, related to issues such as reduced mobility, disfigurement and fatigue, may result in depression.

Classification Juvenile rheumatoid arthritis (Still's disease) may be a variant of rheumatoid arthritis affecting children and characterised by chronic synovitis with or without extra-articular involvement.

Diagnosis ■ Clinical findings – arthritis persisting for at least 6 weeks ■ Radiology – reduced joint space, erosions, subluxations ■ Serology – rheumatoid factor (RF) ■ Blood tests – raised ESR, anaemia, occasionally leukocytosis and hypergammaglobulinaemia.

Treatment ■ Exercise ■ Intralesional corticosteroids ■ Systemic drugs: ● for symptomatic relief, mainly NSAIDs ● disease-modifying drugs, mainly immunomodulators (steroids, methotrexate, azathioprine and cyclophosphamide, anakinra, etanercept, infliximab, lefunomide) and others such as gold, penicillamine or hydroxychloroquine ■ Surgery – in the case of severe osseous deformities or nerve compression.

Prognosis ■ RA is a chronic disease with intermittent exacerbations ■ Bad prognostic indicators include: ● women with insidious onset RA ● constitutional symptoms ● presence of rheumatoid nodules ● high rheumatoid factor levels ■ Life expectancy is shortened by 10–15 years.

Oral findings

■ Sjögren's syndrome is the main oral complication of RA ■ There is a predilection for RA to affect small joints, including the TMJ (Table 3.139). However, although there may be limitation of TMJ opening or stiffness, this is often painless. Radiographic changes are common in the TMJ and consist of erosions, flattening of the joint surfaces and marginal proliferation. Even when the disease is severe, pain from the TMJ appears to trouble only a minority. ■ Occasionally an anterior open bite or even sleep apnoea may result ■ The drugs used in RA may be associated with oral side effects such as lichenoid reactions and ulcers (Box 3.25) ■ Low-dose methotrexate may cause ulceration.

Table 3.139 **Rheumatoid arthritis of the temporomandibular joint: subtypes**

Type	TMJ disease	TMJ symptoms	TMJ radiographic findings	Occlusal and facial features
I	Early adult	Continuous dull pain	Erosive changes	Normal
II	Advanced	Variable pain; crepitus	Gross erosive changes	Open bite. Decreased ramus height. Increased anterior facial height
III	Arrested	Often none	Loss of condylar shape	Open bite. Decreased ramus height. Increased anterior facial height
IV	Idiopathic	Variable symptoms	Flattened, shortened condylar stump	Open bite. Decreased ramus height. Increased anterior facial height

Box 3.25 Oral adverse effects of drugs used in rheumatoid arthritis

- Antimalarials – lichenoid reactions
- Corticosteroids – candidosis
- Gold – lichenoid reactions, ulceration
- Leflunomide – taste disturbance, candidosis, salivary swelling
- Methotrexate – ulceration
- NSAIDs – lichenoid reactions, ulceration
- Pencillamine – loss of taste, lichenoid reactions, severe ulceration

Dental management

Risk assessment ■ The patient may seem uncooperative but this is commonly associated with the psychosocial implications of RA, and the strong association with depression in advanced disease ■ In some patients, weakness of the ligaments can result in dislocation of the atlanto-axial joint or fracture of the odontoid peg can follow sudden jerking extension of the neck – disastrous accidents of this sort have been known to follow adjustment of the head-rest of older types of dental chair, or sudden extension of the neck during the induction of general anaesthesia.

Appropriate health care ■ There is no reliable evidence of a need for antibiotic prophylaxis before most dental treatment in most patients with prosthetic joints; the British Society for Antimicrobial Chemotherapy does not recommend it ■ The risks from adverse reactions to antibiotics, were they to be given routinely to all patients with prosthetic joints, would probably exceed any benefit ■ However, guidelines issued by the American Dental Association advocate the use of antibiotic prophylaxis for dental at-risk procedures in certain cases (Box 3.26) ■ Although these do not agree with current practice in the UK, some UK orthopaedic surgeons nevertheless insist upon it – careful negotiation is required in these cases, with the risk to the patient evaluated on an individual basis ■ a few patients are treated with corticosteroids ■ some therapies induce neutropenia or thrombocytopenia or a bleeding tendency.

Pain and anxiety control **Local anaesthesia** LA may be given with routine precautions. **Conscious sedation** CS may be given with the routine precautions. **General anaesthesia** Caution is required to protect the neck during induction.

Patient access and positioning **Timing of treatment.** Appointments should be short and are generally better in the afternoon.
Patient positioning Sometimes patients with RA have to be treated upright, avoiding the supine position, and possibly supplementary cushions maybe needed to achieve stability. In advanced stages some patients use a wheelchair.

Treatment modification **Preventive dentistry** Patients may also have severely restricted manual dexterity and consequent difficulty maintaining

Box 3.26 Prophylactic antibiotics in patients with prosthetic joints: based on AAOS/ADA guidelines*

Dental at-risk procedure

● Tooth removal ● Oral or periodontal surgery or raising mucogingival flaps for any other purpose (including implants) ● Subgingival procedures including probing, scaling, root planing, subgingival fibre placement or any form of periodontal surgery ● Intraligamentary injections ● Reimplantation of avulsed teeth ● Endodontic manipulation beyond the root apex ● Orthodontic banding

Joint at risk

● Joint placed within previous 2 years ● Joint with history of previous infection ● Joint in patient with haemophilia ● Joint in patient with type 1 diabetes ● Joint in patient with rheumatoid arthritis ● Joint in patient on immunosuppressive therapy

Antibiotic prophylaxis regimens

Cephalexin 2 g *or* Clindamycin 600 mg *or* Azithromycin 500 mg *or* Clarithromycin 500 mg *or* Amoxicillin 2 g

*Modified from 1997 American Association of Orthopedic Surgeons & American Dental Association

adequate oral hygiene. Toothbrushes may need specially adapted handles, e.g. by adding a plastic or rubber ball to help the patient grip the brush. Electric toothbrushes may be of benefit. **Surgery** ■ Consider any bleeding tendency, and the need for steroid or antibiotic cover ■ Orthognathic surgery may be necessary in patients with severe malocclusion (anterior open bite) ■ TMJ ankylosis and severe condyle destruction may also require surgical management. **Implantology** Implants are not recommended in RA patients with severe disability, limited mouth opening or painful TMJ, and in those having difficulty maintaining good oral hygiene. **Fixed prosthetics and conservation** Complex treatment is not recommended in patients with severe disability, and in those having difficulty maintaining good oral hygiene. **Orthodontics** Orthodontics is not recommended, because unpredictable occlusal changes related to TMJ disturbances have been described.

Drug use ■ Avoid NSAIDs with platelet antiaggregant effect in patients with drug-induced thrombocytopenia or a bleeding tendency ■ Patients receiving steroid therapy may require supplementation before operative treatment or GA.

Further reading ● Ahmed N, Bloch-Zupan A, Murray K J, Calvert M, Roberts G J, Lucas V S 2004 Oral health of children with juvenile idiopathic arthritis. J Rheumatol 31:1639–1643 ● Bathi R J, Taneja N, Parveen S 2004 Rheumatoid arthritis of TMJ – a diagnostic dilemma? Dent Update 31:167–174 ● Gleissner C, Kaesser U, Dehne F, Bolten W W, Willershausen B 2003 Temporomandibular joint function in patients with longstanding rheumatoid arthritis – I. Role of periodontal status and prosthetic care – a clinical study. Eur J Med Res 8:98–108 ● Miranda L A, Fischer R G, Sztajnbok F R, Figueredo C M, Gustafsson A 2003 Periodontal conditions in patients with juvenile idiopathic arthritis. J Clin Periodontol 30:969–974.

Table 3.140 **Key considerations for dental management in rheumatoid arthritis (see text)**

	Management modifications*	Comments/possible complications
Risk assessment	1	Atlanto-axial joint dislocation or fracture; drug related bleeding tendency
Appropriate dental care	2	Corticosteroid supplementation and possibly antibiotic cover
Pain and anxiety control		
– Local anaesthesia	0	
– Conscious sedation	0	
– General anaesthesia	3/4	Protect the neck
Patient access and positioning		
– Access to dental office	0	
– Timing of treatment	1	Afternoon; short
– Patient positioning	1	Upright; supplementary cushions
Treatment modification		
– Preventive dentistry	1	Adapted toothbrushes
– Oral surgery	1	Bleeding tendency; infections
– Maxillofacial surgery	4	TMJ and orthognathic surgery
– Implantology	2	Possibly not recommended
– Conservative/Endodontics	1	Only single procedures
– Fixed prosthetics	2	Possibly not recommended
– Removable prosthetics	0	
– Non-surgical periodontology	1	Bleeding tendency
– Surgical periodontology	1	Bleeding tendency; infection
Hazardous and contraindicated drugs	1	Avoid NSAIDs which increase bleeding tendency

*0 = No special considerations. 1 = Caution advised. 2 = Specialised medical advice recommended in some cases. 3 = Specialised medical advice mandatory. 4 = Only to be performed in hospital environment. 5 = Should be avoided.

RICKETS AND OSTEOMALACIA

Definition Rickets and osteomalacia are characterised by normal bone amount but low mineral (calcium and phosphorus) content.

General aspects

Aetiopathogenesis Rickets and osteomalacia are caused by vitamin D deficiency. This may be related to: ■ dietary deficiency – there are few dietary sources of vitamin D, the best ones are fatty fish such as salmon and sardines, and margarines supplemented with vitamin D (milk contains added vitamin D in the USA but not in the UK) ■ lack of sunlight exposure – most people in the UK get much of their vitamin D from exposure of the skin to sunlight ■ malabsorption ■ renal disease causing deficiency of 1,25 di-hydroxycholecalciferol ■ liver disease reducing 25-hydroxy vitamin D ■ vitamin D resistance.

Clinical presentation ■ Rickets – starts in the period of bone growth; patients usually show knock-knees and bow legs, a knobby deformity of the chest (rachitic rosary), and possibly seizures due to hypocalcemia ■ Osteomalacia – starts after bone growth ceases, and is characterised by bone pain, fractures and myopathy.

Diagnosis Diagnosis is based on: ■ low serum calcium ■ low phosphate ■ high alkaline phosphatase ■ radiographic changes (low density, thin cortical and hypomineralisation lines or Milkman's lines).

Treatment Treatment is with vitamin D, sunlight exposure and calcium.

Prognosis In untreated patients, both rickets and osteomalacia may cause a severe disability.

Oral findings

Rickets ■ Dental defects are seen only in unusually severe cases ■ Eruption may be retarded ■ The jaws may show abnormal radiolucency and loss of cortical bone ■ In malabsorption syndromes there may be: ● secondary hyperparathyroidism or vitamin K deficiency, with endocrine or bleeding disorders respectively ● oral manifestations of malabsorption ■ In vitamin D-resistant rickets (familial hypophosphataemia): ● the skull sutures are wide ● there may be frontal bossing ● dental complaints frequently bring notice to the disease – large pulp chambers, abnormal dentine calcification liable to pulpitis, and multiple, apparently spontaneous, dental abscesses.

Dental management

Risk assessment Potential complications are due to any underlying disease, including renal disease, endocrine or bleeding disorders.

Pain and anxiety control **Local anaesthesia** LA may be used with routine precautions. **Conscious sedation** Respiratory-depressant drugs are contraindicated in children with a rachitic chest. **General anaesthesia** GA should be undertaken with specialist advice and a thorough preoperative assessment in conjunction with the anaesthetist. It should be avoided in children with a rachitic chest.

Treatment modification **Preventive dentistry** Since even minimal caries or attrition can lead to pulpitis in vitamin D-resistant rickets, comprehensive preventive care and prophylactic occlusal coverage are needed. **Surgery** Jaw fractures during tooth extraction have been described. **Implantology** Due to the reduced mineral content of the bone,

Table 3.141 Key considerations for dental management in rickets/osteomalacia (see text)

	Management modifications*	Comments/possible complications
Risk assessment		Due to the underlying disease
Pain and anxiety control		
– Local anaesthesia	0	
– Conscious sedation	2	Avoid respiratory depressants
– General anaesthesia	3/4	Avoid if rachitic chest
Patient access and positioning		
– Access to dental office	0	
– Timing of treatment	0	
– Patient positioning	0	
Treatment modification		
– Preventive dentistry	1	Prophylactic occlusal coverage
– Oral surgery	1	Jaw fracture
– Implantology	1/5	Compromised osseointegration
– Conservative/Endodontics	0	
– Fixed prosthetics	0	
– Removable prosthetics	0	
– Non-surgical periodontology	0	
– Surgical periodontology	0	
Hazardous and contraindicated drugs	1	Underlying disease

*0 = No special considerations. 1 = Caution advised. 2 = Specialised medical advice recommended in some cases. 3 = Specialised medical advice mandatory. 4 = Only to be performed in hospital environment. 5 = Should be avoided.

osseointegration could be compromised. As a consequence, dental implants are not recommended.

Drug use Drugs prescription will be modified in patients with underlying malabsorption, renal or liver disease.

Further reading

- Alexander S, Moloney L, Kilpatrick N 2001 Endodontic management of a patient with X-linked hypophosphataemic rickets. Aust Endod J 27:57–61
- Chaussain-Miller C, Sinding C, Wolikow M, Lasfargues J J, Godeau G, Garabedian M 2003 Dental abnormalities in patients with familial hypophosphatemic vitamin D-resistant rickets: prevention by early treatment with 1-hydroxyvitamin D. J Pediatr 142:324–331
- Seow W K 2003 Diagnosis and management of unusual dental abscesses in children. Aust Dent J 48:156–168
- Zambrano M, Nikitakis N G, Sanchez-Quevedo M C, Sauk J J, Sedano H, Rivera H 2003 Oral and dental manifestations of vitamin D-dependent rickets type I: report of a pediatric case. Oral Surg Oral Med Oral Pathol Oral Radiol Endod 95:705–709.

SCHIZOPHRENIA

Definition ■ Schizophrenia is the most common psychotic disorder (or a group of disorders), marked by severely impaired thinking, emotions, and behaviours ■ Disorders of perception (hallucinations) and thought (delusions) and disintegration of the personality cause thoughts and behaviour that can be totally inappropriate and incomprehensible ■ Approximately 1% of the world's population is affected by schizophrenia.

General aspects

Classification The fourth (1994) edition of the *Diagnostic and Statistical Manual of Mental Disorders* (*DSM-IV*) specifies five subtypes of schizophrenia: **Paranoid** ■ The key feature of this subtype is the combination of false beliefs (delusions) and hearing voices (auditory hallucinations), with more nearly normal emotions and cognitive functioning (cognitive functions include reasoning, judgment, and memory) ■ The delusions of paranoid schizophrenics usually involve thoughts of being persecuted or harmed by others or exaggerated opinions of their own importance, but may also reflect feelings of jealousy or excessive religiosity ■ Paranoid schizophrenics function at a higher level than other subtypes, but are at risk for suicidal or violent behaviour under the influence of their delusions. **Disorganised (formerly called hebephrenic)** ■ Disorganised speech, thinking, and behaviour ■ Flat or inappropriate emotional responses to a situation (affect). **Catatonic** ■ Disturbances of movement that may include rigidity, stupor, agitation, bizarre posturing, and repetitive imitations of the movements or speech of other people ■ These patients are at risk of malnutrition, exhaustion, or self-injury. **Undifferentiated** ■ Characteristic positive and negative symptoms of schizophrenia but not meeting the specific criteria for the paranoid, disorganised, or catatonic subtypes. **Residual** ■ At least one acute schizophrenic episode occurs but these individuals do not presently have strong positive psychotic symptoms, such as delusions and hallucinations ■ They may have negative symptoms, such as withdrawal from others, or mild forms of positive symptoms, which indicate that the disorder has not completely resolved.

Aetiopathogenesis The aetiology of schizophrenia remains unclear: ■ genetic predisposition has been implicated in about 10% of cases (involving chromosomes 5 and 10) ■ stress and some organic diseases may trigger an acute phase.

Clinical presentation ■ *Acute schizophrenia* may develop in previously unaffected individuals and appears to be precipitated by organic disorders or external stress ■ *Chronic schizophrenia* is more common and characterised by inappropriate affect, disordered thought processes, delusions and hallucinations ■ The first signs of schizophrenia often appear as confusing, or even shocking, changes in behaviour – the person's speech and behaviour can be so disorganised that they may be incomprehensible or frightening to others because of (4 Ds): ● distorted perceptions of reality ● delusions, hallucinations and illusions ('positive' symptoms) ● disordered thinking ● diminished emotional expression ('negative' symptoms).

Diagnosis The average time between the onset of schizophrenia and diagnosis is one year. There is no laboratory test and diagnosis is made from the clinical presentation.

Treatment Treatment includes: ■ rehabilitation ■ individual psychotherapy ■ family education ■ self-help groups ■ admission to hospital (may be necessary if behaviour causes disturbance in the home or society) ■ antipsychotics (neuroleptics or major tranquilisers) (Table 3.142). Antipsychotic medications used in the treatment of schizophrenia alter the

Table 3.142 **Main antipsychotic drugs used to treat schizophrenia**

Antipsychotic drug	Examples	Features
Phenothiazines with pronounced sedative effects, but moderate antimuscarinic and extrapyramidal effects	Chlorpromazine Methotrimeprazine Promazine	If there is considerable anxiety or hyperactivity, chlorpromazine is most commonly used but parenteral use of fluphenazine enanthate or decanoate, pipothiazine palmitate or zuclopenthixol decanoate by bi-weekly injection overcomes compliance difficulties
Phenothiazines with low extrapyramidal effects, moderate sedative and antimuscarinic effects	Pericyazine Pipotiazine Thioridazine	Fewer extrapyramidal effects than other phenothiazines. Thioridazine may be cardiotoxic
Piperazine phenothiazines, with low sedative and antimuscarinic activity but high extrapyramidal effects	Fluphenazine Perphenazine Prochlorperazine Trifluoroperazine	If no sedation is needed piperazine phenothiazines may be given but may have pronounced extrapyramidal effects and may worsen depression
Butyrophenones	Benperidol Droperidol Haloperidol	Useful mainly for violent patients
Thioxanthines	Flupenthixol/ flupentixol Zuclopenthixol	Extrapyramidal effects common
Atypical antipsychotics	Clozapine Amisulpride Olanzapine Quetiapine Risperidone Sertindole Zotepine	All, apart from clozapine, are first-line treatment for newly diagnosed schizophrenia. Clozapine is used for resistant cases; it does not produce tardive dyskinesia but has significant antimuscarinic effect and can cause agranulocytosis
Diphenylbutylpiperidines	Fluspirilene Pimozide	Danger of sudden unexplained, probably cardiac, death

dopamine/cholinergic balance in the basal ganglia so that extrapyramidal and anticholinergic effects are common and can be disabling. Extrapyramidal features from medication are most common with the piperazine phenothiazines, butyrophenones and use of depot preparations, and include: • dystonia and dyskinesia (abnormal movements) • akathisia (restlessness) • Parkinsonism • tardive dyskinesia – characterised by involuntary movements most often affecting the mouth, lips, and tongue, and sometimes the trunk or other parts of the body such as arms and legs; it affects about 15–20% of patients who have been receiving phenothiazines for many years, but may also develop in patients who have been treated with these drugs for shorter periods of time • neuroleptic malignant syndrome – a rare, but potentially life-threatening, drug-induced disorder.

Oral findings

■ Poor oral hygiene and a high prevalence of caries and periodontal disease are common findings in patients living alone or in psychiatric hospitals ■ Smoking is strongly associated with schizophrenia; most individuals have heavily stained teeth ■ Individuals with schizophrenia often have decreased salivary flow, particularly if on long-term neuroleptics (with an increased susceptibility to candidosis and caries) ■ Attrition may occur in patients with tardive dyskinesia ■ The long-term use of neuroleptics can lead to oral pigmentation ■ Haloperidol and clozapine can cause hypersalivation ■ Muscular rigidity or tonic spasms frequently involve the bulbar or neck muscles, with subsequent difficulties in speech or swallowing. Alternatively, there may be uncontrollable facial grimacing (orofacial dystonia), which may start after only a few doses. This may be controlled by stopping the neuroleptic and giving anti-Parkinsonian/antimuscarinic drugs. ■ Schizophrenic patients may have delusional oral symptoms, the treatment of which is beyond the expertise of the dental surgeon.

Dental management

Risk assessment ■ Extrapyramidal symptoms related to neuroleptic drugs may make dental management difficult ■ The airway should be protected during dental treatment because of the patient's propensity to have an impaired gag reflex ■ Phenothiazines can cause dose-related impaired temperature regulation; they may also occasionally cause obstructive jaundice, leucopenia or ECG changes that can influence dental management.

Appropriate health care ■ Patients should be approached slowly in a non-threatening manner and should be advised of what to expect during the procedure ■ The dental staff should adopt an open manner, with no whispering or talking quietly to staff, as this may induce a paranoid episode ■ Appropriate behavioural control techniques should be selected on an individual patient basis ■ Mild schizophrenic features (which are often unrecognised) include loss of social contact, flatness of mood or inappropriate social behaviour, which may appear at first as mere tactlessness or stupidity. Thus the patient, when asked to sit down in the surgery, sits in the operator's

Table 3.143 **Key considerations for dental management in schizophrenia (see text)**

	Management modifications*	Comments/possible complications
Risk assessment	2	Phenothiazines adverse effects; extrapyramidalism; impaired gag reflex
Appropriate dental care	2	Behaviour control; consent issues
Pain and anxiety control		
– Local anaesthesia	1	Drug induced epinephrine reversal or block
– Conscious sedation	4	Drug interactions; hallucinations
– General anaesthesia	3/4	Avoid barbiturates
Patient access and positioning		
– Access to dental office	0	
– Timing of treatment	1	Short appointments
– Patient positioning	1	Avoid orthostatic hypotension
Treatment modification		
– Oral surgery	1	
– Implantology	3/5	Usually not recommended
– Conservative/Endodontics	1	
– Fixed prosthetics	1	
– Removable prosthetics	1	Possibly not recommended
– Non-surgical periodontology	1	
– Surgical periodontology	1	
Hazardous and contraindicated drugs	1	Avoid tramadol

*0 = No special considerations. 1 = Caution advised. 2 = Specialised medical advice recommended in some cases. 3 = Specialised medical advice mandatory. 4 = Only to be performed in hospital environment. 5 = Should be avoided.

rather than the dental chair; attempts at communication may be met by a response that indicates a failure to get through, or are interrupted by totally irrelevant remarks. Psychiatric help must be sought through the patient's medical practitioner. ■ Consent issues may need to be addressed, particularly when the patient is having an acute episode ■ Elective dental treatment should not be undertaken during acute episodes ■ Care must be taken to avoid injury to the patient/self due to sudden movements related to tardive dyskinesia and/or orofacial dyskinesia.

Preventive dentistry Most patients show impaired ability to plan and perform oral hygiene. However, obsessive toothbrushing has been described in some cases.

Pain and anxiety control **Local anaesthesia** ■ Phenothiazines have alpha-adrenergic blocking activity and can thus cause epinephrine reversal in patients given epinephrine in a local anaesthetic. There is vasodilatation instead of the anticipated vasoconstriction. The importance of this in relation to local anaesthesia is unclear but it may be prudent to avoid vasoconstrictors. ■ Haloperidol and droperidol also reportedly block the vasoconstrictor activity of epinephrine. **Conscious sedation** Sedatives should be used with caution because of their synergic effects with some neuroleptics and propensity to cause hallucinations. **General anaesthesia** ■ In some patients, general anaesthesia will represent the only available behavioural control technique ■ However, general anaesthesia, especially with intravenous barbiturates, may lead to severe hypotension and should therefore be avoided if possible.

Patient access and positioning **Timing of treatment** Shorter appointments are recommended. **Patient positioning** Haloperidol and phenothiazines may cause orthostatic hypotension and thus patients should be raised slowly and carefully assisted from the dental chair.

Treatment modification **Implantology** Dental implants are usually not recommended due to neglected oral hygiene and the high prevalence of heavy smokers. **Removable prosthetics** Removable appliance may be misplaced or ingested.

Drug use With tramadol, there is a risk of seizures.

Further reading
● McCreadie R G, Stevens H, Henderson J et al 2004 The dental health of people with schizophrenia. Acta Psychiatr 110:306–310 ● Ramon T, Grinshpoon A, Zusman S P, Weizman A 2003 Oral health and treatment needs of institutionalised chronic psychiatric patients in Israel. Eur Psychiatry 18:101–105 ● Stanfield M 2004 Schizophrenia and oral healthcare. Dent Update 31:510–515 ● Tang W K, Sun F C, Ungvari G S, O'Donnell D 2004 Oral health of psychiatric in-patients in Hong Kong. Int J Soc Psychiatry 50:186–191 ● Yaltirik M, Kocaelli H, Yargic I 2004 Schizophrenia and dental management: review of the literature. Quintessence Int 35:317–320.

SCLERODERMA

Definition ■ Scleroderma is an uncommon connective tissue disease characterised by degenerative changes and hypertrophy of collagenous tissue with sclerosis of skin and other tissues ■ Diffuse systemic sclerosis also causes renal, gastrointestinal, myocardial disease and malignant hypertension.

General aspects

Aetiopathogenesis The aetiology remains unknown. Autoimmune reactions, endocrine disorders and vascular and neural disturbances have been suggested to play a role but genetics and some drugs have also been implicated.

Clinical presentation The main clinical findings (Fig. 3.36) include: ■ sclerodactyly (fibrosis and contracture of fingers) ■ arthralgia ■ Raynaud's phenomenon ■ skin pigmentation (ivory colour) and

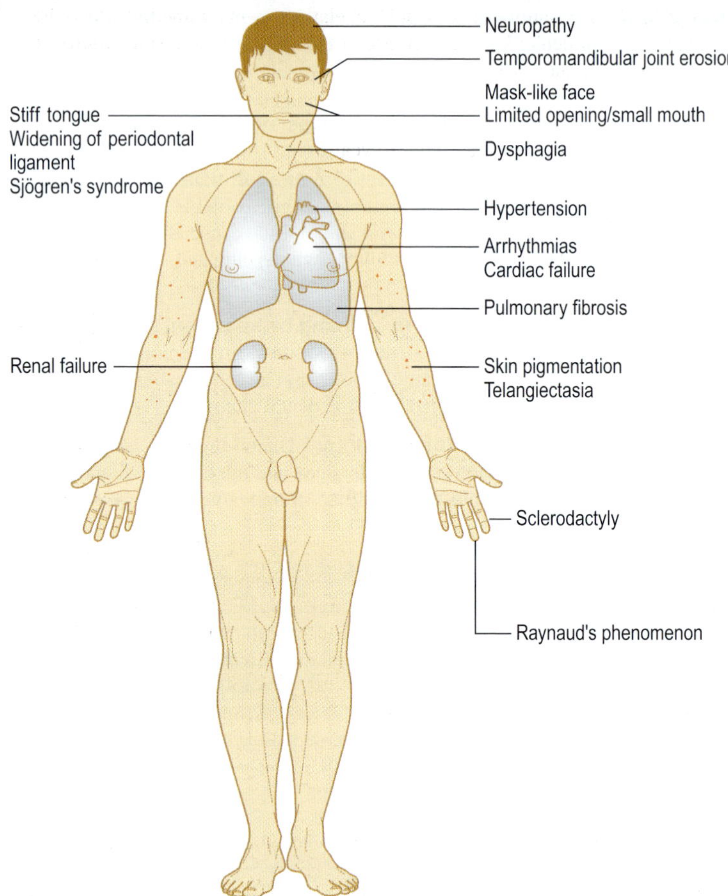

Figure 3.36 **Clinical presentation of scleroderma**

telangiectasia ■ neuropathy ■ pulmonary fibrosis ■ dysphagia ■ hypertension and possibly renal failure ■ arrhythmias and possibly cardiac failure ■ Sjögren's syndrome.

Classification There are two main groups: ■ Localised scleroderma (localised cutaneous fibrosis); rare and restricted, includes morphoea ■ Systemic scleroderma (cutaneous and non-cutaneous involvement); this includes CREST syndrome (calcinosis, Raynaud's, oesophageal hypofunction, sclerodactyly, telangiectasia of face and extremities).

Diagnosis Patients with systemic involvement have autoantibodies to: ■ topoisomerase (Scl-70) ■ RNA polymerase ■ centromeres.

Treatment Para-aminobenzoic acid, chelating agents, dimethylsulphoxide, azathioprine and penicillamine have been used with limited results. Steroids may be useful in the early stages.

Prognosis Systemic scleroderma with visceral involvement has a poor prognosis, with 50% mortality over 10 years.

Oral findings

■ Some 80% of individuals have manifestations in the head and neck region; in 30% the symptoms start there – involvement of the face causes characteristic changes in appearance: ● notably narrowing of the eyes and mask-like restriction of facial movement (Mona Lisa face) ● constriction of the oral orifice can cause progressively limited opening of the mouth (fish-mouth) ● the submucosal connective tissue may also be affected and the tongue may become stiff and less mobile (chicken tongue) ■ A typical manifestation of morphoea is involvement of one side of the face causing an area of scar-like contraction aptly described as coup de sabre; morphoea in childhood is believed to be a cause of facial hemiatrophy ■ A recognised but uncommon feature seen in fewer than 10% of cases of systemic sclerosis is widening of the periodontal membrane space without tooth mobility ■ The mandibular angle may be resorbed or, rarely, there is gross extensive resorption of the jaw ■ TMJ erosion is a common radiographic finding ■ Sjögren's syndrome also develops in a significant minority, but very frequently when systemic sclerosis is associated with primary biliary cirrhosis ■ There is often an increase in the number of decayed, missing or filled teeth ■ Penicillamine therapy may cause loss of taste, oral ulceration, lichenoid reactions and other complications.

Dental management

Risk assessment The risk of complications during dental treatment is conditioned by the underlying disease, especially when there is visceral involvement. Occasionally there is involvement of the periarticular tissues of the temporomandibular joint together with the microstomia, limiting access to the mouth so as to make dental treatment more or less impracticable.

Appropriate health care/Preventive dentistry ■ Limited mouth opening and sclerodactyly contributes to difficult oral hygiene ■ Children's toothbrushes may be more appropriate but may need to be adapted if there is extensive sclerodactyly ■ Occasionally, electric toothbrushes with small heads may be of benefit.

Pain and anxiety control **Local anaesthesia** LA may be used with routine precautions. **Conscious sedation** Associated pulmonary, cardiac and renal disease are potential contraindications for conscious sedation. Nitrous oxide methods are preferred. **General anaesthesia** ■ Dysphagia and pulmonary, cardiac or renal disease are potential contraindications for general anaesthesia ■ There is an increased risk of regurgitation and pulmonary aspiration during GA.

Table 3.144 **Key considerations for dental management in scleroderma (see text)**

	Management modifications*	Comments/possible complications
Risk assessment	1	Visceral involvement; limited oral access
Pain and anxiety control		
– Local anaesthesia	0	
– Conscious sedation	3	Visceral involvement
– General anaesthesia	4/5	Visceral involvement
Patient access and positioning		
– Access to dental office	0	
– Timing of treatment	0	
– Patient positioning	1	Avoid supine position
Treatment modification		
– Oral surgery	1	Access may be limited
– Implantology	1	
– Conservative/Endodontics	1	Paediatric handpieces/ burs
– Fixed prosthetics	1	
– Removable prosthetics	1	Difficult oral insertion
– Non-surgical periodontology	1	
– Surgical periodontology	1	
Hazardous and contraindicated drugs	1	Renal failure

*0 = No special considerations. 1 = Caution advised. 2 = Specialised medical advice recommended in some cases. 3 = Specialised medical advice mandatory. 4 = Only to be performed in hospital environment. 5 = Should be avoided.

Patient access and positioning **Patient positioning** In patients with pulmonary involvement, avoid the supine position.

Treatment modification **Conservative/Endodontics** Paediatric handpieces/burs may be of help. **Removable prosthetics** Insertion of removable prosthesis may be progressively difficult due to restricted mouth opening. Indeed, access for taking impressions for construction of the prosthesis may be very limited. Some articulated and flexible devices have been successfully used. When possible, fixed prostheses are the treatment of choice.

Drug use Drug use may need to be modified in patients with renal failure.

Further reading
● Kurian K, Shanmugam S, Mathew B, Elongavan 2003 Facial hemiatrophy – a report of 5 cases. Indian J Dent Res 14:238–245 ● Phoa K H, de Baat P, de Baat C 2003 Microstomia as a complication of scleroderma. Ned Tijdschr Tandheelkd 110:457–459 ● Scardina G A, Messina P 2004 Systemic sclerosis: description and diagnostic role of the oral phenomena. Gen Dent 52:42–47 ● Spackman G K 2004 Scleroderma: what the general dentist should know. Gen Dent 47:576–579.

SJÖGREN'S SYNDROME

Definition Sjögren's syndrome (SS) is an autoimmune exocrinopathy, the essential changes of which are infiltration of the lacrimal, salivary and other exocrine glands by lymphocytes and plasma cells, with progressive acinar destruction and often multi-system disease. SS mainly affects middle-aged or older women.

General aspects

Aetiopathogenesis ■ SS is characterised by an excessive activity of B-lymphocytes and hypergammaglobulinaemia with an increased production of antibodies against the SS-A (Ro: Robair) and SS-B (La: Lattimer) antigens ■ A genetic predisposition has been suggested in patients with HLA-DR3 and HLA-B8. Hormones, drugs, viruses and environmental factors have been implicated.

Clinical presentation ■ Dry mouth and dry eyes are the most common findings ■ Raynaud's phenomenon or other autoimmune manifestations are frequent ■ Multi-system disease can manifest with skin and vaginal dryness, lung, renal, peripheral nervous system and gastrointestinal problems, and autoimmune thyroid disorders.

Classification ■ The 'sicca syndrome' (primary Sjögren's syndrome) is the association of dry mouth (xerostomia) with dry eyes (keratoconjunctivitis sicca) in the absence of any connective tissue disease ■ The term 'Sjögren's syndrome' (secondary Sjögren's syndrome: SS-2) refers to the association of dry mouth and dry eyes with a connective tissue disease, usually rheumatoid arthritis.

Diagnosis ■ Drugs, irradiation, and infections (hepatitis C, HIV and HTLV-1), should be excluded as the cause of xerostomia ■ No single investigation will reliably establish the diagnosis of SS, but the following are useful: ● presence of serum autoantibodies, especially antinuclear antibodies SS-A and SS-B ● an ophthalmological examination; a Schirmer test shows impaired lacrimation ● salivary flow rates – confirm the presence and degree of xerostomia but are non-specific ● labial salivary gland biopsy: this is more specific than the other tests, but it is invasive and may be associated with postoperative scarring/paraesthesia ● sialography ● scintigraphy ● ultrasound.

Treatment Management is largely symptomatic though there have been attempts at immunosuppression to control the disease process.

Prognosis ■ Women who have SS can pass autoantibodies across the placenta into the fetal circulation, which can lead to heart block ■ About 5% of people with SS develop lymphoma.

Oral findings

■ Oral involvement in SS results in discomfort caused by the reduced salivary flow, obvious dryness of the mucosa in severe cases, and erythema and lobulation of the tongue – apart from its dryness, the oral mucosa appears normal unless infected ■ The other effects of persistent xerostomia include: ● difficulty in speaking or swallowing ● difficulty wearing dentures ● disturbed taste sensation ● accelerated caries ● susceptibility to oral candidosis ● susceptibility to ascending (bacterial) sialadenitis ● swelling of the parotid or other salivary glands – seen in a minority and, rarely, these glands can also be persistently painful. Late onset of salivary gland swelling, especially in sicca syndrome, may indicate development of a MALT (mucosa-associated lymphoid tissue) lymphoma.

Dental management

Risk assessment Risk during dental procedures is limited to patients with multi-system involvement, and those with underlying connective tissue diseases.

Appropriate health care ■ Cotton wool rolls should be moistened to avoid adherence to the oral mucosa ■ Dry mouth may be helped symptomatically by simple methods, such as frequently sipping water or drinks, sucking ice, or using frequent, liberal rinses of a salivary substitute containing carboxymethyl cellulose or mucin ■ Salivation may be stimulated by chewing sugar-free gum or sucking citrus or malic acid lozenges. Sialogogues such as pilocarpine 5 mg three times daily with meals, or an anticholinesterase such as pyridostigmine may increase salivation if any functional tissue remains, but systemic effects such as diarrhoea and blurred vision may be troublesome and there may be arrhythmias. Cevimeline is a newer alternative. ■ Infections should be treated. Antifungal treatment is given as rinses of nystatin or amphotericin mixture. Acute complications such as ascending parotitis should be treated with a penicillinase-resistant penicillin such as flucloxacillin in combination with metronidazole, because of the possible presence of anaerobes. Pus should be sent for culture and antibiotic susceptibilities. ■ Some patients with secondary SS are treated with corticosteroids and may require supplementation before dental treatment; some may have thrombocytopenia or a bleeding tendency, which needs to be considered before undertaking invasive treatment.

Preventive dentistry ■ Preventive dental care is vital ■ Patients have a tendency to consume a cariogenic diet because of the impaired sense of taste: this must be avoided ■ Caries should also be controlled by fluoride applications ■ Improved oral hygiene and the use of a 0.2% chlorhexidine mouthwash will help to control periodontal disease and other infections ■ Denture hygiene is important because of susceptibility to candidosis; antifungal treatment is often needed.

Pain and anxiety control **Local anaesthesia** LA may be used with routine precautions. **Conscious sedation** Multi-system involvement is potentially a contraindication for CS. **General anaesthesia** ■ Patients with SS who need dental treatment may not be good candidates for GA because of their increased risk of respiratory infections ■ It is important to: ● lubricate the eyes and throat ● humidify the gases ● avoid drying

Table 3.145 **Key considerations for dental management in Sjögren's syndrome (see text)**

	Management modifications*	Comments/possible complications
Risk assessment	1	Multi-system involvement
Appropriate dental care	1	Possibly corticosteroid supplementation
Pain and anxiety control		
– Local anaesthesia	0	
– Conscious sedation	1	Multi-system involvement
– General anaesthesia	3/4	Respiratory infections
Patient access and positioning		
– Access to dental office	0	
– Timing of treatment	1	See Rheumatoid arthritis
– Patient positioning	1	See Rheumatoid arthritis
Treatment modification		
– Oral surgery	0	
– Implantology	1	Evaluate oral hygiene
– Conservative/Endodontics	0	
– Fixed prosthetics	1	Delay until 1 year caries free
– Removable prosthetics	1	Minimise acrylic–mucosa contact
– Non-surgical periodontology	0	
– Surgical periodontology	0	
Hazardous and contraindicated drugs	1	Trimethoprim allergy

*0 = No special considerations. 1 = Caution advised. 2 = Specialised medical advice recommended in some cases. 3 = Specialised medical advice mandatory. 4 = Only to be performed in hospital environment. 5 = Should be avoided.

agents (atropine, phenergan) • be conscious of the possibility of cervical spine involvement in rheumatoid arthritis • maintain body heat (because of Raynaud's disease) • consider renal function.

Treatment modification **Implantology** Some patients benefit from implant-retained prostheses, but systematic studies have not been published. **Fixed prosthetics and conservation** No crowns should be constructed until caries is controlled and there are no new lesions for more than one year. **Removable prosthetics** Removable prostheses, particularly those manufactured with acrylic, may cause oral discomfort due to trauma of the dry oral mucosa.

Drug use There is an increased incidence of drug allergies, especially to trimethoprim – which may induce a systemic reaction of fever, headache, backache and meningeal irritation (trimethoprim-induced aseptic meningitis).

Further reading • Cassolato S F, Turnbull R S 2003 Xerostomia: clinical aspects and treatment. Gerodontology 20:64–77 • Mandel L, Sunwoo J 2003 Primary Sjögren's syndrome. NY State Dent J 69:34–36 • Mignogna M D, Fedele S, Russo L L, Muzio L L,

Wolff A 2005 Sjögren's syndrome: the diagnostic potential of early oral manifestations preceding hyposalivation/xerostomia. J Oral Pathol Med 34:1–6 ● Porter S R, Scully C, Hegarty A M 2004 An update of the etiology and management of xerostomia. Oral Surg Oral Med Oral Pathol Oral Radiol Endod 97:28–46 ● Rhodus N L 1999 An update on the management for the dental patient with Sjögren's syndrome and xerostomia. Northwest Dent 78:27–34 ● Soto-Rojas A E, Kraus A 2002 The oral side of Sjögren syndrome. Diagnosis and treatment. A review. Arch Med Res 33:95–106.

SPINA BIFIDA

Definition Spina bifida is failure of fusion of vertebral arches, an important cause of spinal cord disease and severe physical handicap.

General aspects

Aetiopathogenesis Deficiency of folic acid in pregnancy may predispose to spina bifida in the fetus; most cases are of unknown aetiology.

Clinical presentation and classification **Spina bifida occulta** Spina bifida occulta rarely causes any obvious clinical or neurological disorder but can be detected by a small naevus or tuft of hair over the lumbar spine in some patients, and radiographically in about 50% of normal children. **Spina bifida cystica** Spina bifida cystica is an extensive vertebral defect through which the spinal cord or its coverings protrude, presenting as:

■ *Meningocele*: protrusion of the meninges as a sac covered by skin, rarely causing neurological defect but 20% have hydrocephalus

■ *Myelomeningocele*: ten times as common as meningocele, and characterised by meninges and nerve tissue which are protruded and exposed and liable to infection, particularly meningitis. It causes severe neurological defects, typically complete paralysis of and loss of sensation and reflexes in the lower limbs (paraplegia), followed by deformities (club foot or dislocated hip). Patients with myelomeningocele therefore tend also to suffer from: ● inability to walk ● liability to develop pressure sores ● urinary incontinence ● faecal retention ● other problems such as hydrocephalus, cerebral complications (epilepsy or learning impairment), other vertebral or renal anomalies.

Diagnosis Diagnosis can be made by amniocentesis, looking for raised levels of alpha-fetoprotein and acetylcholinesterase.

Treatment ■ Patients with myelomeningocele are severely handicapped and require specialist paediatric attention to manage urinary tract, bowel and locomotion disabilities ■ Surgical closure of myelomeningocele and decompression of hydrocephalus is often carried out, usually in early infancy ■ Hydrocephalus is typically drained by ventriculo-atrial (V/A) or, more frequently nowadays, by ventriculo-peritoneal (V/P) shunts.

Prognosis The prognosis is influenced by the severity of the defect (e.g. complete open spine or rachischisis is incompatible with life).

Dental management

Risk assessment There is a high prevalence of latex allergy in these patients and the risk increases with the: ■ number of previous surgical procedures ■ use of bladder catheters ■ existence of a ventriculo-peritoneal shunt ■ presence of symptoms when blowing up a toy balloon ■ familial history of atopic diseases.

Appropriate health care ■ Dental care of patients with spina bifida (Fig. 3.37) should be performed in a latex-free environment using latex-free dental appliances ■ Care must be taken not to traumatise the patient who is unable to respond protectively ■ Bowel and bladder are best emptied before dental treatment ■ In patients with hydrocephalus bypassed by a shunt, antibiotic prophylaxis may be necessary if there is a V/A shunt but not for the newer V/P shunts.

Preventive dentistry It is important to minimise the necessity for dental treatment due to the risk of developing latex allergy.

Pain and anxiety control **Local anaesthesia** LA may be used with routine precautions, although care must be taken to use cartridges that do not have a latex bung/stopper. **Conscious sedation** Latex-free equipment should be used. **General anaesthesia** General anaesthesia should be performed in a latex-free operating theatre.

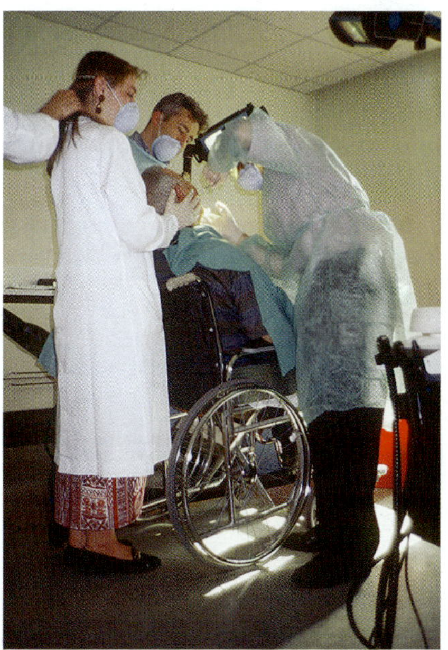

Figure 3.37 **Dental treatment of a patient with spina bifida**

Table 3.146 **Key considerations for dental management in spina bifida (see text)**

	Management modifications*	Comments/possible complications
Risk assessment	2	Latex allergy
Appropriate dental care	2	Latex-free appliances; latex-free environment; antibiotic prophylaxis (shunt)
Pain and anxiety control		
– Local anaesthesia	1	Latex-free cartridges
– Conscious sedation	1	Latex-free equipment
– General anaesthesia	3/4	Latex-free operating theatre
Patient access and positioning		
– Access to dental office	1	Many are chairbound
– Timing of treatment	1	Early morning
– Patient positioning	1	Avoid supine position
Treatment modification		
– Oral surgery	0	
– Implantology	0	
– Conservative/Endodontics	0	
– Fixed prosthetics	0	
– Removable prosthetics	0	
– Non-surgical periodontology	0	
– Surgical periodontology	0	
Hazardous and contraindicated drugs	1	Many are given anticoagulants; possibly antibiotic resistance

*0 = No special considerations. 1 = Caution advised. 2 = Specialised medical advice recommended in some cases. 3 = Specialised medical advice mandatory. 4 = Only to be performed in hospital environment. 5 = Should be avoided.

Patient access and positioning **Timing of treatment** Preferably in the early morning to minimise the concentration of latex particles in the air. **Patient positioning** Postural hypotension is likely, and thus the patient is best not treated supine. In any event, many are chairbound, and it is better just to tilt the wheelchair back slightly if there are facilities for this, or transfer the patient to the dental chair using a board between wheelchair and dental chair, and then treat the patient in the semi-reclined position.

Drug use ■ Some patients are on anticoagulants or other appropriate medication ■ Because many patients are often administered antibiotics (e.g. for urinary infections) there may be selection of resistant bacteria, and therefore an appropriate antibiotic regimen should be prescribed for prophylaxis or treatment of oral infections.

Further reading
● Hamann C P, Rodgers P A, Sullivan K 2002 Management of dental patients with allergies to natural rubber latex. Gen Dent 50:526–536 ● Hudson M E 2001 Dental surgery in pediatric patients with spina bifida and latex allergy. AORN J 74:57–70 ● Proctor R, Kumar N, Davies R, Porter S 2004 Cerebrospinal fluid shunts

and dentistry – a short review of relevant literature. J Dent Disability 5:27–30 ● Ugar D A
Semb G 2001 The prevalence of anomalies of the upper cervical vertebrae in subjects with cleft lip, cleft palate, or both. Cleft Palate Craniofac J 38:498–503.

STEROIDS (CORTICOSTEROIDS)

General aspects

Background ■ The adrenal glands secrete three main types of steroids: ● glucocorticoids ● mineralocorticoids ● sex hormones. ■ Cortisol is the major glucocorticoid. Secretion is regulated via the hypothalamic–pituitary–adrenal (HPA) axis by a biological feedback involving adrenocorticotrophic hormone (ACTH). Cortisol is involved in: ● metabolic processes ● vascular tonicity ● inflammatory responses ● control of the body's response to stresses such as trauma, infection, general anaesthesia or surgery – at such times there is normally an increased adrenal corticosteroid response related to the degree of stress, but in patients given exogenous steroids, this response may not occur.

Classification Glucocorticoids are classified based on their potency and their duration of action (Box 3.27).

Indications Synthetic (cortisol-like) glucocorticoids are used frequently for immunosuppression, and occasionally to replace missing hormones (in Addison's disease or after adrenalectomy), or to treat many other diseases (Box 3.28).

Side effects ■ Long-term systemic use of corticosteroids can cause many side effects, and can cause significant morbidity or mortality (Fig. 3.38, Box 3.29) including: ● adrenal suppression (see below) ● cushingoid weight gain around the face (moon face) and upper back (buffalo hump), and hirsutism, which are the most immediately obvious effects ● growth retardation in children ● diabetes ● hypertension ● infections ● perforated or bleeding peptic ulcers ● mood changes/psychoses ● cataracts ● muscle weakness ● osteoporosis ● tumours, if given long term ■ These complications may be reduced but not abolished if steroids are given on alternate days, thus, once the desired therapeutic effect of the steroid is achieved by daily administration, there should be a transition to giving the entire 48-hour dose as a single early-morning dose on alternate

Box 3.27 Approximate potencies of systemic corticosteroids relative to cortisol*

- *Short acting*: Cortisone = 1, Methylprednisolone = 5, Prednisolone = 4, Prednisone = 4
- *Medium acting*: Triamcinolone = 5
- *Long acting*: Betamethasone = 25, Dexamethasone = 30

*Cortisol (hydrocortisone) = 1.

Box 3.28 Some uses of systemic corticosteroids

- *Allergic disorders*: asthma
- *Connective tissue disorders*: rheumatoid arthritis (rarely), systemic lupus erythematosus
- *Renal disorders*: nephrotic syndrome, renal transplants
- *Gastrointestinal disorders*: ulcerative colitis, Crohn's disease
- *Blood dyscrasias*: idiopathic thrombocytopenia, lymphocytic leukaemia, lymphoma
- *Adrenal insufficiency*: Addison's disease, adrenalectomy, hypopituitarism
- *Mucocutaneous diseases*: pemphigus
- *Post-transplantation*: any organ transplant

days ■ In order to minimise the complications, patients on systemic steroids are usually also given: ● ranitidine ● calcium.

Adrenal suppression ■ Suppression of the HPA axis becomes deeper if treatment with exogenous steroids is prolonged and the dose of corticosteroids exceeds physiological levels (more than about 7.5 mg/day of prednisolone) ■ Adrenal suppression is less when the exogenous steroid is given on alternate days or as a single morning dose (rather than as divided doses through the day) ■ Corticotrophin (ACTH) was formerly used in the hope of reducing adrenal suppression, but the response is variable and unpredictable, and wanes with time ■ Topical steroids should always be used in preference to systemic steroids provided that the desired therapeutic effect is achievable, however, there can also be adrenocortical suppression from extensive application of steroid skin preparations – particularly if occlusive dressings are used ■ Systemic corticosteroids cause the greatest risk of adrenocortical suppression, such that adrenocortical function is likely to be suppressed if the patient is currently on daily systemic corticosteroids at doses of/above 10 mg prednisolone, or has been in the last 3 months.

Prognosis Acute adrenal insufficiency (adrenal crisis) may result as the adrenal cortex is unable to produce the necessary steroid response to stress. This is characterised by: ■ vomiting ■ headache ■ fever ■ rapidly developing hypotension ■ collapse and possibly death.

Oral findings

■ Susceptibility to infection is increased by systemic steroid use and there is a predisposition to: ● herpes virus infections (particularly herpes simplex); chickenpox is an especial hazard to those patients who are not immune and fulminant disease has resulted ● candidosis and bacterial infections also tend to be more frequent and severe ■ Wound healing is impaired in systemic corticosteroid therapy and wound infections are more frequent ■ Long-term and profound immunosuppression may lead to the appearance of hairy leukoplakia, Kaposi's sarcoma, lymphomas, lip cancer or oral keratoses ■ Topical corticosteroids for use in the mouth are unlikely to have any systemic effect but predispose to oral candidosis.

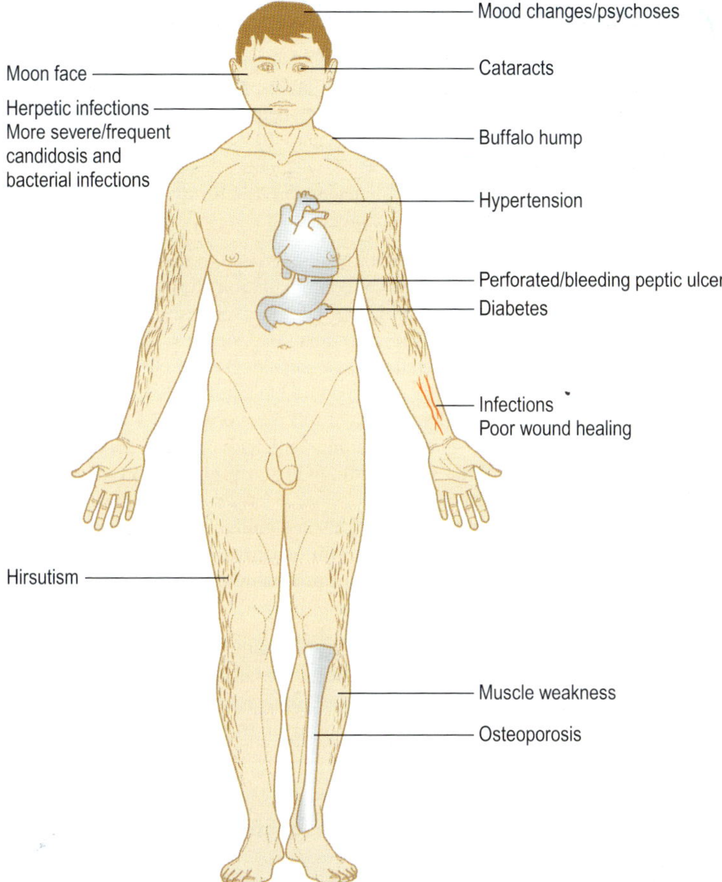

Figure 3.38 **Long-term effects of systemic corticosteroids**

Box 3.29 Complications of systemic corticosteroid therapy

- *Metabolic*: hypothalamic–pituitary–adrenal suppression, impaired glucose tolerance, diabetes mellitus, growth retardation, loss of sodium and potassium, osteoporosis, fat redistribution (moon face and buffalo hump)
- *Immunosuppressive*: increased susceptibility to infections
- *Cardiovascular*: hypertension, myocardial infarction, cerebrovascular accidents
- *Gastrointestinal*: peptic ulcer
- *Neurological*: mood changes, psychosis
- *Ophthalmological*: cataracts
- *Dermatological*: acne, striae, bruising, neoplasms

Dental management

Risk assessment ■ Prevent adrenal crisis in patients at risk, although prediction of suppression is sometimes unreliable ■ Treatment of an adrenal crisis includes: ● call for immediate help ● lay patient supine ● give hydrocortisone 200mg IM ● oxygen 10L/min ● if IV access can be obtained, give 1 litre dextrose saline ● check blood pressure ■ Patients may also require special management as a result of diabetes, hypertension, poor wound healing, or infections.

Appropriate health care In 1998, Nicholson et al reviewed all the available evidence and published new recommendations for steroid cover, where hydrocortisone supplementation is given intravenously. Patients who have taken steroids in excess of 10mg prednisolone, or equivalent, within the last 3 months, should be considered to have some degree of HPA suppression and will require supplementation. Patients who have not received steroids for more than 3 months are considered to have full recovery of HPA axis and require no supplementation. These recommendations have been adopted by anaesthetists in the UK (Table 3.147) and are increasingly used by other specialties, including dentists.

However, the implementation of Nicholson's guidelines is not universal amongst the dental profession. Some are still using regimens such as doubling the normal daily steroid dose on the day of procedure (Gibson & Ferguson 2004) (Table 3.148).

Pain and anxiety control **Local anaesthesia** LA may be used with routine precautions. **Conscious sedation** Sedatives should be avoided. **General anaesthesia** Drugs, especially sedatives and general anaesthetics, are a hazard and it is extremely important to avoid hypoxia, hypotension or haemorrhage.

Table 3.147 **Current recommendations for steroid cover (Nicholson et al 1998)**

Amount of steroid (prednisolone or equivalent) currently taken	Type of surgery*	Cover needed
< 10mg per day	No cover required	No cover required
> 10mg per day	Minor surgery	25mg hydrocortisone IV at start of treatment
	Moderate surgery	Usual preop steroids, 25mg hydrocortisone IV plus 100mg/day for 24 h
	Major surgery	Usual preop steroids, 25mg hydrocortisone IV plus 100mg/day for 48–72h

*Minor surgery: extractions under LA. Moderate surgery: reduction of a fractured mandible/zygoma. Major surgery: head and neck surgery/orthognathic surgery.

Table 3.148 **Alternative management of patients with a history of systemic corticosteroid therapy (Gibson and Ferguson 2004)**

Amount of steroid (prednisolone or equivalent) taken (currently or within 2 months)	Type of surgery	Steroid supplementation
<10 mg per day	All procedures	Do not warrant supplementation
10–50 mg per day*	Surgical procedures under LA	Double the usual steroid dose on the day
	Surgical procedure under GA	Minor surgery: 100 mg hydrocortisone IM preop Major surgery: 100 mg hydrocortisone IM preop followed by 50 mg 8-hourly for 48 h

*Patients taking more than 50 mg prednisolone are close to the innate maximum cortisol level seen in patients when stressed and do not require steroid supplementation.

Patient access and positioning **Patient positioning** Osteoporosis introduces the danger of fractures when handling the patient.

Treatment modification **Surgery** Dentoalveolar or maxillofacial surgery may result in stress and a cortisol response, but most other forms of dental treatment cause little response. Steroid supplementation should be considered (Tables 3.147, 3.148). The blood pressure must be carefully monitored during operative care and recovery. **Implantology** There is no evidence that corticosteroid therapy is a contraindication to implants, but previous medical advice is recommended.

Drug use Aspirin and other non-steroidal anti-inflammatory agents should be avoided as they may increase the risk of peptic ulceration in those on corticosteroids.

Further reading • Alexander R E, Throndson R R 2000 A review of perioperative corticosteroid use in dentoalveolar surgery. Oral Surg Oral Med Oral Pathol Oral Radiol Endod 90:406–415 • Gibson N, Ferguson J W 2004 Steroid cover for dental patients on long-term steroid medication: proposed clinical guidelines based upon a critical review of the literature. Br Dent J 197:681–685 • Greenwood M, Meechan J G 2003 General medicine and surgery for dental practitioners. Part 6: The endocrine system. Br Dent J 195:129–133 • Lorenzo-Calabria J, Grau D, Silvestre F J, Hernandez-Mijares A 2003 Management of patients with adrenocortical insufficiency in the dental clinic. Med Oral 8:207–814 • Nicholson G, Burrin J M, Hall G M 1998 Peri-operative steroid supplementation. Anaesthesia 53:1091–1104 • Perry R J, McLaughlin E A, Rice P J 2003 Steroid cover in dentistry: recommendations following a review of current policy in UK dental teaching hospitals. Dent Update 30:45–47 • Seymour R A 2003 Dentistry and the medically compromised patient. Surgeon 1:207–214.

Table 3.149 **Key considerations for dental management in patients treated with systemic corticosteroids (see text)**

	Management modifications*	Comments/possible complications
Risk assessment	2	Adrenal crisis; underlying diseases
Appropriate dental care	2	Steroid supplementation
Pain and anxiety control		
– Local anaesthesia	0	
– Conscious sedation	3	Avoid sedatives
– General anaesthesia	4	
Patient access and positioning		
– Access to dental office	0	
– Timing of treatment	0	
– Patient positioning	1	Osteoporosis
Treatment modification		
– Oral surgery	2	Steroid supplementation; antimicrobials required; impaired wound healing
– Implantology	2	See oral surgery
– Conservative/Endodontics	0	
– Fixed prosthetics	0	
– Removable prosthetics	0	
– Non-surgical periodontology	1	
– Surgical periodontology	2	See oral surgery
Hazardous and contraindicated drugs	1	Avoid aspirin and NSAIDs

*0 = No special considerations. 1 = Caution advised. 2 = Specialised medical advice recommended in some cases. 3 = Specialised medical advice mandatory. 4 = Only to be performed in hospital environment. 5 = Should be avoided.

STROKE AND OTHER CEREBROVASCULAR ACCIDENTS

STROKE

Definition Stroke or cerebrovascular accident (CVA) is characterised as sudden, or rapidly progressing, focal CNS signs and symptoms that do not resolve within 24 hours, which result in impaired motor function, speech and mental damage, and sometimes death.

General aspects

Classification Strokes have been classified based on their aetiology, namely strokes caused by: ■ thrombosis ■ emboli ■ haemorrhage.

Aetiopathogenesis ■ Risk factors for a CVA are similar to those of ischaemic heart disease and include advanced age, hypertension, smoking, diabetes and heart disease ■ CVA is mainly caused by cerebrovascular thrombosis or by emboli from heart or great vessels – in these cases interruption of blood supply produces focal necrosis (infarction) of the brain ■ CNS bleeding following hypertension, ruptured aneurysm, or trauma, may also produce a stroke.

Clinical presentation ■ The person who has had a stroke involving the brain's cerebral cortex or middle capsule and survives may have a variety of motor, cognitive, and sensory deficits as well as confusion, memory loss, and emotional distress including ● contralateral hemiplegia ● contralateral sensory loss ● visual defect (homonymous hemianopia) ● dysphasia ■ Strokes affecting the brainstem may compromise the gag and swallowing reflexes ■ Many recent stroke survivors are overwhelmed by too much stimulation ● others have diminished sensations of touch, pressure, sight or pain – causing them to suffer a constant level of sensory deprivation, leading to psychological stress ■ Psychosocial changes: ● the patient's anxiety, fear, and frustration are enormous ● many stroke survivors initially suffer confusion that makes it impossible to do the simplest mental tasks ● emotional lability is common ● victims often feel helpless and dependent, and their sense of self-worth is diminished ● depression is the most common emotional sequela, reported in up to 40% of survivors within several months of an acute stroke.

Diagnosis Diagnosis is from clinical findings and on cerebral imaging techniques including MRI, CT and Doppler ultrasound.

Treatment ■ During acute episodes, anticoagulant therapy – anticoagulants or platelet anti-aggregants – is prescribed to prevent new episodes of thrombosis (unless haemorrhage is present) ■ Occasionally, surgical management (carotid endarterectomy, placement of internal carotid artery stents or haematoma removal) is required ■ Rehabilitation may require assistance with walking, or the use of a Zimmer frame ■ Psychosocial support: ● encouragement is an extremely important motivating factor for stroke survivors ● caregivers should avoid being critical ● while inappropriate behaviour should be pointed out, nagging tends to upset and anger stroke survivors, and discourages rather than encourages effort ● on a survivor's return home, the following guidelines will encourage a positive recovery – set attainable goals (the road to recovery is built of simple achievements); involve the survivor in daily activities and routines; encourage independent activities, while recognising the survivor's limitations; try to maintain social contacts within the family and community. It is important to understand the survivor's limitations and allow an appropriate time for recovery – self-worth, confidence and enjoyment of life will gradually return.

Prognosis ■ The mortality rate ranges from 30% when stroke is caused by cerebrovascular thrombosis, to 80% when it is due to intracerebral haemorrhage ■ Overall, about 50% of patients will survive at least 5 years without or with minimal residual disability.

TRANSIENT ISCHAEMIC ATTACKS (TIA)

Definition ■ Transient ischaemic attacks are sudden, or rapidly progressing, focal CNS signs and symptoms that fully resolve within 24 hours ■ They must always be taken seriously, as they are a clear warning that further TIAs may occur, and a second episode often causes more damage than the first ■ They may also precede: ● stroke ● myocardial infarction ■ Around 30000 people a year in the UK experience a TIA – that is one person in every 2000.

General aspects

Aetiopathogenesis A transient ischaemic attack results from a temporary reduction in blood and oxygen supply to part of the brain. The underlying pathology is usually carotid atherothromboembolism.

Clinical presentation Variable features, resembling strokes.

Diagnosis ■ MRI/CT ■ Chest radiograph ■ ECG ■ Carotid Doppler ultrasound.

Treatment ■ Aspirin ■ Treat underlying cause.

Prognosis Without treatment, one in 10 people who have had a TIA will have a full stroke within the next year. TIAs should therefore always be investigated, the cause found and, where possible, treated.

SUBARACHNOID HAEMORRHAGE

Definition ■ Spontaneous arterial haemorrhage into the subarachnoid space of the brain from a burst saccular aneurysm (Berry aneurysm) ■ It appears in younger patients than those having typical strokes.

General aspects

Aetiopathogenesis Risk factors include: ■ smoking ■ alcohol abuse ■ hypertension ■ bleeding disorder ■ genetic tendency (type 3 collagen deficiency, polycystic kidneys, coarctation of aorta, Ehlers–Danlos syndrome).

Clinical presentation ■ Acute intense headache ■ Vomiting ■ Collapse ■ Neck stiffness or pain ■ Coma ■ Death.

Diagnosis ■ CT ■ ± lumbar puncture.

Treatment Neurosurgery (urgent).

Prognosis About 35% of patients die from the initial haemorrhage, and a further 15% from subsequent haemorrhages in the ensuing weeks.

SUBDURAL HAEMORRHAGE

Definition Venous haemorrhage between dura and arachnoid – mostly caused by trauma (which can be long before and/or mild and forgotten).

General aspects

Aetiopathogenesis Predisposed by: ■ advanced age ■ anticoagulation ■ falls.

Clinical presentation Intracranial pressure rises slowly, causing: ■ fluctuating consciousness ■ headache ■ personality changes ■ unsteadiness ■ stroke-like symptoms.

Diagnosis ■ Papilloedema ■ CT.

Treatment ■ Neurosurgery.

EXTRADURAL HAEMORRHAGE

Definition Arterial and/or venous haemorrhage between skull bone and dura mater.

General aspects

Aetiopathogenesis ■ Mainly caused by fracture of the temporal or parietal bone ■ Sometimes caused by a tear in the dural venous sinus.

Clinical presentation ■ Deteriorating consciousness after a lucid interval after head injury ■ Worsening headache ■ Vomiting ■ Convulsions ■ Hemiparesis ■ Coma ■ Death.

Diagnosis ■ Bradycardia ■ Hypertension ■ CT.

Treatment Neurosurgery (urgent).

Oral findings in CVA

■ Unilateral paralysis of the face and orofacial musculature ■ Loss of oral sensations (i.e. taste) ■ Deviated tongue on extrusion, showing flaccidity and multiple folds ■ Dysphagia ■ Gag reflex may be reduced.

Dental management

Risk assessment ■ A person who has had a TIA or stroke is at greater risk of another ■ Difficulties in dental management in a patient with a stroke may include: ● access and impaired mobility ● communication difficulties, since there may be cognitive and visual defects as well as dysarthria, aphasia, confusion, memory loss and emotional distress ● psychosocial changes/depression ● loss of protective reflexes, such as the swallowing and gag reflexes in brainstem lesions; oropharyngeal dysphagia post-stroke occurs in around half the patients, and has a significant contribution to morbidity and mortality, since it predisposes to respiratory infection, malnutrition and weight loss; multidisciplinary care is required ● patients after a CVA may not be able to provide proper consent ● systemic conditions: anticoagulation, hypertension, diabetes mellitus, old age, cardiovascular disease and the possible placement of stents requiring endocarditis prophylaxis ■ Hospital-based care is recommended for patients at high risk of CVA, and for stressful or surgical procedures in patients with hypertension or poorly controlled haemostasis ■ Patients who have headaches, dizzy spells, and transient ischaemic episodes should be referred to the physician for investigation ■ Strokes are a possible cause of sudden loss of consciousness in the dental surgery and should be recognisable by the features already described, especially the sudden loss of consciousness and, usually, signs of one-sided paralysis. Protection of the airway, oxygen administration and a call for an ambulance are the only really useful immediate measures.

Appropriate health care ■ Elective/invasive dental care should be deferred for 6 months after a stroke; however support with preventive care is critical ■ Elective dental care is not recommended in patients suffering TIA episodes ■ Treatment goals should be adapted to take into account the patient's changing needs/eventual recovery ■ Take care to communicate clearly with the patient who has had a CVA, by not wearing a mask, and by facing the patient, and speaking slowly, clearly and in language which is not complex ■ Monitor blood pressure ■ Monitor anticoagulation status ■ Antibiotic prophylaxis for coronary artery stents is *not* required.

Pain and anxiety control **Local anaesthesia** ■ Use minimum amount of epinephrine in local anaesthesia ■ Avoid using epinephrine-containing gingival retraction cords ■ Some advise not using electronic dental analgesia. **Conscious sedation** ■ Opiates are best avoided in strokes as they may cause CNS depression ■ Nitrous oxide may be administered without adverse effects. **General anaesthesia** ■ General anaesthesia should be avoided for 6 months after a stroke ■ Barbiturates are contraindicated as they may cause severe hypotension.

Patient access and positioning **Access to dental surgery** The treatment plan must consider physical limitations; paralysis often results from CVA. Impaired mobility may make access difficult; some patients are chairbound. **Timing of treatment** Short treatment sessions in mid-morning are desirable. **Patient positioning** ■ Patients are best treated in the upright position, and extra care must be taken to avoid foreign bodies entering the pharynx ■ Good suction must be at hand ■ If the patient has been supine or reclined, raise slowly to avoid hypotension.

Treatment modification **Preventive dentistry** ■ Patients after a stroke may have unilateral (upper motor neurone) facial palsy affecting mainly the lower face but emotional facial responses may be retained ■ Oral hygiene tends to deteriorate on the paralysed side and impaired manual dexterity may interfere with toothbrushing ■ An electric toothbrush or adapted holders may therefore help. **Implantology** May be compromised by impaired oral hygiene. **Fixed prosthetics and conservation** Only simple bridgework is recommended. Dysphagia compromises protection of the airway, so consider: ■ using rubber dam ■ limiting the use of the handpiece and other water sprays ■ rapidly evacuating oral fluids. **Removable prosthetics** Removable prostheses may be difficult to insert and remove by the patient, who may be unable anyway to use dentures due to the neuromuscular deficits.

Table 3.150 **Key considerations for dental management in stroke (see text)**

	Management modifications*	Comments/possible complications
Risk assessment	2	Further strokes; anticoagulation; hypertension; loss of gag reflex; consent issues
Appropriate dental care	3/4	Deferred 6 months; no elective care in TIA; monitor blood pressure; monitor anticoagulation
Pain and anxiety control		
– Local anaesthesia	1	Avoid epinephrine and electronic dental analgesia
– Conscious sedation	1	Avoid opiates
– General anaesthesia	4	Deferred 6 months; avoid barbiturates
Patient access and positioning		
– Access to dental office	1	Impaired mobility
– Timing of treatment	1	Mid-morning; short visits
– Patient positioning	1	Upright position
Treatment modification		
– Preventive dentistry	1	Electric toothbrush
– Oral surgery	1	Anticoagulation
– Implantology	1	Poor oral hygiene; anticoagulation
– Conservative/Endodontics	1	Only simple procedures
– Fixed prosthetics	1	Difficult to place
– Removable prosthetics	1	Anticoagulation
– Non-surgical periodontology	1	Anticoagulation; poor oral hygiene
– Surgical periodontology	1	Anticoagulation
Imaging	1	Carotid plaques
Hazardous and contraindicated drugs	1	Acetaminophen – drug of choice; avoid hypertensive drugs

*0 = No special considerations. 1 = Caution advised. 2 = Specialised medical advice recommended in some cases. 3 = Specialised medical advice mandatory. 4 = Only to be performed in hospital environment. 5 = Should be avoided.

Imaging Calcified atherosclerotic plaques may sometimes be detected on dental panoramic radiographs and may identify patients at risk for stroke.

Drug use ■ Acetaminophen is the drug of choice for postoperative pain ■ Hypertension must be avoided, since it can precipitate subarachnoid or cerebral haemorrhage ■ Fatal subarachnoid haemorrhage has resulted from the use of norepinephrine in local anaesthetic solutions ■ Cerebral haemorrhage can also result from hypertension caused by interactions of monoamine oxidase inhibitors with other drugs, particularly pethidine.

Further reading ● August M 2001 Cerebrovascular and carotid artery disease. Oral Surg Oral Med Oral Pathol Oral Radiol Endod 92:253–256 ● Almog D M, Illig K A, Carter L C, Friedlander A H, Brooks S L, Grimes R M 2004 Diagnosis of non-dental conditions. Carotid artery calcifications on panoramic radiographs identify patients at risk for stroke. NY State Dent J 70:20–25 ● Meurman J H, Sanz M, Janket S J 2004 Oral health, atherosclerosis, and cardiovascular disease. Crit Rev Oral Biol Med 15:403–413 ● Maupome G, Gullion C M, White B A, Wyatt C C, Williams P M 2003 Oral disorders and chronic systemic diseases in very old adults living in institutions. Spec Care Dentist 23:199–208 ● Niessen L C, Fedele D J 2002 Aging successfully: oral health for the prime of life. Compend Contin Educ Dent 23:4–11 ● Rose L F, Mealey B, Minsk L, Cohen D W 2002 Oral care for patients with cardiovascular disease and stroke. J Am Dent Assoc 133:37S–44S.

THROMBOCYTOPENIA

Definition A platelet count below 100×10^9/L is termed thrombocytopenia and can lead to purpura and a prolonged bleeding tendency.

General aspects

Aetiopathogenesis The main causes are: ■ altered platelet production (i.e. myelosuppressive chemotherapy, radiation, leukaemia, viruses) ■ disturbed platelet distribution (i.e. splenomegaly) ■ increased platelet destruction (i.e. idiopathic [autoimmune] thrombocytopenic purpura: ITP).

Classification Based on the platelet count, thrombocytopenia has been classified as mild, moderate, severe and life-threatening (Table 3.151).

Clinical presentation ■ Thrombocytopenia is usually asymptomatic in patients where the platelet counts do not fall below 50×10^9/L ■ Severe thrombocytopenia can cause: ● petechiae ● ecchymoses ● postoperative haemorrhage ● spontaneous bleeding in/from inflamed tissues.

Diagnosis Diagnosis is made based on clinical findings, reduced platelet count and prolonged bleeding time.

Treatment ■ Most patients are managed mainly with corticosteroids or other immunosuppressive agents ■ Sometimes splenectomy is required

Table 3.151 **Manifestations of thrombocytopenia and management in relation to oral surgery**

Platelet count (× 10^9/L)	Severity of thrombocytopenia	Manifestations	Management in relation to type of oral surgery	
			Dentoalveolar	**Major**
100–150	Mild	Mild purpura sometimes Slight increase in postoperative bleeding	No platelet transfusion Local haemostatic measures* Observe	Consider platelet transfusion Local haemostatic measures* Observe
50–100	Moderate	Purpura, postoperative bleeding	Platelets may be needed Local haemostatic measures* Consider postoperative tranexamic acid mouthwash for 7 days	Platelets needed Local haemostatic measures* Postoperative tranexamic acid mouthwash for 7 days
30–50	Severe	Purpura, postoperative bleeding, and even from venepuncture	Platelets needed Local haemostatic measures* Postoperative tranexamic acid mouthwash for 7 days	Platelets needed Local haemostatic measures* Avoid surgery where possible Postoperative tranexamic acid mouthwash for 7 days
<30	Life-threatening	Purpura, spontaneous bleeding	Platelets needed Local haemostatic measures* Avoid surgery where possible Postoperative tranexamic acid mouthwash for 3 days	Platelets needed Local haemostatic measures* Avoid surgery where possible Postoperative tranexamic acid mouthwash for 3 days

*Local haemostatic measures = compressive packing, sutures, and microfibrillar collagen or oxidised cellulose.

■ About 20% of cases are resistant to treatment ■ Platelets may need to be given to cover operative procedures.

Prognosis Prognosis is conditioned by the severity of the thrombocytopenia and the underlying disease (i.e. thrombotic thrombocytopenic purpura has a 75% mortality rate within 3 months).

Oral findings

■ Gingival bleeding ■ Blood-filled bullae ■ Palatal petechiae ■ Prolonged bleeding following surgery.

Dental management

Risk assessment ■ The main danger in dental treatment is haemorrhage ■ Splenectomy predisposes to infections, typically with pneumococci, and especially within the first 2 years ■ Long-term, corticosteroids can cause well-recognised problems.

Appropriate health care **Platelet replacement/supplementation** ■ In patients with platelet counts below 50×10^9/L, operative procedures associated with bleeding are best performed in hospital or other specialist centre under platelet cover – this is mandatory if the platelet levels are below 30×10^9/L ■ Platelets can be replaced or supplemented by platelet transfusions, but sequestration of platelets is very rapid ■ One unit of platelets should raise the count by around 10×10^9/L ■ Platelet transfusions are therefore best used for controlling already established thrombocytopenic bleeding ■ When given prophylactically, platelets should be given in two halves – the first half before surgery to control capillary bleeding, and the second half at the end of the operation to facilitate the placement of adequate sutures ■ Platelets should be used within 6–24 hours of collection ■ Suitable preparations include: ● platelet-rich plasma (PRP), which contains about 90% of the platelets from a unit of fresh blood in about half this volume ● platelet-rich concentrate (PRC), which contains about 50% of the platelets from a unit of fresh whole blood in a volume of only 25 mL; PRC is thus the best source of platelets per unit volume ■ Platelet infusions carry the risk of isoimmunisation, infection with blood-borne viruses and, rarely, graft-versus-host disease ■ Where there is immune destruction of platelets (e.g. in ITP), platelet infusions are less effective.
Local measures to minimise bleeding The need for platelet transfusions can be reduced by: ■ Local haemostatic measures: ● placement of sutures ● absorbable haemostatic agents such as oxidised regenerated cellulose (Surgicel®), synthetic collagen (Instat®) or microcrystalline collagen (Avitene®) may be put in the socket to assist clotting ■ Desmopressin ■ Tranexamic acid ■ Topical administration of platelet concentrates. **Splenectomy** Occasional reports of systemic infection post-splenectomy, involving oral streptococci, have prompted some to suggest that antimicrobial prophylaxis should be given before invasive dental procedures. However this is not recommended by the British Society for Antimicrobial Chemotherapy.

Table 3.152 **Key considerations for dental management in thrombocytopenia (see text)**

	Management modifications*	Comments/possible complications
Risk assessment	2	Haemorrhage; infections; long-term corticosteroids
Appropriate dental care	1–4	According to procedure and platelet count
Pain and anxiety control		
– Local anaesthesia	1	Regional block
– Conscious sedation	1	Haematoma
– General anaesthesia	3/4	Airway
Patient access and positioning		
– Access to dental office	0	
– Timing of treatment	0	
– Patient positioning	0	
Treatment modification		
– Oral surgery	1–4	According to procedure and platelet count
– Implantology	3	
– Conservative/Endodontics	1	
– Fixed prosthetics	1	
– Removable prosthetics	0	
– Non-surgical periodontology	1–4	According to platelet count
– Surgical periodontology	1–4	According to platelet count
Hazardous and contraindicated drugs	1	Avoid aspirin and NSAIDs, amoxicillin, ampicillin; consider steroid supplementation

*0 = No special considerations. 1 = Caution advised. 2 = Specialised medical advice recommended in some cases. 3 = Specialised medical advice mandatory. 4 = Only to be performed in hospital environment. 5 = Should be avoided.

Pain and anxiety control **Local anaesthesia** Regional anaesthetic block injections should be minimised, and can be given only if the platelet levels are above 30 × 10^9/L. **Conscious sedation** CS may be given safely, although care must be taken if an intravenous cannula is placed, as a large haematoma may result. **General anaesthesia** The airway may be compromised due to persistent bleeding associated with intubation. Specialist advice from the haematologist and a thorough preoperative assessment in close consultation with the anaesthetist are required.

Treatment modification **Surgery** ■ Haemostasis after dentoalveolar surgery is usually adequate if platelet levels are above 50 × 10^9/L ■ Major surgery requires platelet levels above 75 × 10^9/L (Table 3.151). **Periodontology** The need for platelet transfusions can be reduced by local haemostatic measures and with a 5% tranexamic mouthwash postoperatively – 10 mL used 4 times a day for 7 days.

Drug use Acetaminophen and codeine are recommended analgesics. Drugs that impair platelets must be avoided; these include: ■ Aspirin and other NSAIDs: ● the aspirin effect is *not* dose-dependent; even very low doses can affect the platelet cyclo-oxygenase irreversibly for their lifetime (approximately a week) ● other NSAIDs may have a reversible effect and act for only up to 48 hours ■ COX-2 inhibitors (e.g. celecoxib) have no such effect on platelets but may be cardiotoxic ■ Other drugs often used in dentistry that may affect platelet function include beta-lactam antibiotics (amoxicillin, ampicillin, cephalosporins) and diazepam.

Further reading ● Barnard N, Scully C 1993 Epstein's syndrome. Implications for oral surgery. Oral Surg Oral Med Oral Pathol 76:32–34 ● Fleming P 1991 Dental management of the pediatric oncology patient. Curr Opin Dent 1:577–582 ● Porter S R, Sugerman P B, Scully C, Luker J, Oakhill A 1994 Orofacial manifestations in the Wiskott–Aldrich syndrome. ASDC J Dent Child 61:404–407 ● Schramm A, Schon R, Gellrich N C 1999 Therapy refractory idiopathic thrombocytopenia. Contraindication for dental surgery interventions. Mund Kiefer Gesichtschir 3:43–45 ● Scully, C, Diz Dios P, Shotts R 2004 Oral health care in patients with the most important medically compromising conditions; 1. Platelet disorders. CPD Dentistry 5:3–7.

TRANSPLANT PATIENTS

General aspects

■ Transplantation is a life-saving procedure for many patients with end-stage diseases, and is often the only viable treatment available ■ The organs, tissues, and cells transplanted can include: kidneys, heart, lungs, pancreas, liver, and small bowel; bone marrow, cornea, bone, and skin; and cells of muscle, bone, and pancreas ■ General features of transplantation are considered here; specific transplants are discussed under the organ in question.

Indications Transplants are generally indicated under the following circumstances: ■ untreatable end-stage disease ■ substantial limitation of daily activities ■ limited life expectancy ■ ambulatory patient with rehabilitation potential ■ acceptable nutritional status ■ satisfactory psychosocial profile and emotional support system ■ absence of other severe concomitant underlying diseases.

Sources of organs ■ Transplants can be living donors or sometimes from donors who are 'brain dead', or from cadaveric donors ■ An irreversible cessation of all brain and brainstem function is defined as brain death in a potential donor.

Outcomes ■ As surgical methods to transplant grafts improve, rejection becomes the major cause of graft failure ■ The major barrier to successful transplantation is immunological rejection since, except for transplants between identical twins, all transplant donors and recipients are immunologically incompatible. This causes the recipient to try to destroy or reject the new organ, tissue or cells. In graft-versus-host disease, rejection occurs when the transplanted donor haematopoietic cells try to destroy or reject recipient tissues. ■ Rejection episodes may be mild or severe but, with time, will lead to graft failure or patient death ■ Success rates vary for the different types of organs transplanted and can be as high as 90% or as low as 50% at one year ■ Of those people awaiting organ transplantation, more than 25% of patients have already had at least one graft failure.

Immunological evaluation ■ Recipients of transplants undergo an extensive immunological evaluation that primarily serves to avoid transplants that are at risk for antibody-mediated hyperacute rejection ■ The immunological evaluation includes: ● ABO blood group determination ● human leucocyte antigen (HLA) typing ● serum screening for antibody to HLA phenotypes ● crossmatching.

Complications ■ Graft dysfunction ■ Recurrent organ disease ■ Cardiac disease: ● increased risk of coronary heart disease (10–20 times more prevalent) ● arterial hypertension may develop as an adverse effect of immunosuppressive medications ■ Endocrine problems: ● adrenal suppression ● diabetes mellitus may be caused by some immunosuppressive medications such as corticosteroids ■ Gingival swelling in association with ciclosporin (used typically in heart, liver and lung transplant patients) occurs commonly and is dose-related; it is usually reversible within 6 months after withdrawal of ciclosporin ■ Graft-versus-host disease, after bone marrow transplantation.

Infections ■ Patients on immunosuppressive drugs are clearly immunocompromised by virtue of the drugs taken to prevent rejection ■ Infections may spread rapidly, may be opportunistic (involving microorganisms that are normally commensal) and may be clinically silent or atypical ■ Even mild infections are a serious threat in immunosuppressed patients and immunosuppression must then be reduced or even completely stopped temporarily ■ Viral, fungal, mycobacterial and protozoal infections are a particular problem, though the infections experienced also depend on which microorganisms are in the environment and, to some extent, on other concurrent treatments ■ Viral infections account for substantial morbidity and mortality: ● Herpes simplex and herpes zoster infections are common and usually treated with a 10–14-day course of aciclovir ● Cytomegalovirus (CMV) infection is common, usually observed 3 or more weeks after transplantation and treated with ganciclovir ● Epstein–Barr virus (EBV) may be responsible for post-transplant lymphoproliferative disease (see below) ■ Fungi can cause severe locally or systematically invasive infections in immunosuppressed patients: ● Candida species (i.e. *Candida albicans*, *Candida tropicalis*, *Candida parapsilosis*, *Candida krusei*) are most common ● *Aspergillus niger*, *Aspergillus flavus* or *Aspergillus fumigatus* infections may involve the lungs, the upper respiratory tract, the skin, the soft tissues, and the CNS ● *Cryptococcus neoformans* infections may cause pulmonary, CNS and disseminated cutaneous disease in immunosuppressed patients ● *Mucor* and *Rhizopus* infections (phycomycoses) are rarely encountered but can produce destructive CNS or soft tissue infections that are difficult to eliminate ■ Bacterial infections are less of a problem in general, and are better tolerated in persons receiving ciclosporin than azathioprine, but still must be treated aggressively. *Legionella* and *Pneumocystis* infections are more common in immunosuppressed patients and must be treated early.

Post-transplant malignancies ■ Transplant recipients have an increased risk of some malignant neoplasms after transplantation as a consequence of the immunosuppressive drug therapy ■ The neoplasms may be recurrence of pre-existing cancers in recipients, donor-transmitted, or *de novo* malignancies ■ Skin cancer, including squamous cell carcinoma, melanoma, and basal cell carcinoma, occurs up to 20 times more frequently in transplant recipients than in the general population ■ *De novo* malignancies include Kaposi's sarcoma, lymphomas and squamous cell carcinomas of the skin and lip, and carcinoma of the cervix, external genitalia, and perineum ■ These malignancies can be virally induced, such as HPV-associated carcinoma of the cervix, HHV-8 associated Kaposi's sarcoma, and EBV-associated post-transplant lymphoproliferative disease (PTLD) and lymphomas ■ Some malignancies are seen more frequently in certain subpopulations of transplant recipients, according to pre-existing risk factors or behaviours, such as oropharyngeal and lung cancer in those with alcoholism and those who smoke, or colon cancer in patients with pre-existing inflammatory bowel disease transplanted for primary sclerosing cholangitis.

Post-transplant lymphoproliferative disorder (PTLD) ■ Post-transplant lymphoproliferative disorder (PTLD) is a relatively uncommon but serious complication of transplantation ■ PTLD forms a heterogeneous group of tumours, ranging from benign B-cell hyperplasia to immunoblastic malignant lymphoma ■ The incidence of PTLD varies with the type of transplanted allograft but is generally about 2%, and most cases develop within the first year after transplantation ■ The more intense the immunosuppression used, the higher the incidence of PTLD, and the earlier it appears ■ PTLD is usually associated with Epstein–Barr virus (EBV) infection. Risk factors include recipient pre-transplant EBV seronegativity and donor EBV seropositivity. ■ Clinical presentation of PTLD is very variable and includes fever, lymphadenopathy, gastrointestinal symptoms, infectious mononucleosis-like syndrome that can be fulminant, pulmonary symptoms, CNS symptoms and weight loss ■ The presentation and clinical course are variable; at one end of the spectrum is aggressive disease with diffuse involvement, at the other end of the spectrum are localised lesions that are indolent and slow, growing over months, as opposed to days or weeks ■ The most common sites involved are lymph nodes, liver, lung, kidney, bone marrow, small intestine, and spleen. *Diagnosis* A diagnosis of PTLD is made by having: ■ a high index of suspicion in the appropriate clinical setting ■ histopathological evidence of lymphoproliferation ■ EBV-DNA, RNA, or viral protein in the biopsy tissue. *Treatment* ■ Treatment is reduction or withdrawal of immunosuppression, plus ganciclovir therapy ■ Other treatment modalities that can be employed additionally include: ● rituximab – a new anti-CD20 monoclonal antibody ● interferon alpha ● immunoglobulin ● surgical excision ● radiation therapy ● chemotherapy.

Oral findings in patients having transplants

■ Oral candidosis may be persistent, and can usually be managed with topical nystatin, amphotericin or miconazole ■ Herpes simplex or zoster, cytomegalovirus, and Epstein–Barr virus can be prevented, deferred or ameliorated by prophylactic low-dose oral antiviral drugs ■ Rarely, dental infections may spread, with serious complications such as cavernous sinus thrombosis or metastatic infections; oral bacteria are an important source of bacteraemias. Mixed bacterial oral mucosal plaques may respond to the appropriate antibiotic and possibly to an aqueous chlorhexidine (0.2%) mouthwash. ■ Mucositis and large aphthous ulcers may be suggestive of over-immunosuppression ■ Routine cancer surveillance is mandatory to assure rapid diagnosis and treatment of any malignancy.

Dental management in patients having transplants

Risk assessment ■ Any invasive dental treatment should only be carried out after consultation with the responsible physician and with due consideration to the bleeding tendency related to anticoagulation, corticosteroid cover, any infectious risk and impaired drug metabolism – this applies probably for at least 2 years post-transplantation ■ Pre-existing illnesses of the transplant candidate may need to be considered ■ Viral hepatitis B and C infections may be present, especially in older patients who have received blood transfusions before blood was routinely screened.

Appropriate health care ■ Before transplantation there should be a full oral and dental evaluation and treatment provided to eliminate orodental disease, bearing in mind that after transplantation the patient will be chronically immunosuppressed and at increased risk from infection (Box 3.30) ■ During the immediate post-transplant and chronic rejection phases only emergency dental care is recommended (Box 3.30) ■ Dental treatment guidelines include attention to prevent risk of infection, using antibiotic

Box 3.30 Oral health care of transplant patients

Pre-transplantation
• Examination • Treatment planning • Remove unsaveable teeth after consultation with physician • Evaluate bleeding tendency • Institute preventive oral health care

Peri-transplantation
• Continue preventive oral health care • Prophylaxis for viral infections • Prophylaxis for fungal infections • Evaluate bleeding tendency • Consider prophylaxis for invasive oral procedures

Post-transplantation
• Continue preventive oral health care • Prophylaxis for viral infections • Prophylaxis for fungal infections • Care of gingival swelling • Emergency dental care only for the first 6 months • Evaluate bleeding tendency • Consider prophylaxis for invasive oral procedures

Box 3.31 Drug use in transplanted patients

Drugs that increase ciclosporin levels
- Amphotericin
- Clarithromycin
- Erythromycin
- Ketoconazole
- Norfloxacin

Drugs that decrease ciclosporin levels
- Carbamazepine
- Phenytoin
- Sulphamethoxazole

Drugs that increase nephrotoxicity
- Amphotericin
- Clarithromycin
- Diclofenac
- Erythromycin
- Indometacin
- Sulphamethoxazole
- Vancomycin

Drugs that increase hepatotoxicity
- Aminoglycosides
- Co-trimoxazole
- Erythromycin
- Halothane
- Quinolones
- Tetracyclines

Table 3.153 **Key considerations for dental management in transplant patients (see text)**

	Management modifications*	Comments/possible complications
Risk assessment	3	Bleeding; infection; corticosteroids; viral hepatitis; pre-existing disease
Appropriate dental care	3	Postpone elective care; consider antibiotic prophylaxis; possibly corticosteroid cover
Pain and anxiety control		
– Local anaesthesia	1	Chlorhexidine
– Conscious sedation	2	Avoid sedatives
– General anaesthesia	4/5	Avoid where possible
Patient access and positioning		
– Access to dental office	0	
– Timing of treatment	0	
– Patient positioning	0	
Treatment modification		
– Oral surgery	2	Bleeding; infection
– Implantology	2	
– Conservative/Endodontics	1	
– Fixed prosthetics	1	
– Removable prosthetics	0	
– Non-surgical periodontology	1	
– Surgical periodontology	2	Bleeding; infection
Hazardous and contraindicated drugs	2	Avoid sedatives, aspirin, acetaminophen, and drugs interfering with ciclosporin

*0 = No special considerations. 1 = Caution advised. 2 = Specialised medical advice recommended in some cases. 3 = Specialised medical advice mandatory. 4 = Only to be performed in hospital environment. 5 = Should be avoided.

prophylaxis for invasive dental procedures – particularly if provided within 6 months post-transplantation.

Preventive dentistry A full preventive oral health care programme, including diet modification, brushing, antiseptic mouth rinses and topical fluorides, should be instituted before transplantation and maintained at a high standard thereafter.

Pain and anxiety control **Local anaesthesia** LA should be given with caution due to the bleeding and infection risk. A rinse with chlorhexidine mouthwash (0.2%) prior to administration is advisable. **Conscious sedation** Sedative drugs should be avoided, but if unavoidable must only be given in hospital with appropriate expertise and facilities. **General anaesthesia** General anaesthesia should be avoided, but if unavoidable must only be given in hospital with appropriate expertise and facilities.

Treatment modification **Surgery** A full blood count and coagulation status should be tested before surgical procedures. **Fixed prosthetics and conservation** Extensive caries in patients with poor oral hygiene is an indication for tooth extraction before transplantation. **Periodontology** A preoperative full blood count and bleeding test may be required. Advanced periodontal disease is an indication for tooth extraction before transplantation.

Drug use ■ Drug selection and adequate doses should be determined in consultation with the physician in patients with end-stage liver or kidney disease ■ Drugs such as sedatives, aspirin and paracetamol/acetaminophen are best avoided ■ Ciclosporin, nifedipine and basiliximab may induce gingival swelling ■ Several drugs, especially erythromycin and azole antifungals, may interfere with ciclosporin (Box 3.31) ■ Corticosteroid supplementation may be indicated.

Further reading
● Fernandez de Preliasco M V, Viera M J, Sebelli P, Rodriguez Rilo L, Sanchez G A 2002 Compliance with medical and dental treatments in child and adolescent renal transplant patients. Acta Odontol Latinoam 15:21–27 ● Golder D T, Drinnan A J 1993 Dental aspects of cardiac transplantation. Transplant Proc 25:2377–2380 ● Niederhagen B, Wolff M, Appel T, von Lindern J J, Berge S 2003 Location and sanitation of dental foci in liver transplantation. Transpl Int 16:173–178 ● Thomason J M, Girdler N M, Kendall-Taylor P, Wastell H, Weddel A, Seymour R A 1999 An investigation into the need for supplementary steroids in organ transplant patients undergoing gingival surgery. A double-blind, split-mouth, cross-over study. J Clin Periodontol 26:577–582.

TRAUMATIC INJURY TO CNS (BRAIN AND SPINAL CORD)

Definition Brain or spinal cord injury is severe, sometimes with irreversible, functional consequences – when the injury is to the brain only, it is known as traumatic brain injury (Fig. 3.39) ■ Traumatic brain injury occurs when a sudden physical assault on the head causes damage to the brain ■ The damage can be focal, confined to one area of the brain, or diffuse, involving more than one area of the brain ■ It can result from: ● closed head injury ● penetrating head injury ■ The severity can range from a mild concussion to the extremes of coma or even death.

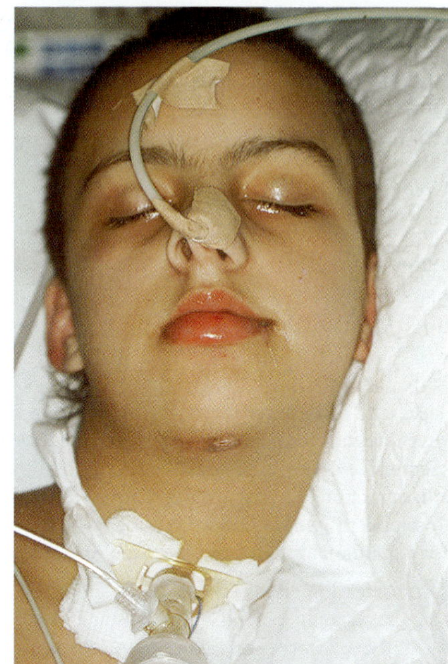

Figure 3.39 **An individual with traumatic brain injury affecting the central nervous system**

General aspects

Aetiopathogenesis ■ Mainly caused by road traffic accidents, assaults, and war injuries ■ Occasionally caused by other accidents, particularly sports, or by surgery.

Clinical presentation **Traumatic brain injury** ■ Symptoms may include: ● headache ● nausea ● confusion or other cognitive problems ● a change in personality ● depression ● irritability ● other emotional and behavioural problems ● seizures ■ The part of the brain damaged determines the extent of motor and sensory deficits and other sequelae ■ Of those with traumatic brain injury, 12% die within 2 days, while approximately 50% have permanent after-effects such as paralyses, loss of speech, impaired vision, epilepsy ■ Delayed effects may result from ischaemia, hypoxia, cerebral oedema, intracranial hypertension, and/or abnormalities of cerebral blood flow. **Spinal cord injury** The level at which the spinal cord is injured determines the extent of sensory and motor deficits. Individuals with higher spinal cord injury may have: ■ impaired ventilation ■ reduced gag and cough reflex ■ difficulty controlling oral fluids.

Classification/grading of injury **Traumatic brain injury** The level of consciousness is graded according to the Glasgow coma scale (Table 3.154). **Spinal cord injury** The level of spinal cord injury is used to assist in determining the clinical features that may be expected (Table 3.155).

Diagnosis ■ CT ■ MRI.

Treatment of CNS trauma ■ Protection of the airway, oxygen administration and a call for an ambulance are the most useful immediate measures ■ The possibility of cervical spine damage should always be considered in patients involved in road traffic accidents since movement of the neck may then cause serious cord damage, spastic quadriplegia or death – the neck must not be extended or rotated, and a support collar should be fitted prophylactically ■ Hospitalisation is needed ■ Neurosurgery (urgent) ■ In severe cases diaphragmatic pacemakers and mechanical ventilation devices may be necessary ■ Hyperbaric oxygen may help in recovery ■ Experienced psychologists, cognitive therapists, and vocational therapists work with the patients to educate and orient them, improve their reading and writing skills, and help restore and ensure their mental and psychological wellbeing ■ Most patients will need wheelchairs ■ Most patients with injuries at or below the lumbar level are wheelchair-independent and may be able to walk independently with long leg braces and crutches

Table 3.154 **Glasgow Coma or Responsiveness Scale**

Event	Score
Eye opening (E)	
– Spontaneous	4
– To speech	3
– To pain	2
– Nil	1
Motor response (M)	
– Obeys	6
– Localises	5
– Withdraws	4
– Abnormal flexion	3
– Extends	2
– Nil	1
Verbal response (V)	
– Orientated	5
– Confused conversation	4
– Inappropriate words	3
– Incomprehensible sounds	2
– Nil	1
EMV score or responsiveness sum	3–15 = range 7 or less = coma in 100% 9 or more = absence of coma

Table 3.155 **Effects of spinal cord injuries at different levels**

Level of spinal cord damage	Features
C1–C5	Quadriplegia (tetraplegia) or death
C5–C6	Paraplegia Hands paralysed Arms paralysed except for abduction and flexion
C6–C7	Paraplegia Hands, but not arms, paralysed
T1	Paraplegia Normal hand function Patients can perform all functions of a non-injured person, with the exception of standing and walking
T2–T5	Paraplegia Patients have partial trunk movement and may be able to stand, with long leg braces and a walker, and may be able to walk short distances with assistance
T6–T12	Paraplegia Patients have partial abdominal muscle strength, and may be able to walk independently for short distances with long leg braces and a walker or crutches
T11–T12	Paraplegia Sensory loss T12 and below
T12–L1	Legs paralysed below knees
L2	Patients have all movement in the trunk and hips
L3	Patients have knee extension
L4	Patients have ankle dorsification
L5	Patients have extensor hallucis longus function. They are able to walk independently with ankle braces and canes, and may use wheelchairs only for long distances
S1–S2	Patients have function of the gastrocnemius and soleus muscles and walk independently on all surfaces, usually without bracing

Orofacial findings

■ Unilateral paralysis of the face and orofacial musculature ■ Maxillofacial injuries ■ Loss of oral sensations (i.e. taste) ■ Deviated tongue on extrusion, showing flaccidity and multiple folds ■ Dysphagia ■ Salivary incontinence/drooling ■ Extensive calculus deposits may be present ■ Gag reflex possibly reduced ■ Cranial nerve lesions in patients with head injuries may indicate a basal skull fracture or other lesion; cranial nerves I, II, III, V, VII and VIII are most vulnerable to damage ■ Lip and tongue-biting may be seen in patients with profound neurodisability – this may be associated with extensive tissue loss and scarring.

Dental management

Risk assessement Difficulties that may be encountered when providing dental management in a patient with CNS injury include: ■ Access and impaired mobility ■ Communication difficulties – there may be cognitive and sensory defects as well as dysarthria, aphasia, confusion, memory loss and emotional distress ■ Consent issues – it is important to assess each patient on an individual basis ■ Calculus deposits – may be a hazard to the airway ■ Individuals with brain or higher spinal cord injury may have: ● impaired ventilation ● reduced gag and cough reflex with a liability to aspiration of material into the lungs ● difficulty controlling oral fluids ■ Oropharyngeal dysphagia – occurs in many patients, and has a significant contribution to morbidity and mortality since it predisposes to respiratory infection, malnutrition and weight loss; multidisciplinary care is required ■ Patients with spinal cord injury experience a loss of bowel and bladder control – these patients should void urine and carry out their bowel programme before the dental appointment.

Appropriate health care ■ Preventive care should be introduced early, particularly as calculus deposits may be a hazard to the airway ■ Invasive dental care should be deferred for 6 months after trauma ■ Effective high-speed suction is mandatory during operative dentistry, to avoid compromising the airway ■ Individuals with higher spinal cord injury receiving dental treatment may require: ● special treatment areas (hospital) ● additional personnel ● attentive and rapid evacuation of fluids ● blood pressure monitoring ● other specific monitoring ■ Individuals with lower spinal cord injury usually require no special preparation for dental care other than attention to bowels/bladder unless they become latex allergic ■ Take care to communicate clearly with the patient, by not wearing a mask, facing the patient, and speaking slowly, clearly and in language that is not complex – caregivers may help to communicate with the patient ■ Some patients may not be able to provide consent.

Pain and anxiety control **Local anaesthesia** ■ Use minimum amount of epinephrine in local anaesthesia ■ Avoid using epinephrine-containing gingival retraction cords ■ Some advise not using electronic dental analgesia. **Conscious sedation** ■ Opiates are best avoided as they may cause CNS depression ■ Nitrous oxide may be administered without adverse effects. **General anaesthesia** ■ General anaesthesia should be avoided for 6 months after trauma ■ Barbiturates are contraindicated as they may cause severe hypotension ■ Patients with quadriplegia are at risk from respiratory infections so that general anaesthesia should be avoided if possible ■ Muscle relaxants should be avoided.

Patient access and positioning **Access to dental surgery** ■ The treatment plan must consider physical limitations as paralysis is often present. Impaired mobility may make access difficult; some patients are chairbound or bedbound. When it is necessary to place the patient in the dental chair, proper wheelchair transfer technique is essential to prevent injury to patient or dental staff. ■ Since paralysed patients may develop

Table 3.156 **Key considerations for dental management in traumatic injury to CNS (see text)**

	Management modifications*	Comments/possible complications
Risk assessment	2	Mobility; communication; consent; loss of cough and gag reflexes
Appropriate dental care	3/4	Defer elective treatment for 6 months; monitor blood pressure
Pain and anxiety control		
– Local anaesthesia	1	Avoid epinephrine and electronic dental analgesia
– Conscious sedation	1	Avoid opiates
– General anaesthesia	4	Avoid barbiturates and muscle relaxants
Patient access and positioning		
– Access to dental office	1	Impaired mobility
– Timing of treatment	1	Mid-morning; short visits
– Patient positioning	1	Upright position if possible
Treatment modification		
– Preventive dentistry	1	Electric toothbrush
– Oral surgery	1	Poor oral hygiene
– Implantology	1	Only simple procedures
– Conservative/Endodontics	1	Only simple procedures
– Fixed prosthetics	1	Only simple procedures
– Removable prosthetics	1	Difficult to place
– Non-surgical periodontology	1	Poor oral hygiene
– Surgical periodontology	1	Only simple procedures
Hazardous and contraindicated drugs	1	Acetaminophen – drug of choice; avoid hypertensive drugs

*0 = No special considerations. 1 = Caution advised. 2 = Specialised medical advice recommended in some cases. 3 = Specialised medical advice mandatory. 4 = Only to be performed in hospital environment. 5 = Should be avoided.

ischaemia in weight-bearing areas causing decubitus ulcers (bed sores), the patient must not be left in the same position for extended periods. **Timing of treatment** Treatment sessions should be short and scheduled for mid-morning. **Patient positioning** ■ Patients are best treated in the upright position, and extra care must be taken to avoid anything entering the pharynx. Good suction must be at hand. ■ If the patient has been supine or reclined, raise slowly to avoid hypotension.

Treatment modification **Preventive dentistry** Oral hygiene tends to deteriorate on the paralysed side and impaired manual dexterity may also interfere with toothbrushing. An electric toothbrush or adapted holders may therefore help. **Implantology** May be compromised by impaired oral hygiene. **Fixed prosthetics and conservation** ■ Only simple bridgework is recommended; however, it may be a very useful alternative to often poorly retained/tolerated dentures, and can help restore aesthetics anteriorly, thereby dramatically improving social interaction ■ Dysphagia compromises protection of the airway, so consider: ● maintaining the patient in an upright position ● using rubber dam ● limiting the use of handpiece and other water sprays ● rapidly evacuating oral fluids.

Removable prosthetics ■ Removable prostheses may be difficult to insert and remove by the patient, who may be unable anyway to use dentures due to neuromuscular deficits ■ Removable shields may be useful to help limit lip biting; however they are often poorly tolerated.

Drug use ■ Acetaminophen is the drug of choice for postoperative pain ■ Hypertension must be avoided, since it can precipitate subarachnoid or cerebral haemorrhage; fatal subarachnoid haemorrhage has resulted from the use of norepinephrine in local anaesthetic solutions. Cerebral haemorrhage can also result from hypertension caused by interactions of monoamine oxidase inhibitors with other drugs, particularly pethidine.

Treatment in patients with spinal damage Dental management may be uncomplicated in spinal injuries, although postural hypotension in the early stages may necessitate treatment in the upright position and latex allergy should be considered.

Further reading

● Gilmore R, Aram J, Powell J, Greenwood R 2003 Treatment of oro-facial hypersensitivity following brain injury. Brain Inj 17:347–354 ● Kleint G, Kanitz G, Harzer W 2002 Orthodontic treatment in handicapped children: report of four cases. ASDC J Dent Child 69:31–38 ● Millwood J, Fiske J 2001 Lip-biting in patients with profound neuro-disability. Dent Update 28:105–108.

TUBERCULOSIS

Definition ■ Tuberculosis (TB) is an infectious chronic disease caused mainly by *Mycobacterium tuberculosis*, an acid-fast non-motile aerobic rod, which mainly infects the lungs ■ One-third of the world population is infected, most coming from the developing world.

General aspects

Aetiopathogenesis ■ Humans are the only reservoir for *M. tuberculosis* (*M. bovis* and *M. africanum* are very uncommon) ■ Primary infection mainly spreads to lungs by droplets or occasionally to ileocaecum ■ After an asymptomatic latency, post-primary TB due to reactivation may develop if the patient becomes immuno-incompetent (e.g. in diabetes, HIV, corticosteroids, cancer) ■ Of particular concern is the emergence of multi-drug resistant TB (MDR-TB), where transmission via a dental setting has been recorded ■ Atypical mycobacteria include species such as *M. avium*, *M. intracellulare* (*M. avium-intracellulare* complex: MAC), *M. kansasii*, *M. scrofulaceum*, *M. fortuitum*, *M. marinum*, *M. ulcerans*, *M. chelonae* and *M. xenopi*. They are widely distributed in water, soil, animals and man, usually without causing disease. Most infections with such non-tuberculous mycobacteria (NTM) are believed to come from environmental exposure.

Clinical presentation ■ TB is often self-limiting and may go undiagnosed ■ Primary infection is usually asymptomatic but patients may have fever, night sweats, cough, anorexia and weakness ■ Post-primary TB may be pulmonary, or can spread widely (e.g. to meninges, bone, renal tract, etc.) to cause organ-specific symptoms.

Diagnosis ■ Radiology (chest films) ■ Sputum smear is cheap and quick, but it has low sensitivity ■ Sputum culture gives definitive diagnosis but it takes 4–8 weeks ■ PCR on sputum may facilitate a prompt diagnosis ■ Skin reactions – tuberculin test or Mantoux; a positive test means that a person has been infected but it does not mean active TB ■ Histology of infected organs.

Treatment ■ Rifampicin, isoniazid plus pyrazinamide are the antimicrobials of choice ■ Drug-resistant TB is increasingly common, especially in AIDS ■ Ethambutol, streptomycin, amikacin, kanamycin or capreomycin are added in cases of drug resistance ■ Most NTM are resistant to standard anti-tubercular medication and, though it is possible that clarithromycin or clofazimine may have some effect, excision of affected tissues is recommended.

Prognosis ■ About 5% of patients with primary infection will develop active TB during the first 2 years after infection ■ Every year almost 3 million people die of TB associated complications.

Oral findings

Oral ulceration ■ Chronic ulcers, usually on the dorsum of the tongue, are the main oral manifestation of TB but are rare. ■ Occasionally the diagnosis of pulmonary tuberculosis is made from the biopsy of an oral ulcer after granulomas are seen microscopically. Acid-fast bacilli are rarely seen in oral biopsies, even with the help of special stains. Such cases (usually middle-aged males) may result from neglect of symptoms, or default from treatment for TB. Unfixed material should also be sent for culture if possible. However, the diagnosis needs to be confirmed by sputum culture and chest radiographs.

Tuberculous cervical lymphadenopathy ■ Tuberculous cervical lymphadenopathy is the next most common form of the infection to pulmonary disease ■ It is particularly common among those from South Asia.

TB lymphadenitis ■ Cervical and submandibular lymphadenitis due to NTM (e.g. MAC, *M. scrofulaceum* and *M. kansasii*) may affect otherwise healthy young children under 12 years, but is also seen in HIV disease ■ Most TB lymphadenitis is painless, with several enlarged matted nodes – systemic symptoms are seen only in a minority ■ Only about 15% have pulmonary manifestations on radiography ■ Absence of fever or tuberculosis, a positive tuberculin test, and failed response to conventional antimicrobials are highly suggestive – but definitive diagnosis is by culture or polymerase chain reaction of biopsy material obtained by fine needle aspiration or removal of the nodes

Dental management

Risk assessment ■ Tuberculosis can be transmitted to staff during oral health care if the person being treated has active pulmonary TB ■ The risk is greater if the dental staff are immunocompromised ■ MDR-TB is of particular concern ■ Person-to-person transmission of NTM is not important in acquisition of infection with these organisms, except for skin infections. Individuals with respiratory disease from NTM do not readily infect others and, therefore, do not need to be isolated. ■ Mycobacteria proliferate in biofilms forming within dental units. Studies of water from dental units have revealed NTM species including *Mycobacterium gordonae*, *M. flavescens*, *M. chelonae*, '*M. chelonae*-like organism' and *M. simiae*. Other mycobacteria such as *M. simiae* and *M. mucogenicum* have even been isolated from units that were being routinely treated intermittently with a chemical cleaner.

Appropriate health care ■ Patients with pulmonary TB are contagious and dental treatment is thus best deferred until the TB has been treated, although 2 weeks of therapy has been considered adequate to consider a patient as non-infectious ■ If patients with active pulmonary TB must be treated, special precautions should be used to prevent the release of mycobacteria into the air, to remove any that are present, and to stop the inhalation by other persons: • reduction of splatter and aerosols, by minimising coughing and avoiding ultrasonic instruments, and use of high volume suction and rubber dam, are important • improved ventilation (open window rather than air-conditioning) • ultraviolet germicidal light • new masks; ideally with a

Table 3.157 **Management of patients with known or suspected TB**

History of TB	Potential infectivity	Comment
Active sputum positive for TB	High	Defer elective dental care until TB treatment complete or use special infection control precautions
Recent history of TB and sputum known positive for TB	High	Defer elective dental care until TB treatment complete or use special infection control precautions
Past history of TB	Needs confirmation	Defer elective dental care until medical advice received
No history of TB but signs or symptoms suggestive	Needs confirmation	Defer elective dental care until medical advice received. Use special infection control precautions for emergency dental care
No history of TB but positive tuberculin test	Needs confirmation	Defer elective dental care until medical advice received. Use special infection control precautions for emergency dental care

Table 3.158 **Key considerations for dental management in tuberculosis (see text)**

	Management modifications*	Comments/possible complications
Risk assessment	1	Transmission
Appropriate dental care	2	Active TB, defer elective dental care; infection control precautions
Pain and anxiety control		
– Local anaesthesia	0	
– Conscious sedation	3	Avoid nitrous oxide
– General anaesthesia	5	Risk of contamination
Patient access and positioning		
– Access to dental office	0	
– Timing of treatment	1	End of session; minimise staff exposed
– Patient positioning	0	
Treatment modification		
– Oral surgery	0	
– Implantology	0	
– Conservative/Endodontics	1	Minimise aerosols; use barriers
– Fixed prosthetics	1	Minimise aerosols; use barriers
– Removable prosthetics	0	
– Non-surgical periodontology	0	
– Surgical periodontology	0	
Hazardous and contraindicated drugs	1	Avoid acetaminophen, aspirin and azoles

*0 = No special considerations. 1 = Caution advised. 2 = Specialised medical advice recommended in some cases. 3 = Specialised medical advice mandatory. 4 = Only to be performed in hospital environment. 5 = Should be avoided.

visor to enhance eye-protection ● in cases of MDR-TB, other personal protective devices, such as high-efficiency particulate air filters (HEPA) and personal respirators, may be used ● Mycobacteria are very resistant to disinfectants, so that heat sterilisation should be used wherever possible ■ Other factors such as alcoholism or intravenous drug use, hepatitis or HIV disease may also influence dental management.

Pain and anxiety control **Local anaesthesia** LA is the method of choice and may be given with routine precautions.
Conscious sedation Nitrous oxide is contraindicated because of the risk of contamination of the apparatus. Caution is advised with oral sedation as the clearance of diazepam is enhanced by rifampicin.
General anaesthesia ■ General anaesthesia is also contraindicated for dental treatment because of the risk of contamination of the anaesthetic apparatus or because of impaired pulmonary function ■ Aminoglycosides

such as streptomycin enhance the activity of some neuromuscular blocking drugs and in large doses may cause a myasthenic syndrome during general anaesthesia.

Patient access and positioning For patients with active TB who require urgent care, this should be scheduled at the end of the treatment session, taking care to minimise the number of staff in contact/exposed.

Drug use ■ The clearance of diazepam and the hepatotoxicity of paracetamol/acetaminophen are enhanced by rifampicin ■ Paracetamol/acetaminophen should be avoided in patients on isoniazid ■ Aspirin should be avoided in patients on streptomycin, amikacin, kanamycin or capreomycin because it increases the risk of ototoxicity ■ Azole antifungals and clarithromycin also interact with rifampicin.

Further reading ● Lassiter T E, Panagakos F S 2003 Tuberculosis. NY State Dent J 69:23–26 ● Porteous N B, Redding S W, Jorgensen J H 2004 Isolation of non-tuberculosis mycobacteria in treated dental unit waterlines. Oral Surg Oral Med Oral Pathol Oral Radiol Endod 98:40–44 ● Yepes J F, Sullivan J, Pinto A 2004 Tuberculosis: medical management update. Oral Surg Oral Med Oral Pathol Oral Radiol Endod 98:267–273.

ULCERATIVE COLITIS

Definition Ulcerative colitis is a chronic inflammatory bowel disease, characterised by ulceration of the large intestine, involving mainly the rectum (proctitis) or colon (total colitis).

General aspects

Aetiopathogenesis Although allergy, infective agents, stress and immunologic factors have been suggested to play a role, the aetiology remains unknown.

Clinical presentation ■ Bloody diarrhoea (mainly) ■ Sometimes fever, anorexia, weight loss ■ Extra-intestinal features (Fig. 3.40) include: ● oral – ulceration ● eyes – conjunctivitis, episcleritis, iritis ● skin – pyoderma or erythema nodosum ● joints – arthritis, sacroiliitis, clubbing ● liver – various ■ Since uveitis, skin lesions and mouth ulcers can be found in ulcerative colitis, it is important to differentiate it from Behçet's and Sweet's syndrome where similar lesions may appear.

Diagnosis ■ Full blood count, haemoglobin and haematocrit (iron anaemia) ■ Abdominal radiograph ■ Sigmoidoscopy/colonoscopy ■ Rectal biopsy ■ Barium enema.

Treatment ■ Corticosteroids ■ Sulphasalazine or olsalazine ■ ± Surgery (colectomy).

Prognosis ■ The risk of epithelial dysplasia and colonic cancer is increased ■ Up to 25% require colectomy within 5–10 years ■ Overall mortality rate is twice that of the general population.

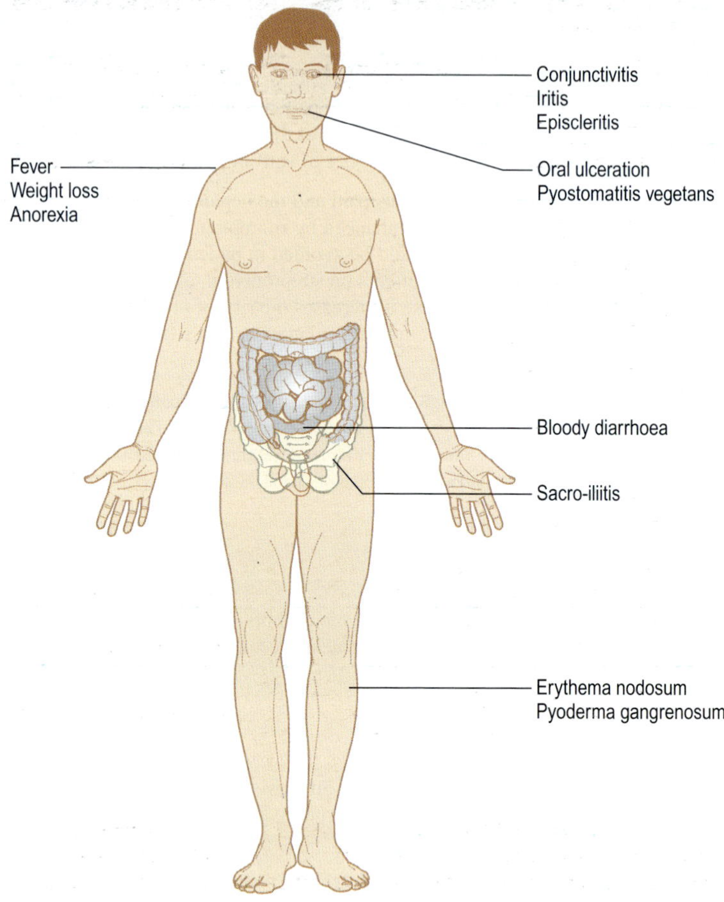

Figure 3.40 **Clinical presentation of ulcerative collitis**

Oral findings

Oral manifestations in ulcerative colitis are rare but include: ■ pyostomatitis gangrenosum (chronic ulceration) ■ pyostomatitis vegetans (multiple intra-epithelial microabscesses) ■ discrete haemorrhagic ulcers or lesions related to anaemia. Although most lesions resolve when the systemic disease is controlled, topical steroids may help.

Dental management

Risk assessment ■ Management complications may include anaemia and those associated with corticosteroid therapy ■ Sulphasalazine may cause leucopenia, anaemia and thrombocytopenia.

Table 3.159 **Key considerations for dental management in ulcerative colitis (see text)**

	Management modifications*	Comments/possible complications
Risk assessment	1	Anaemia; steroid therapy
Appropriate dental care	1	Consider disease activity; steroid cover
Pain and anxiety control		
– Local anaesthesia	0	
– Conscious sedation	0	
– General anaesthesia	3/4	Anaemia
Patient access and positioning		
– Access to dental office	0	
– Timing of treatment	0	
– Patient positioning	0	
Treatment modification		
– Oral surgery	1	Therapy side effects
– Implantology	1	Therapy side effects
– Conservative/Endodontics	0	
– Fixed prosthetics	0	
– Removable prosthetics	0	
– Non-surgical periodontology	0	
– Surgical periodontology	1	Therapy side effects
Hazardous and contraindicated drugs	1	Avoid NSAIDs, clavulanate and clindamycin

*0 = No special considerations. 1 = Caution advised. 2 = Specialised medical advice recommended in some cases. 3 = Specialised medical advice mandatory. 4 = Only to be performed in hospital environment. 5 = Should be avoided.

Appropriate health care ■ During acute episodes only emergency dental care should be performed ■ Corticosteroid supplementation may be indicated ■ In patients treated with sulphasalazine, full blood count and bleeding tests are recommended before any procedure associated with bleeding.

Pain and anxiety control **Local anaesthesia** LA may be used with routine precautions. **Conscious sedation** Benzodiazepine and nitrous oxide may be useful to minimise stress. **General anaesthesia** Profound anaemia is a contraindication for GA.

Drug use ■ NSAIDs should be avoided: acetaminophen is recommended ■ Antibiotics that could aggravate diarrhoea should be avoided; these include amoxicillin-clavulanate and clindamycin.

Further reading

● Hegarty A M, Barrett A W, Scully C 2004 Pyostomatitis vegetans. Clin Exp Dermatol 29:1–7 ● Katz J, Shenkman A, Stavropoulos F, Melzer E 2003 Oral signs and symptoms in relation to disease activity and site of involvement in patients with inflammatory bowel disease. Oral Dis 9:34–40 ● Scully C 2001 Gastroenterological diseases and the mouth. Practitioner 245:215–222.

VISUALLY IMPAIRED PATIENTS

Definition ■ Visual difficulties and impairments include: ● blindness ● low vision ● colour blindness ■ Visual impairments (VI) encompass people who have: ● never had any visual function ● those who had normal vision for some years before becoming gradually or suddenly partially or totally blind ● those with disabilities in addition to the visual loss ● those with selective impairments of parts of the visual field ● those with a general degradation of acuity across the visual field.

General aspects

Blindness ■ A person is considered blind if they see clearly at 20 feet what someone with very good vision can see at 200 feet, and if glasses or contact lenses cannot make them see better – this is called 20/200 vision ■ 'Legally blind' indicates that a person has less than 20/200 vision in the better eye or a very limited field of vision (20 degrees at its widest point) ■ In the UK, the statutory definition of 'blind' is: 'so blind as to be unable to perform any work for which eyesight is essential' (the Blind Persons Act 1920).

Partial sight There is no statutory definition of 'partial sight' although the guideline is 'substantially and permanently handicapped by defective vision caused by congenital defect, illness, or injury' (the National Assistance Act 1948).

Low vision ■ 'Low vision' generally refers to a severe VI, not necessarily limited to distance vision ■ Low vision applies to all individuals with sight who are unable to read the newspaper at a normal viewing distance, even with the aid of eyeglasses or contact lenses.

Aetiopathogenesis ■ VI happens when there is a problem with one or more parts of the eyes or the parts of the brain needed to process the visual images, or a problem with the eye–brain connections ■ It can be hereditary or acquired – a fetus might develop a VI if infected *in utero* (e.g. rubella); VI can also be caused by trauma to the eye, infections (e.g. toxoplasmosis) or systemic problems such as diabetes ■ Specific eye problems can cause VI, and typically are seen in older people; they include conditions such as: ● *macular degeneration*, which tends to run in families, suggesting heredity is involved in some cases ● *glaucoma*, where pressure builds up inside the eye (normal intraocular pressure is between 12 and 21 mmHg) ● *cataracts*, when cloudy spots in the lens block light and change vision – irradiation, diabetes, steroids, hypercalcaemia and excessive sunlight exposure may cause cataracts to form at a younger age in adults.

Clinical presentation ■ Some people are totally blind; others who may be considered to be blind can still see a little light or shadows, but are unable to see objects clearly ■ Blindness or defects of visual fields can be caused by ocular, optic nerve or cortical damage but the type of defect varies according to the site and extent of the lesion ■ A complete lesion of one optic nerve causes that eye to be totally blind. There is no direct reaction of the pupil to light (loss of constriction) and, if a light is shone into the affected eye, the pupil of the unaffected eye also fails to respond (loss of the consensual reflex).

However, the nerves to the affected eye responsible for pupil constriction run in the IIIrd cranial nerve and should be intact. If, therefore, a light is shone into the unaffected eye, the pupil of the affected eye also constricts – even though that eye is sightless. ■ Lesions of the optic tract, chiasma, radiation or optic cortex cause various visual field defects involving both visual fields but without total field loss on either side. An ophthalmological opinion should always be obtained if there is any suggestion of a visual field defect.

Diagnosis ■ VI should be suspected when the patient: ● has difficulty in recognising people ● holds books or reading material close to face or at arm's length ● has over-cautious driving habits ● finds lighting either too bright or too dim ● has frequent spectacle prescription changes ● squints or tilts the head to see ● changes leisure time activities, personal appearance or table etiquette ● moves about cautiously or bumps into objects ● acts confusedly or is disoriented.

■ Eye charts ● Vision is tested by visual acuity testing using the Snellen eye chart or a similar standard eye chart. This has a series of letters or letters and numbers, with the largest at the top. As the person being tested reads down the chart, the letters gradually become smaller. ● When checking visual acuity, one eye is covered at a time and the vision of each eye is recorded separately, as well as both eyes together. Normal vision is 20/20, which means that the eye being tested can read a certain size letter when it is 20 feet away. If a person sees 20/40, then at 20 feet from the chart that person can read letters that a person with 20/20 vision could read from 40 feet away. The 20/40 letters are twice the size of 20/20 letters; however, if 20/20 is considered 100% visual efficiency, 20/40 visual acuity is 85% efficient. ● For people who have worse than 20/400 vision, a different eye chart can be used. It is common to record vision worse than 20/400 as Count Fingers (CF at a certain number of feet), Hand Motion (HM at a certain number of feet), Light Perception (LP), or No Light Perception (NLP).

■ Ophthalmoscopy – after the pupils have been dilated, direct ophthalmoscopy provides a wider, magnified view of the retina.

■ Tonometry – measures pressure inside the eye and is one of several tests necessary to detect glaucoma.

■ A slit lamp examination – allows examination of the front of the eye.

■ A phoropter – detects refractive errors.

■ Visual field examination (perimetry) – tests the total area where objects can be seen in the peripheral vision while the eye is focused on a central point.

■ Confrontation visual field examination – a quick and basic evaluation of the visual field done by an examiner sitting directly in front of the patient who is asked to look at the examiner's eye and tell when they can see the examiner's hand.

■ Tangent screen exam – the patient looks at a central target and tells the examiner when an object brought into the peripheral vision can be seen.

■ Automated perimetry – the patient sits in front of a computer-driven programme that flashes small lights at different locations, and presses a button whenever the lights in the peripheral vision are seen.

Treatment ■ Totally blind people learn via Braille or other non-visual media ■ People with low vision use a combination of vision and other senses to learn, although they may require adaptations in lighting or the size of print, and, sometimes, Braille ■ Assistive technology for computer users includes:

- *Screen enlargers* (or screen magnifiers) work like a magnifying glass.
- *Screen readers* are software programmes that present graphics and text as speech. A screen reader is used to verbalise, or 'speak', everything on the screen including names and descriptions of control buttons, menus, text, and punctuation.
- *Speech recognition systems* (voice recognition programmes), allow people to give commands and enter data using their voices rather than a mouse or keyboard.
- *Speech synthesisers* (text-to-speech [TTS] systems) receive information going to the screen in the form of letters, numbers, and punctuation marks, and then 'speak' it out loud. Using speech synthesisers allows blind users to review their input as they type.
- *Refreshable Braille* displays provide tactile output of information represented on the computer screen. The user reads the Braille letters with their fingers, and then, after a line is read, refreshes the display to read the next line.
- *Braille embossers* transfer computer-generated text into embossed Braille output. Braille translation programmes convert text scanned in or generated via standard word processing programmes into Braille, which can be printed on the embosser (Fig. 3.41).
- *Talking word processors* are software programmes that use speech synthesisers to provide auditory feedback of what is typed.
- *Large-print word processors* allow the user to view everything in large text without added screen enlargement.

Prognosis The prognosis of VI varies depending on its cause.

Oral findings

■ The oral health of people with VI can be disadvantaged, since they are not in a position to detect and recognise early oral disease and may be unable to take immediate action unless informed of the situation ■ The number of dental fractures in children with VI however, is similar to those without VI. As a consequence, mouth-guards are not recommended for everyday life activities.

Dental management

Risk assessment ■ Congenital VI is often found in polymalformative syndromes (e.g. Crouzon, Ehlers–Danlos, hydrocephalus) where systemic involvement may influence dental management (e.g. infective endocarditis prophylaxis in patients with 'at risk' heart disease) ■ Diabetes is not uncommon in adults with VI ■ Unexpected noises or sensations may provoke sudden movements, making the use of sharp and rotatory instruments hazardous.

Appropriate dental care ■ It can be helpful if medical history and consent forms have large font/Braille (Fig. 3.41) ■ Postoperative instructions may be taped ■ The patient should be invited to touch and feel

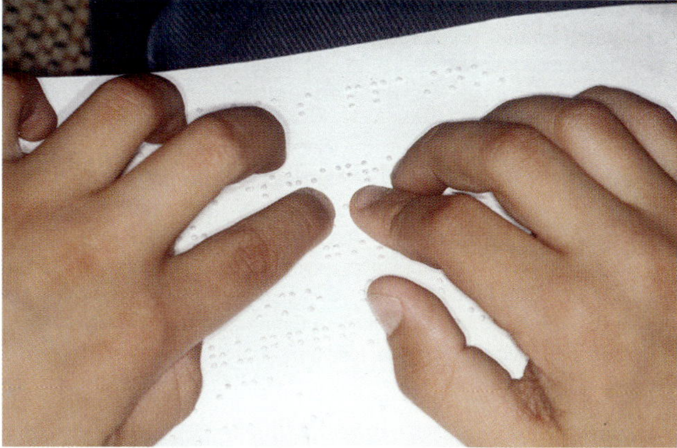

Figure 3.41 **Braille**

the chair and equipment to familiarise themselves ■ Dental staff should use a verbally oriented approach, explaining clearly procedures before performing them, especially anything that makes a noise or causes discomfort. Comment on textures, odours, vibrations and tastes that the patient will notice (Fig. 3.42).

Preventive dentistry People with VI may benefit from adapted oral health education programmes. It has been shown that DMF index, plaque accumulation and the prevalence of gingivitis in children with VI under controlled oral hygiene programmes are the same as in children with normal vision.

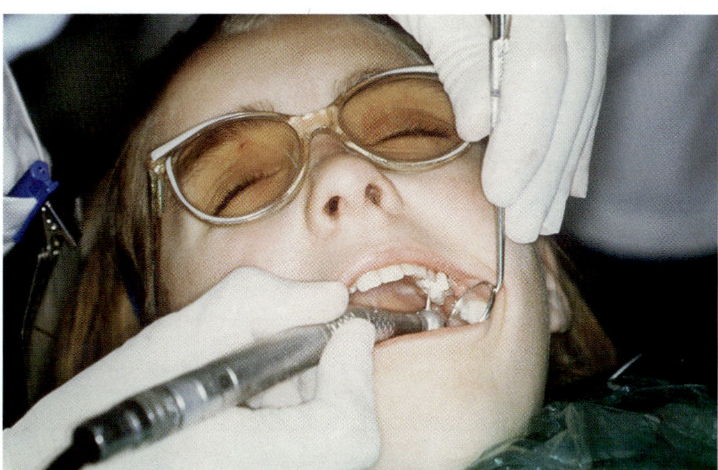

Figure 3.42 **Dental treatment of a patient with visual impairment**

Pain and anxiety control **Local anaesthesia** Sometimes patients show low pain tolerance (even to LA), which could be due to increased tactile sensitivity. **Conscious sedation** Avoid diazepam and other benzodiazepines in patients with glaucoma. **General Anaesthesia** Avoid atropinics in patients with glaucoma.

Patient access and positioning **Access to dental surgery** It can be helpful to people with VI if : ■ they are told before they are touched; people with visual impairments may have an increased sense of touch – verbally advise them of your presence, as an unexpected touch on the face or arm can be startling to the patient ■ when guiding the patient, staff offer an arm and let them hold and do not push them; describe obstacles ■ they are told before staff leave the room ■ notices have large writing ■ the

Table 3.160 **Key considerations for dental management in visual impairment (see text)**

	Management modifications*	Comments/possible complications
Risk assessment	1	Underlying disease; unexpected movements
Appropriate dental care	1	Communication
Pain and anxiety control		
– Local anaesthesia	1	Pain intolerance
– Conscious sedation	0	
– General anaesthesia	0	
Patient access and positioning		
– Access to dental office	1	Assist appropriately
– Timing of treatment	0	
– Patient positioning	0	
Treatment modification		
– Oral surgery	0	
– Implantology	0	
– Conservative/Endodontics	0	
– Fixed prosthetics	1	Impaired oral hygiene
– Removable prosthetics	1	Patient's manual ability; prosthesis tolerance
– Non-surgical periodontology	0	
– Surgical periodontology	0	
Hazardous and contraindicated drugs	1/2	Atropine, scopolamine and glycopyrrolate are contraindicated, especially in open angle glaucoma. Carbamazepine, diazepam, steroids and tricyclics may also be contraindicated

*0 = No special considerations. 1 = Caution advised. 2 = Specialised medical advice recommended in some cases. 3 = Specialised medical advice mandatory. 4 = Only to be performed in hospital environment. 5 = Should be avoided.

edges of steps are painted in a bright colour ■ bright colours are used for doors or pillars ■ any guide dog is not touched, petted or interfered with.

Treatment modification **Fixed prosthetics** Consider the patient's ability to perform oral hygiene. **Removable prosthetics** ■ Consider the patient's ability to recognise, insert and remove appliances ■ Mucous membrane supported prostheses may be poorly tolerated due to increased tactile sensibility, and the results of repeated polishing or relines to overcome this may not be satisfactory.

Drug use Drugs that may cause visual deterioration are contraindicated: namely, atropine, scolamine and glycopyrrolate, and to some extent steroids, tricyclics, diazepam and carbamazepine.

Further reading

● Al-Sarheed M, Bedi R, Hunt N 2000 The development of a tactile graphic version of IOTN for visually impaired patients. Clin Orthod Res 3:94–100 ● Al-Sarheed M, Bedi R, Hunt N P 2004 The views and attitudes of parents of children with a sensory impairment towards orthodontic care. Eur J Orthod 26:87–91 ● Diz Dios P 1995 Oral care in the blind and visually impaired. In: Porter S, Scully C (eds) Oral health care for those with HIV infection and other special needs. Science Reviews, Northwood ● O'Donnell D, Crosswaite M A 1990 Dental health education for the visually impaired child. J R Soc Health 110:60–61 ● Schembri A, Fiske J 2001 The implications of visual impairment in an elderly population in recognising oral disease and maintaining oral health. Spec Care Dentist 21:222–226 ● http://www.microsoft.com/enable/guides/vision.aspx ● http://www.spedex.com/napvi/ ● http://www.nichcy.org/pubs/factshe/fs13txt.htm ● http://www.rnib.org.uk/xpedio/groups/public/documents/code/InternetHome.hcsp

VON WILLEBRAND DISEASE

Definition ■ Von Willebrand disease (vWD) is typically due to inherited deficiency in von Willebrand factor (vWF: see below) ■ vWD affects about 1% of the population, females as well as males, and is the most common inherited bleeding disorder of humans ■ Rare cases are acquired, as in some people with hypothyroidism.

General aspects

Aetiopathogenesis vWF, synthesised in endothelium and megakaryocytes, has binding sites for collagen and for platelet glycoprotein (Gp) receptors, and thus normally acts in three ways, by: ■ binding to glycoprotein Ib and acting as a carrier for Factor VIII, protecting it from proteolytic degradation ■ mediating platelet adhesion to damaged endothelium ■ mediating platelet aggregation.

Clinical presentation ■ vWD causes bleeding that has features more similar to those caused by platelet dysfunction than by haemophilia A or B ■ The common pattern in vWD is bleeding from mucous membranes, which results in menorrhagia, gastrointestinal bleeding and epistaxis, with purpura of mucous membranes and the skin.

Classification There are various types of vWD: 1, 2A, 2B, 2C, 2M, 2N, 3 (Table 3.161) and the severity in each varies from patient to patient, and from time to time.

Diagnosis vWD is characterised by: ■ a prolonged bleeding time ■ usually a prolonged APTT ■ low levels of von Willebrand factor (Factor VIIIR:Ag) ■ low Factor VIIIC ■ low VIIIR:RCo (ristocetin co-factor) levels; platelets usually fail to aggregate in the presence of ristocetin so that, unlike haemophilia, the bleeding time is prolonged – but the best assay is the ristocetin co-factor assay.

Treatment ■ Desmopressin (DDAVP), given via a nasal spray, is: ● used in type 1 vWD ● contraindicated in type 2B and type 3 vWD, which require clotting factor replacement. Desmopressin is contraindicated in type 2B because it stimulates release of dysfunctional von Willebrand factor, which leads, in turn, to platelet aggregation and severe but transient thrombocytopenia. Desmopressin is contraindicated in type 3 vWD where so little vWF is formed that essentially the same management is required as for haemophilia A. ■ Intermediate purity Factor VIII, cryoprecipitate and fresh frozen plasma are effective, though pure Factor VIII may be ineffective.

Oral findings

■ The common pattern in vWD is bleeding from, and purpura of, mucous membranes. Gingival haemorrhage is more common than in haemophilia. ■ Prolonged bleeding following tooth exfoliation or dental manipulation may be the first sign of disease.

Dental management

Risk assessment Patients with vWD have an increased risk of haemorrhage from any dental manipulation that injures soft tissues or bone.

Appropriate health care ■ Most of the comments on management in haemophilia apply equally to patients with vWD (see p 186) ■ Haematologist advice is mandatory before any dental procedure

Table 3.161 **Types of von Willebrand disease**

Type	% vWD	Defect in vWF	Factor VIIIc
1	80	Partial quantitative decrease of vWF	May be normal
2A	15	Predominantly qualitative defect of vWF	Reduced
2B	Rare	Predominantly qualitative defect of vWF	Reduced
2C	Rare	Predominantly qualitative defect of vWF	Reduced
2M	Rare	Predominantly qualitative defect of vWF	Reduced
2N	Rare	Predominantly qualitative defect of vWF	Reduced
3	5	Complete lack of vWF	Reduced

associated with bleeding ■ Desmopressin, via nasal spray, and factor VIII replacement may be required.

Preventive dentistry Minimising gingivitis is important to prevent excessive bleeding during dental care.

Table 3.162 Von Willebrand disease: cover for operations*

VW disease type	Desmopressin	Factor VIII replacement
1	Given via a nasal spray	–
2A	Given via a nasal spray	±
2B	Contraindicated	+
2C	Given via a nasal spray	±
2M	Contraindicated	+
2N	Given via a nasal spray	±
3	Contraindicated	+

*Plus local haemostatic measures.

Table 3.163 Key considerations for dental management in Von Willebrand disease

	Management modifications*	Comments/possible complications
Risk assessment	3	Haemorrhage
Appropriate dental care	3	DDAVP; factor VIII
Pain and anxiety control		
– Local anaesthesia	1	Avoid regional blocks
– Conscious sedation	2	Avoid nitrous oxide
– General anaesthesia	3/4	Factor VIII
Patient access and positioning		
– Access to dental office	0	
– Timing of treatment	0	
– Patient positioning	0	
Treatment modification		
– Oral surgery	3	Bleeding
– Implantology	3	Bleeding
– Conservative/Endodontics	1	
– Fixed prosthetics	1	
– Removable prosthetics	0	
– Non-surgical periodontology	3	Bleeding
– Surgical periodontology	3	Bleeding
Hazardous and contraindicated drugs	1	Avoid NSAIDs

*0 = No special considerations. 1 = Caution advised. 2 = Specialised medical advice recommended in some cases. 3 = Specialised medical advice mandatory. 4 = Only to be performed in hospital environment. 5 = Should be avoided.

Pain and anxiety control **Local anaesthesia** Regional block anaesthesia and injections in the floor of the mouth should be avoided. **Conscious sedation** Nitrous oxide is not recommended since it may affect platelet aggregation. **General anaesthesia** Endotracheal intubation during general anaesthesia may require prior intermediate purity Factor VIII, cryoprecipitate or fresh frozen plasma.

Treatment modification **Surgery** Before surgery, patients with Von Willebrand's disease need treatment to ensure haemostasis (Table 3.162). Local haemostatic agents are also recommended. **Implantology** There is no evidence that Von Willebrand disease represents a contraindication to implants, but these patients may not be a good risk group, and medical advice should be taken first. **Fixed prosthetics and conservation** Rubber dam is recommended to minimise soft tissue injury. **Periodontology** The same bleeding control protocol as in oral surgery should be applied.

Drug use Aspirin and NSAIDs should be avoided.

Further reading ● Federici A B, Sacco R, Stabile F, Carpenedo M, Zingaro E, Mannucci P M 2000 Optimising local therapy during oral surgery in patients with von Willebrand disease: effective results from a retrospective analysis of 63 cases. Haemophilia 6:71–77 ● Piot B, Sigaud-Fiks M, Huet P, Fressinaud E, Trossaert M, Mercier J 2002 Management of dental extractions in patients with bleeding disorders. Oral Surg Oral Med Oral Pathol Oral Radiol Endod 93:247–250 ● Schardt-Sacco D 2000 Update on coagulopathies. Oral Surg Oral Med Oral Pathol Oral Radiol Endod 90:559–563 ● Scully C, Diz Dios P, Giangrande P, Lee C 2002 Oral Health Care in Hemophilia and Other Bleeding Tendencies. World Federation on Hemophilia Treatment of Hemophilia Monograph Series, No. 27. Faculty of General Dental Practitioners, London ● Stubbs M, Lloyd J 2001 A protocol for the dental management of von Willebrand's disease, haemophilia A and haemophilia B. Aust Dent J 46:37–40.

WARFARINISATION

Definition ■ Coumarins such as warfarin are drugs administered in order to decrease blood coagulability ■ Warfarin and the coumarin drugs antagonise vitamin K, thus reducing the vitamin K-dependent synthesis of several coagulation factors, especially factors II (prothrombin), VII, IX and X and proteins C, S and Z ■ Warfarin effects begin after 8–12 hours, are maximal at 36 hours, but persist for 72 hours. In patients receiving warfarin, the prothrombin time (PT) and activated partial thromboplastin time (APTT) are prolonged.

General aspects

Indications Warfarin is commonly prescribed for patients who have had cardiac surgery, organ transplants, pulmonary embolism or deep vein thrombosis.

Laboratory tests The International Normalised Ratio (INR) is the prothrombin time (PT) ratio (patient's PT/control PT) that would have been obtained if an international reference thromboplastin reagent had been used and is recommended by the World Health Organization (WHO) for reporting PT values. Warfarin increases the INR ■ in a person with a PT within the normal range, the INR is approximately 1 ■ an INR above 1 indicates that clotting will take longer than normal ■ an INR of 2 to 3 is the usual therapeutic range for deep vein thrombosis ■ an INR of up to 3.5 is required for patients with prosthetic heart valves.

Dental management

Risk assessment ■ Surgery is the main oral health care hazard to the patient on warfarin ■ Systemic conditions that may aggravate the bleeding tendency include any condition or drug that affects the vascular, platelet or coagulation phases of haemostasis. This is a wide range of disorders, including coagulopathies, thrombocytopenias, vascular disorders such as Ehlers–Danlos syndrome, liver disease, renal disease, malignancy, and HIV infection.

Appropriate health care ■ Any surgical intervention can cause problems and thus the possibility of alternatives to surgery, e.g. endodontics (root canal therapy), should always be considered ■ Be sure to warn the patient in advance of the procedure of the increased risk of intra- and postoperative bleeding and intra- and extraoral bruising ■ The management of patients on anticoagulants should take into consideration: ● type of dental procedure ● INR value ● underlying condition for which anticoagulation is used ● other risk factors ■ The INR should be used as a guideline to care, not a commandment (Box 3.32) ■ The INR should be checked on the day of operation or, if that is not possible, within 24 hours ■ A point of care device, the *CoaguChek* (Roche Diagnostics), may be used; an independent study showed that, although there were statistically significant INR differences between *CoaguChek* and the

Box 3.32 Protocol for warfarinised patients undergoing procedures associated with bleeding

Preoperatively

Check INR within 24 hours of op:

- If INR < 3.0, and no liver disease, do not change warfarin
- If INR < 3.0, and liver disease, or
- If INR > 3.0, consult physician about heparin or warfarin reduction

Perioperatively

● Minimise trauma ● Use regional block LA only if essential ● Local haemostatic measures*

Postoperatively for 24 hours

● Rest ● No mouth rinsing ● No hot food or drink ● No chewing ● No NSAIDs

*Local haemostatic measures = compressive packing, sutures, and microfibrillar collagen or oxidised cellulose.

international reference preparations, these test strips achieved a clinically acceptable level of accuracy ■ Stopping warfarin preoperatively is not the best policy since it does not necessarily significantly reduce bleeding but, in contrast, may cause hypercoagulability and lead to rebound thrombosis – which has damaged prosthetic cardiac valves and even caused thrombotic deaths in dental patients ■ Therefore, unless serious bleeding is anticipated, the warfarin should be continued – in any case, anticoagulant treatment should never be altered without the agreement of the clinician in charge ■ Always refer patients to hospital or other specialist centre for care in the presence of either one of the following conditions: ● INR > 3.0 ● need for more than a simple surgical procedure ● presence of additional bleeding risk factors or logistical difficulties ● drug interactions with warfarin.

Preventive dentistry ■ Dental preventive care is especially important, in order to minimise the need for surgical intervention ■ Some patients are reluctant to brush their teeth or accept professional dental care for fear of bleeding. Education protocols involving daily home care and regular professional care must therefore be stressed.

Pain and anxiety control **Local anaesthesia** Local anaesthetic regional block injections, or those in the floor of the mouth, may be a hazard since bleeding into the fascial spaces of the neck can threaten airway patency. Intraligamentary or intrapapillary injections are preferred, although intraligmentary injections should not be used where there is a risk of infective endocarditis. **Conscious sedation** Care should be taken due to the increased risk of a haematoma if giving intravenous sedation. **General anaesthesia** Endotracheal intubation during general anaesthesia may require warfarin reduction or conversion to heparin.

Patient access and positioning **Timing of treatment** Whenever possible, potentially problematic surgical procedures are best carried out in the morning, allowing more time for haemostasis before nightfall, and early in the week, to avoid problems at the weekend when staffing may be less intense.

Treatment modification

Limited oral surgery, INR < 3.0 ■ If oral surgery is to be limited, such as the uncomplicated forceps extraction of 1–3 teeth, and INR < 3.0 (British Committee for Standards in Haematology), and no other risk factors are present, local measures should give satisfactory haemostasis: ● placement of sutures ● absorbable haemostatic agents, such as oxidised regenerated cellulose (Surgicel®), synthetic collagen (Instat®) or microcrystalline collagen (Avitene®), gelatin sponge or fibrin glue, may be put in the socket to assist clotting ● tranexamic acid mouthwash, 5%, 10 mL used qds for 7 days ■ If bleeding is controlled, the patient should be dismissed and given a 7-day follow-up appointment and phone number of the dentist with instructions to call if bleeding occurs.

Moderate oral surgery, INR > 3.0 ■ If surgery is to be more than simple or minor, or INR > 3.0, or other risk factors are present, the patient should be treated in hospital or other specialist centre ■ The haematologist should be consulted and consideration given to whether the anticoagulation will need to be modified by:

- Changing to low molecular weight heparins during the preoperative period; warfarin therapy should be re-initiated simultaneously with heparin, unless a contraindication exists or if the patient is suspected of having a hypercoagulable state. If anticoagulants are to be continued after the operation, vitamin K should be avoided, as it makes subsequent anticoagulation difficult. Generally, heparin and warfarin overlap for approximately 4 days. Discontinue heparin once the INR is at the required therapeutic level. Arrange for follow-up INR with the patient's physician within 3 days of discharge.
- Tranexamic acid – occasionally, the haematologist may prescribe tranexamic acid systemically (1 g qds) to be commenced 1–2 days preoperatively, and typically continued 2 days postoperatively.

Perioperatively ■ Surgery should be carried out with minimal trauma to both bone and soft tissues. ■ Local measures are important to protect the soft tissues and operation area, and minimise the risk of postoperative bleeding ■ The occurrence of additional risk factors for bleeding should prompt the treating clinician to be more cautious ■ In the case of difficult extractions, when mucoperiosteal flaps must be raised, the lingual tissues in the lower molar regions should preferably be left undisturbed since trauma may open up planes into which haemorrhage can track and endanger the airway. The buccal approach to lower third molar removal is therefore safer. ■ Where possible, minimal bone should be removed and the teeth should be sectioned for removal ■ Bleeding should be assessed intraoperatively – if there is concern, an absorbable haemostatic agent should be placed in the extraction site, such as oxidised regenerated cellulose, resorbable gelatin sponge or collagen (synthetic or microcrystalline or porcine). Cyanoacrylate or fibrin glues, which consist mainly of fibrinogen and thrombin, provide rapid haemostasis as well as tissue sealing and adhesion. Commercial, viral-inactivated products are available in Europe, Canada and Japan, but recombinant fibrin products are preferable. ■ Suturing is desirable to stabilise flaps and to prevent postoperative disturbance of wounds when eating. Resorbable sutures are preferred since they retain less plaque. ■ Apply gauze pressure (a tranexamic acid-soaked gauze helps) and, after 10 minutes biting on gauze, assess haemostasis ■ If bleeding is controlled, the patient should be dismissed and given a 7-day follow-up appointment and the phone number of the dentist with instructions to call if bleeding occurs.

Postoperatively ■ Postoperatively, the patency of the airway must always be ensured. Care should be taken to watch for haematoma formation, which may manifest itself by swelling, dysphagia or hoarseness. ■ Many patients can be managed postoperatively with antifibrinolytic agents given topically. The best known agent is tranexamic acid which is not FDA approved for use on the US market, where epsilon amino caproic acid is an alternative. Tranexamic acid, a synthetic derivative of the amino acid lysine, exerts an antifibrinolytic effect through the reversible blockade of lysine binding sites on plasminogen molecules. Systemic tranexamic acid does not result in therapeutic concentrations in saliva. Topical tranexamic acid is effective even when the anticoagulant therapy remains unchanged. Tranexamic acid is used topically as 10 mL of a 5% w/v solution used as a mouthwash for 2 minutes, four times daily for 7 days. Epsilon aminocaproic acid (250 mg/mL) 25% syrup 5–10 mL is an alternative. ■ Infection appears to induce fibrinolysis and therefore antimicrobials, such as oral penicillin V 250–500 mg four times daily (or clindamycin), may be given postoperatively for a full course of 7 days if there is risk of secondary haemorrhage ■ For postoperative pain management, paracetamol (acetaminophen) is recommended as the analgesic and antipyretic of choice for short-term use (see below) in patients on oral anticoagulant therapy, and is preferred to NSAIDs since it does not affect platelets. Codeine is a suitable alternative analgesic. ■ A diet of cool liquid and minced solids should be taken for several days ■ Postoperative prolonged bleeding should be controlled by biting on a moist gauze, or a gauze pad soaked in tranexamic acid, or a moist tea bag with firm pressure for 30 minutes ■ Faced with a patient with persistent bleeding it is important to establish if the situation is urgent, when the patient will require admission for intravenous fluids, or reversal of anticoagulation – this may well be the case if the patient is losing large quantities of blood or hypotensive (hypovolaemic) ● To stop oral bleeding, wash out clots with warm saline and identify the bleeding area. Put in a local anaesthetic injection containing epinephrine and press firmly with a sterile gauze pad soaked with tranexamic acid over the extraction socket for 10–15 minutes. ● If this is unsuccessful, press with fingers on either side of the socket. If the bleeding stops, suture the socket; using silk sutures to enable a tighter suturing. ● If the bleeding does not stop with simple pressure, pack the socket with a resorbable haemostatic agent and then suture ● If the patient continues to bleed, consult a physician about reversal of warfarin since this is best achieved with a prothrombin complex concentrate (PCC) and fresh frozen plasma (FFP). Vitamin K (1 mg) is essential for sustaining the reversal achieved by PCC and FFP.

Implantology There is no evidence that anticoagulation represents a contraindication to implants, but these patients may not be a good risk group, and medical advice should be taken first. **Periodontology** The same bleeding control protocol as for oral surgery should be applied.

Drug use ■ Warfarin effect may be enhanced by many drugs such as aspirin and NSAIDs, antibiotics and azole antifungal agents (Table 3.164): ● Aspirin and other NSAIDs can enhance warfarin by displacing it from plasma proteins, but can interfere with platelet function and also cause gastric bleeding. COX-2 inhibitors such as celecoxib appear not to have a significant effect on platelets or INR, but may be cardiotoxic. ● Paracetamol (acetaminophen) in excessive and prolonged administration can enhance warfarin, presumably by inhibiting its metabolism. An intake of less than 6 tablets of 325 mg of paracetamol per week has little effect on INR; however, 4 tablets a day for a week significantly affects the INR. Paracetamol will affect the INR within 18–48 hours of administration. ● Tramadol occasionally interferes with warfarin and raises the INR ● Where antibiotics are indicated and where a single dose of amoxicillin is required as, for example, in endocarditis prophylaxis, there should be no problem.

Table 3.164 **Drug use in patients on warfarin**

Drug group	Avoid since warfarin is enhanced	No significant interference	Alternatives that can be used
Antibacterials	• Benzylpenicillin • Cephalosporins (2nd, 3rd generation) • Clarithromycin • Clindamycin • Ciprofloxacin • Co-trimoxazole (and other sulphonamides) • Doxycycline • Erythromycin • Isoniazid • Metronidazole • Neomycin • Ofloxacin • Quinolones • Tetracyclines	• Ampicillin • Amoxicillin • Amoxicillin plus clavulanic acid	• Azithromycin • Cephalosporins (others) • Penicillin V
Antifungals	• Azoles (fluconazole, itraconazole, ketoconazole, miconazole) • Griseofulvin		• Amphotericin • Nystatin
Antivirals	• Ritonavir • Saquinavir		
Analgesics	• Aspirin • Indometacin • Ketorolac • Ketoprofen • Naproxen • Piroxicam • Tramadol	• Ibuprofen • Paracetamol/acetaminophen	• Celecoxib • Codeine • Dextropropoxyphene • Diclofenac • Dihydrocodeine
Others	• SSRIs • TCAs		• Benzodiazepines

Table 3.165 **Key considerations for dental management in patients on warfarin (see text)**

	Management modifications*	Comments/possible complications
Risk assessment	2	Bleeding tendency
Appropriate dental care	2/4	Type of procedure; INR guideline; underlying disease
Pain and anxiety control		
– Local anaesthesia	1	Avoid nerve block
– Conscious sedation	1	Haematoma
– General anaesthesia	3/4	Warfarin reduction or heparin
Patient access and positioning		
– Access to dental office	0	
– Timing of treatment	1	Morning; early in the week
– Patient positioning	0	
Treatment modification		
– Oral surgery	3	INR guideline; bleeding control protocol
– Implantology	3	See oral surgery
– Conservative/Endodontics	1	
– Fixed prosthetics	1	
– Removable prosthetics	0	
– Non-surgical periodontology	3	See oral surgery
– Surgical periodontology	3	See oral surgery
Hazardous and contraindicated drugs	2	Avoid some NSAIDs, metronidazole and others

*0 = No special considerations. 1 = Caution advised. 2 = Specialised medical advice recommended in some cases. 3 = Specialised medical advice mandatory. 4 = Only to be performed in hospital environment. 5 = Should be avoided.

Alternative antibacterials are shown in Table 3.164. If infection is present, no elective surgery should be done until the patient has been treated with antibiotics and is free from acute infection. Even topical miconazole gel has caused problems.

■ Warfarin effect can also be influenced by: • irregular taking of the warfarin medication • a diet high in vitamin K (avocado, beet, broccoli, brussel sprouts, cabbage, chick peas, green peas, green tea, kale, lettuce, liver, spinach and turnips) can reduce the INR • alcohol ingestion can inhibit warfarin, but can have the converse effect if there is liver disease • Diseases such as diarrhoea, liver disease and malignant disease can increase the INR.

Further reading

• Baker R I, Coughlin P B, Gallus A S, Harper P L, Salem H H, Wood E M 2004 Warfarin Reversal Consensus Group. Warfarin reversal: consensus guidelines, on behalf of the Australasian Society of Thrombosis and Haemostasis. Med J Aust 181:492–497 • Chugani V 2004 Management of dental patients on warfarin therapy in a primary care setting. Dent Update 31:379–384 • Diz Dios P, Fernández Feijoo J 2001 Tooth removal in patients receiving oral anticoagulants. Oral Surg Oral Med

Oral Pathol Oral Radiol Endod 92: 248–249 ● Jeske A H, Suchko G D 2003 ADA Council on Scientific Affairs and Division of Science; Journal of the American Dental Association. Lack of a scientific basis for routine discontinuation of oral anticoagulation therapy before dental treatment. J Am Dent Assoc 134:1492–1497 ● Padrón N, Limeres J, Tomás I, Diz Dios P 2003 Oral health and health behavior in patients under anticoagulation therapy. Oral Surg Oral Med Oral Pathol Oral Radiol Endod 96:519–520 ● Pemberton M N, Oliver R J, Theaker E D 2004 Miconazole oral gel and drug interactions. Br Dent J 196:529–531 ● Scully C, Diz Dios P, Shotts R 2004 Oral health care in patients with the most important medically compromising conditions; 3. Anticoagulated patients. CPD Dentistry 5:47–49 ● Scully C, Wolff A 2004 Oral surgery in patients on anticoagulant therapy. Oral Surg Oral Med Oral Pathol Oral Radiol Endod 94:57–64. ● www.bschguidelines.com/pdf/OAC_guidelines_190705.pdf

Chapter 4

MAIN OROFACIAL PROBLEMS

TEETH

Trauma

Trauma is common in severe learning disability, severe epilepsy and in abused and vulnerable individuals (Figs 4.1, 4.2). Learning disabilities, cognitive impairment, delirium (common among the acutely ill/frail elderly), and dementia (occurring in as many as 50% of institutionalised elderly) represent serious barriers to trauma and pain assessment. Management of trauma in these special needs groups should involve a coordinated team approach, where carers, and other health care professionals, such as general medical practitioners, may be able to assist in ensuring the correct diagnosis is made and appropriate treatment is offered.

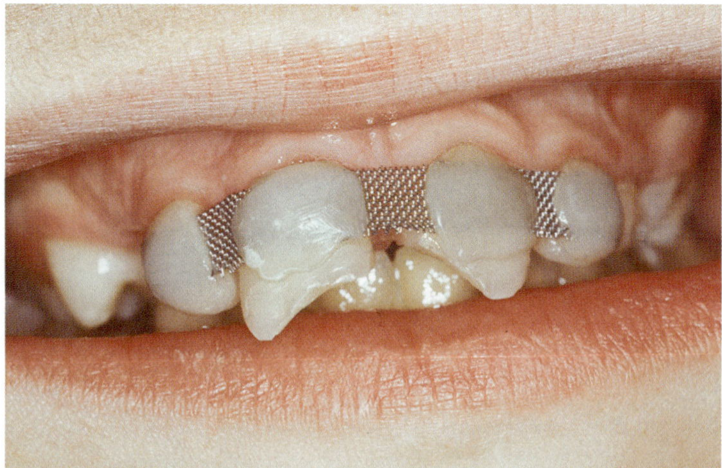

Figure 4.1 **A composite wire mesh splint placed to stabilise the traumatised upper central incisors**

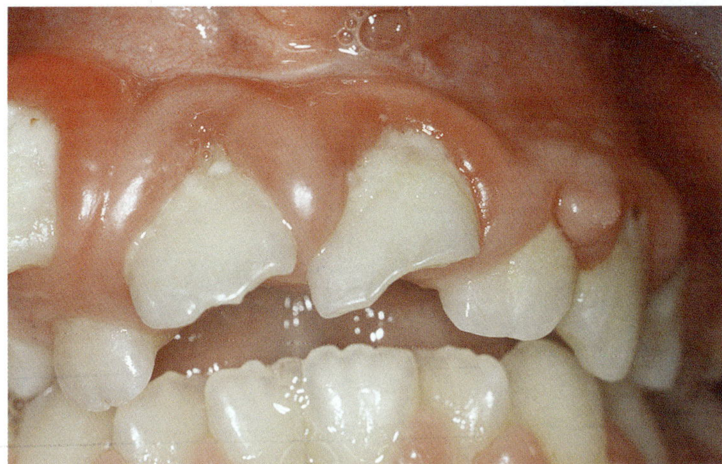

Figure 4.2 **Traumatised upper central incisors**

Further reading ● Glassman P, Miller C, Ingraham R, Woolford E 2004 The extraordinary vulnerability of people with disabilities: guidelines for oral health professionals. J Calif Dent Assoc 32:379–386.

Tooth wear

Attrition (Fig. 4.3) is common (especially in males), where the diet is very coarse, where there is bruxism, or where the teeth are defective, as in dentinogenesis imperfecta or Ehlers–Danlos syndrome. Furthermore, tooth wear may be more common in individuals with intellectual disabilities. Restorative procedures may be needed, including composites and advanced restorative techniques.

Further reading ● Bartlett D W, Smith B G 1998 Etiology and management of tooth wear: the association of drugs and medicaments. Drugs Today (Barc) 34:231–232 ● Bernhardt O, Gesch D, Splieth C et al 2004 Risk factors for high occlusal wear scores in a population-based sample: results of the Study of Health in Pomerania (SHIP). Int J Prosthodont 17:333–339 ● Chu S J, Karabin S, Mistry S 2004 Short tooth syndrome: diagnosis, etiology, and treatment management. J Calif Dent Assoc 32:143–152 ● Rees J S, Jara L, Ondarza A, Mistry P, Laing E, Odell O 2004 A comparison of tooth wear in children with Down syndrome, children with other intellectual disability and children without disability. J Dent Oral Health 5:3–12 ● Yip K H, Smales R J, Kaidonis J A 2004 Differential wear of teeth and restorative materials: clinical implications. Int J Prosthodont 17:350–356.

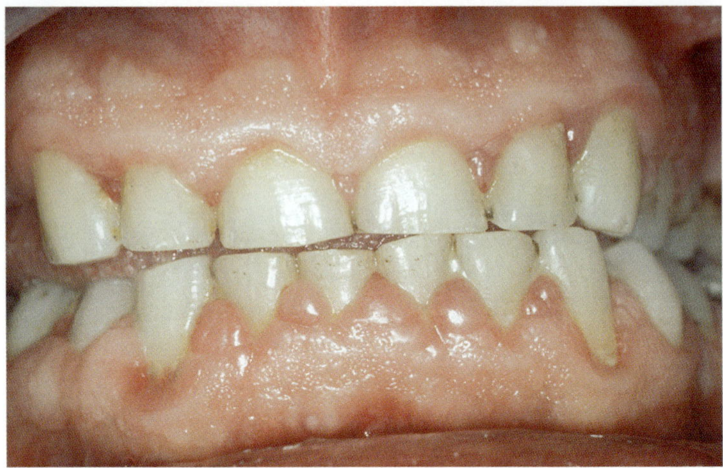

Figure 4.3 **Generalised tooth wear (and gingival hyperplasia)**

Caries

Higher levels of dental caries may be present in some individuals with special needs (Fig. 4.4), with the level of risk dependent on a complex interrelationship between socioeconomic factors and access to oral health care, concurrent illness and its treatment. Examples of factors which may increase caries risk include: ■ xerostomia due to Sjögren's syndrome, radiotherapy, or secondary to the use of tranquilisers or other psychoactive anticholinergic drugs ■ medications containing sugar ■ special diets, including those that require frequent snacking ■ poor motor control of the cheeks, lips and tongue ■ dysfunction in the arms and hands ■ general debilitation/poor motivation due to concurrent illness or chronic depression.

Measures that may be used to help in caries prevention include the use of fluorides, chlorhexidine and xylitol gum.

Further reading ● Anderson M 2003 Chlorhexidine and xylitol gum in caries prevention. Spec Care Dentist 23:173–176 ● Glassman P, Miller C 2003 Dental disease prevention and people with special needs. J Calif Dent Assoc 31:149–160 ● Weintraub J A 2003 Fluoride varnish for caries prevention: comparisons with other preventive agents and recommendations for a community-based protocol. Spec Care Dentist 23:180–186.

Erosion

Frequent exposure to acidic substances may result in the loss of enamel from the tooth surface by chemical erosion (Fig. 4.5). Erosion may be the result of intrinsic or extrinsic sources of acid.

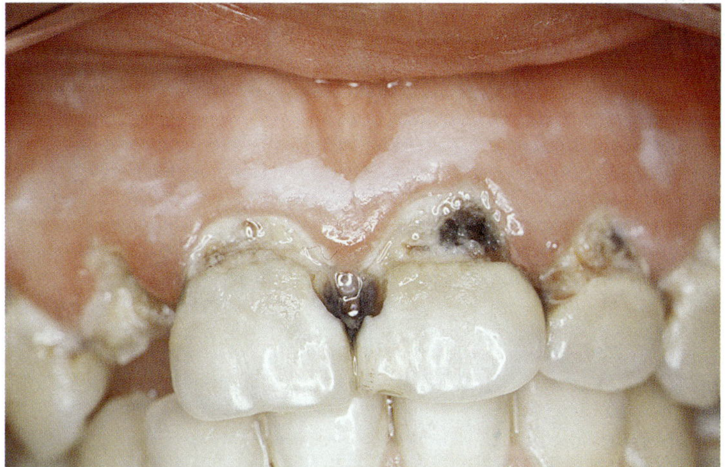

Figure 4.4 **Rampant caries**

The intrinsic sources include: ■ gastro-oesophageal reflux, which may be due to sphincter incompetence, increased gastric pressure (due to obesity) and increased gastric volume ■ vomiting (due to pregnancy, eating disorders) ■ rumination.

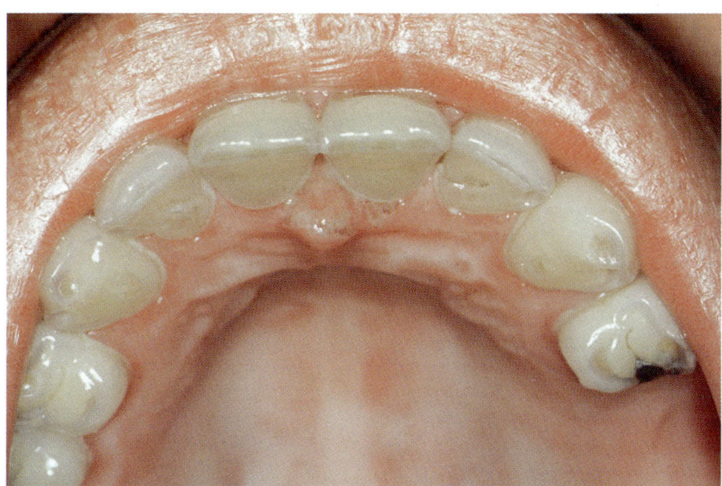

Figure 4.5 **Palatal erosion**

The extrinsic sources include: ■ dietary acids, such as carbonated beverages, alcoholic drinks and citrus foods ■ medication such as vitamin C and iron preparations, ecstasy, anti-asthmatic medication and excessive aspirin ■ some mouthwashes and saliva substitutes that are also acidic ■ environmental contact with acids as part of work or leisure activities.

Immediate management includes desensitisation through the use of fluoride toothpaste and mouthwashes, and implementation of appropriate preventive strategies aimed at reducing the acid exposure. Interim and long-term treatment includes the provision of temporary diagnostic restorations, ongoing monitoring of disease, definitive restorative work where appropriate, and modification and reinforcement of preventive advice.

Further reading
● Deshpande S D, Hugar S M 2004 Dental erosion in children: an increasing clinical problem. J Indian Soc Pedod Prev Dent 22:118–127 ● Grippo J O, Simring M, Schreiner S 2004 Attrition, abrasion, corrosion and abfraction revisited: a new perspective on tooth surface lesions. J Am Dent Assoc 135:1109–1118 ● Kilpatrick N, Mahoney E K 2004 Dental erosion: part 2. The management of dental erosion. NZ Dent J 100:42–47 ● Rees J S 2004 The role of drinks in tooth surface loss. Dent Update 31:318–326.

PERIODONTIUM

Periodontal disease

People who have impaired manual dexterity can find it difficult to achieve good levels of oral hygiene, and thus gingivitis and periodontitis can ensue.

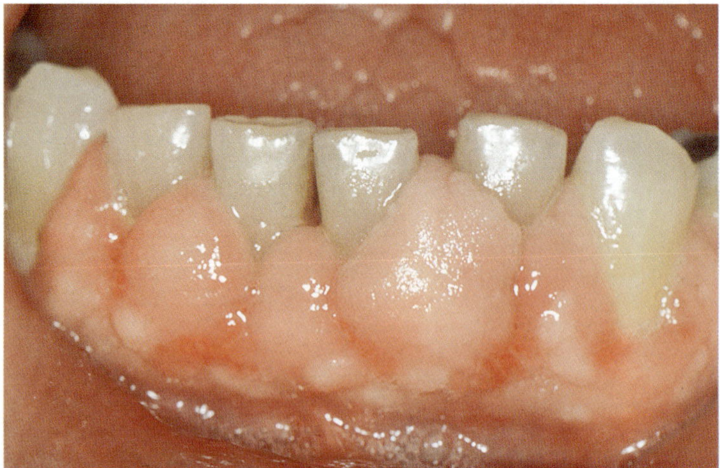

Figure 4.6 **Gingival overgrowth in a renal transplant patient taking ciclosporin**

Furthermore, early, severe periodontal disease can occur in children with impaired immune system or connective tissue disorders, with periodontitis often particularly aggressive in some genetic syndromes (e.g. Down syndrome). Regular professional cleaning by an oral health care provider, local or systemic antibiotics, and modified instructions on home care may be required to control existing periodontal disease. The patient may also need to help with daily toothbrushing, and cleaning aids may need to be adapted. For those patients at increased risk of periodontal disease, frequent appointments with an oral health care provider may be necessary.

Gingival overgrowth is not uncommon in patients receiving immunosuppressant medication (e.g. ciclosporin), antihypertensive calcium-channel blocking drugs (e.g. nifedipine) or anticonvulsants (e.g. phenytoin), and may further compromise periodontal health (Fig. 4.6).

Further reading ● Glassman P 2003 Practical protocols for the prevention of dental disease in community settings for people with special needs: preface. Spec Care Dentist 23(5):157–159 ● Schonfeld S E 2003 Using community-based protocols to prevent dental disease in people with special needs: periodontal prevention and intervention. Spec Care Dentist 23(5):187–188 ● Waldman H B, Perlman S P 2002 What about dental care for people with mental retardation? A commentary. J Am Coll Dent 69(2):35–38.

SALIVARY GLANDS

Drooling

Drooling is usually caused by true excess salivation, but may result from the inability to retain saliva within the mouth, or problems with swallowing. The social implications of drooling include embarrassment, social isolation and alienation for both the individuals and their families. The constant exposure of skin to saliva can cause a rash around the mouth, chin or lips, chapping of lips and infections around the mouth. Not only does it cause discomfort or even pain, but the sores may be considered unsightly. Clothing may need changing several times each day, which can become very laborious for the family or carers. They may opt for the patient to wear a bib, which results in further stigmatisation.

Furthermore, people who drool are at increased risk of inhaling saliva, food, or fluids into the lungs. This may lead to respiratory infection if reflex mechanisms (such as gagging and coughing) are also impaired.

True salivary hypersecretion is usually caused by: ■ food ■ local factors such as teething or oral inflammatory lesions ■ physiological factors such as menstruation or early pregnancy ■ digestive origin, both functional (motility disorders and oesophageal spasm) and organic pathology (ulcers, hiatus hernia) ■ medications (those with cholinergic activity such as pilocarpine, tetrabenazine, clozapine or bethanecol) ■ nasogastric intubation.

False sialorrhoea, or apparent hypersalivation, is caused not by excess saliva production but by an inability to swallow a normal amount of saliva caused by: ■ neuromuscular dysfunction: as a result of muscular incoordination or neurological disorders seen in Parkinson's disease, amyotrophic lateral sclerosis, bulbar palsy, cerebral palsy, learning disability, epilepsy, autonomic neuropathy, Riley–Day syndrome, some psychoses and tumours – especially those near the IVth ventricle ■ poor lip seal and malocclusion, usually linked to learning disability ■ abnormal head position as seen in progressive bulbar palsy ■ pharyngeal or oesophageal obstruction, such as by a neoplasm.

Treatment of drooling involves the management of the underlying cause if possible, and treatment of any concurrent oral disease. Maintaining the patient's head in an upright position may help to minimise symptoms. Additional strategies include:

- Behavioural approaches where appropriate, such as 'anti-drooling lessons'.
- Physiotherapy approaches, such as a modified Andreasen monobloc appliance, Innsbruck Sensory Motor Activators and Regulators (ISMARs) or the Castillo–Morales technique where a palatal appliance encourages lip and tongue control.
- Orthodontics may be indicated if incompetent lips are a possible cause.
- Antisialogogues may be of some benefit and include:
  - *Atropinics* such as benztropine or benzhexol which are theoretically useful to control sialorrhoea, although many, such as scopolamine (hyoscine) or ipatropium bromide, are of little practical value because of adverse effects. However, transdermal scopolamine using dermal patches has been shown to be effective within 15 minutes, and lasts up to 72 hours. Itching under the patch and flushing appear to be the main adverse effects.
  - *Glycopyrrolate*, a quaternary ammonium compound with anticholinergic effects, has minimal side effects to the central nervous system because it penetrates the blood–brain barrier poorly yet has a long-lasting antisialogogue effect. Oral glycopyrrolate 0.4 mg 3× daily is effective in many adults with sialorrhoea though it may cause some flushing and urinary retention.
  - *Antihistamines* are sometimes used. Propantheline bromide 15–30 mg may be effective but is contraindicated in glaucoma, myasthenia gravis and bowel or bladder obstruction. Methantheline is an alternative.
  - *Clonidine* patches 0.1 mg weekly may help.
- Botulinum toxoid injections into the salivary glands may be effective.
- Surgical treatment may be required if the sialorrhoea is severe and unresponsive to the above. Operations that have been devised include: ● bilateral submandibular duct diversion (re-routing the submandibular gland ducts to open posteriorly towards the pharynx) ● unilateral parotid duct ligation ● salivary gland removal ● chorda tympani section ● tympanic neurectomy.
- Radiation of the salivary glands is used in extreme cases by some to decrease salivation.

Further reading ● Calderon J, Rubin E, Sobota W L 2000 Potential use of ipatropium bromide for the treatment of clozapine-induced hypersalivation: a preliminary report. Int Clin Psychopharmacol 15:49–52 ● Davydov L, Botts S R 2000 Clozapine-induced hypersalivation. Ann Pharmacother 34:662–665 ● Kilpatrick N M, Johnson H,

Reddihough D 2000 Sialorrhea: a multidisciplinary approach to the management of drooling in children. J Disability Oral Health 1: 3–9 ● Olsen A K, Sjögren P 1999 Oral glycopyrrolate alleviates drooling in a patient with tongue cancer. J Pain Symptom Manage 18:300–302 ● Pal P K, Calne D B, Calne S, Tsui J K 2000 Botulinum toxin A as treatment for drooling saliva in PD. Neurology 11:244–247 ● Seoane Lestón J M, Diz Dios P, García Pola M J 2000 Hypersecretion and salivary incontinence. In: Alio Sanz J J (ed) Rapport XV Congress of International Association of Disability and Oral Health. Aula Médica, Madrid, p349–365.

Dry mouth

Dry mouth is common in mouth breathers and during periods of anxiety. Other than this, the main causes of dry mouth are iatrogenic and include mainly drugs with anticholinergic or sympathomimetic or diuretic activity. These include: ■ atropine, atropinics and hyoscine ■ antidepressants: tricyclic (e.g. amitriptyline, nortriptyline, clomipramine and dothiepin), selective serotonin reuptake inhibitors (e.g. fluoxetine), lithium and some other antidepressants ■ antihypertensives may also cause a compositional change in saliva; alpha-1-antagonists (e.g. terazosin and prazosin) and alpha-2-agonists (e.g. clonidine) may reduce salivary flow; beta-blockers (e.g. atenolol, propranolol) reduce protein levels ■ phenothiazines ■ antihistamines ■ antireflux agents such as proton-pump inhibitors (e.g. omeprazole) ■ opioids ■ cytotoxic drugs ■ retinoids ■ bupropion ■ others such as: ● protease inhibitors ● didanosine ● diuretics ● ephedrine ● benzodiazepines ● interleukin-2.

Radiotherapy, chemotherapy, graft-versus-host disease and diseases of the salivary glands can also cause salivary dysfunction. Diseases of the salivary glands are mainly: ■ Sjögren's syndrome (dry mouth and dry eyes) ■ sarcoidosis ■ HIV disease ■ hepatitis C virus infection ■ primary biliary cirrhosis ■ cystic fibrosis.

Dehydration, as in diabetes mellitus, diabetes insipidus, hyperparathyroidism or any fever, is an occasional cause of xerostomia. Rarer causes include ectodermal dysplasia, Darier's disease and salivary gland agenesis.

The history and examination may help to determine the cause of dry mouth, but investigations may be indicated to exclude systemic disease, particularly connective tissue disorders: ■ Sjögren's syndrome ■ sarcoidosis ■ diabetes ■ viral infections (hepatitis C, HIV, HTLV-1).

It is important to recognise that some patients complaining of a dry mouth have no evidence of a reduced salivary flow or a salivary disorder. There may then be a psychogenic reason for the complaint.

Management Management measures include:

- *Rectifying any underlying cause of xerostomia*; for example, xerostomia-producing drugs may be changed for an alternative, and causes such as diabetes should be treated.
- *Avoiding factors that may increase dryness* such as: ● dry hot environments ● dry foods such as biscuits ● drugs (e.g. tricyclic antidepressants) ● alcohol (including alcohol-based mouthwashes) ● smoking.

- *Keeping the mouth moist as regularly as possible*. The lips may become dry, atrophic and susceptible to cracking and thus should be kept moist using a water-based lubricant or a lanolin-based product rather than one containing petroleum-derived lubricants (e.g. Vaseline). Olive oil, vitamin E or lip balm may help.

Salivary substitutes may help symptomatically although water or ice chips and frequent sips of water are often more effective than synthetic substitutes. Various are available including:

- Synthetic salivary substitutes, which vary in properties such as patient acceptability, fluoride content and pH (Table 4.1); care must be taken to avoid acidic preparations in dentate patients. These substitutes are usually based on one of the following compounds (Table 4.2): • carboxymethylcellulose – UK: Glandosane®, Luborant® (contains fluoride), Salivace®, Salivix®; USA: Moi-Stir®, Orex®, Salivart®, Xero-Lube®, Mouth-Kote® • mucin – Saliva Orthana®; also contains xylitol and fluoride • glycerate polymer – Oral Balance®; also contains xylitol, glucose oxidase and lactoperoxidase.
- A home preparation can be made using ¼ teaspoon of glycerine in 8 ounces of water. This is best restricted to edentulous patients.

Salivation may be stimulated by:

- Chewing gums (containing sorbitol or xylitol, not sucrose)
- Diabetic sweets
- Cholinergic drugs that stimulate salivation (sialogogues), such as pilocarpine, bethanecol, cevimeline and anetholetrithione
- **Pilocarpine** stimulates M3 cholinergic receptors in exocrine glands and smooth muscle. At doses of 5–10 mg tds with meals (maximum 30 mg daily) it has proved effective in bringing relief in severe salivary dysfunction within about 15 minutes. The sialogogue effect persists for about 3–4 hours. A course of 1–3 months should be tried. Pilocarpine should be used only by a specialist due to the numerous adverse effects which include: • sweating • increased pulse rate and arrhythmias • increased blood pressure • visual problems which interfere with night driving

Table 4.1 **pH of different salivary substitutes**

Preparation®	Approximate pH	
Glandosane	Natural	5.2
	Lemon	5.1
	Peppermint	5.1
Luborant		6.0
Saliva Orthana	Lozenge	6.4
	Spray	5.5
Salivace		6.4
Salivix		4.5

Table 4.2 **Some sialogogues and salivary replacements**

Agent	Use	Comments
Sialogogue		
Pilocarpine (Salagen®)	5 mg up to 3 times daily with food	Patient may be unable to see well enough to drive or operate machinery. Contraindicated in asthma, chronic obstructive airway disease, glaucoma, pregnancy. Care with cardiac disease
Salivix	Malic acid	Pastille
Salivary replacements (artificial salivas)		
Glandosane®	Sodium carboxymethylcellulose base	Spray
Luborant®	Sodium carboxymethylcellulose base	Spray
Oralbalance®	Lactoperoxidase, glucose oxidase and xylitol	Gel
Saliva Orthana®	Mucin	Spray containing fluoride, or lozenge. May be unsuitable if there are religious objections to porcine mucin
Salivace®	Sodium carboxymethylcellulose base	Spray
Saliveze®	Sodium carboxymethylcellulose base	Spray

● headache ● other cholinergic effects such as diarrhoea, bradycardia, and the urge to urinate. Furthermore, pilocarpine is contraindicated in: ● cardiovascular disease ● patients using beta-blockers ● asthma and chronic obstructive airway disease ● peptic ulceration ● gallstones ● iritis ● glaucoma ● pregnancy ● psychiatric disease.

- **Bethanechol** (25 mg, 3 times daily orally) was found to increase the unstimulated and stimulated salivary flow rates of patients with xerostomia secondary to radiotherapy, although objective changes in salivary flow rates did not always correlate with symptomatic improvement. Adverse effects, however, which may include nausea and diarrhoea, are infrequent.
- **Cevimeline** (SnowBrand Pharmaceutics, USA; 30 mg, 3 times daily) is a quinuclidine derivative of acetylcholine with a high affinity for M3 muscarinic receptors on both salivary and lacrimal glands, but a low affinity for cardiac and lung M2 receptors. Metabolised principally in the liver and excreted via the kidneys it has a half-life of approximately

5 hours – greater than for pilocarpine. Cevimeline can have adverse effects including: • sweating • visual problems that interfere with night driving • headache • other cholinergic effects such as diarrhoea, bradycardia, and the urge to urinate. It is contraindicated in: • patients using beta-blockers • asthma and chronic obstructive airway disease • peptic ulceration • gallstones • iritis • glaucoma • pregnancy • psychiatric disease. Cevimeline thus has the advantages over pilocarpine of longer action and possibly fewer adverse effects.

- **Anetholetrithone** increases the availability of muscarinic receptors on the post-synaptic membrane and thus enhances the potential for cholinergic stimulation. It may enhance pilocarpine-induced salivation in patients with radiotherapy-induced xerostomia.

Oral complications such as caries, candidosis and sialadenitis should be prevented and treated.

Further reading • Epstein J B, Stevenson-Moore P, Scully C 1992 Management of xerostomia. J Can Dent Assoc 58:140–143 • Fox P C 1997 Management of dry mouth. Dent Clin N Am 41:863–875 • Mignogna M D, Fedele S, Russo L L, Muzio L L, Wolf A 2005 Sjögren's syndrome: the diagnostic potential of early oral manifestations preceding hyposalivation/xerostomia. J Oral Pathol Med 34:1–6 • Nagler R M, Hershkovich O 2005 Relationships between age, drugs, oral sensorial complaints and salivary profile. Arch Oral Biol 50:7–16 • Porter S R, Scully C, Hegarty A 2004 An update of the etiology and management of xerostomia. Oral Surg Oral Med Oral Pathol Oral Radiol Endod 97:28–46.

MUCOSAL DISEASE

Mucosa

Mucosal trauma may lead to ulceration. Radiotherapy, chemotherapy or combinations can lead to severe mucositis. Lifestyle habits such as drug abuse (which may cause ulceration) and tobacco use (which can cause keratoses) are common in people with mental health problems. Other predisposing factors may include: ■ psychological instability (anxiety or stress) ■ neuroleptic drug-induced immunodeficiency ■ oral infections ■ respiratory and digestive disorders ■ vitamin and folic acid deficiencies.

Further reading • Loh F C, Neo J, Tan P H 1987 The geriatric dental patient. Ann Acad Med Singapore 16(1):88–93 • Scully C, Hegarty A 2003 Prevention of oral mucosal disease. In: Murray J J, Nunn J, Steele J (eds) Prevention of oral disease, 4th edn. Oxford University Press, Oxford p167–185 • Scully C, Epstein J, Sonis S 2003 Oral mucositis: a challenging complication of radiotherapy, chemotherapy, and radiochemotherapy: Part 1, pathogenesis and prophylaxis of mucositis. Head Neck 25:1057–1070 • Scully C, Epstein J, Sonis S 2004 Oral mucositis: a challenging complication of radiotherapy, chemotherapy, and radiochemotherapy: Part 2, diagnosis and management of mucositis. Head Neck 26:77–84 • Tomás I, Diz P, Limeres J, Ocampo A, Vázquez E, Feijoo J F 2000 Oral ulcers in mentally handicapped (original in Spanish). Archivos Odontoestomatología 16(8):551–558.

Biting

Self-mutilation may damage the oral or orofacial tissues, particularly in individuals with mental health problems such as learning disability, dementia, or Tourette's syndrome, or in rare conditions such as in Lesch–Nyhan syndrome where the lips or tongue may be chewed almost to destruction. Rarely, oral self-mutilation is accidental in patients with congenital indifference to pain, including Riley–Day syndrome (familial dysautonomia) and some patients with autism. Biting is also observed in patients with severe CNS damage (Fig. 4.7) following a stroke or cerebral trauma.

Management options include: ■ symptomatic relief, including pain and infection control ■ construction of mouth guards, bite-planes, splints, tongue stents – although these may be poorly tolerated as good patient compliance is required ■ behavioural psychology ■ use of sedative agents ■ selective extraction of teeth involved in the trauma – this should be used as a last resort.

Further reading ● Benz C M, Reeka-Bartschmid A M, Agostini F G 2004 Case report: the Lesch–Nyhan syndrome. Eur J Paediatr Dent 5:110–114 ● Brasic J R, Barnett J Y, Ahn S C, Nadrich R H, Will M V, Clair A 1997 Clinical assessment of self-injurious behavior. Psychol Rep 80:155–160 ● Fardi K, Topouzelis N, Kotsanos N 2003 Lesch–Nyhan syndrome: a preventive approach to self-mutilation. Int J Paediatr Dent 13:51–56 ● Shymoyama T, Horie N, Kato T, Nasu D, Kaneko T 2003 Tourette's syndrome with rapid deterioration by self-mutilation of the upper lip. J Clin Pediatr Dent 27:177–180.

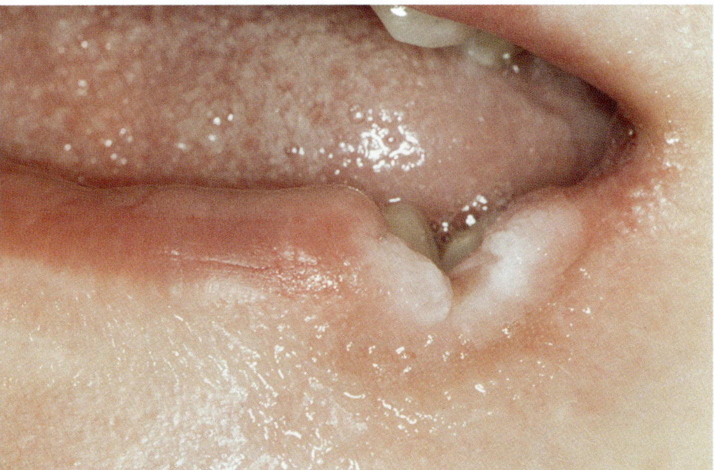

Figure 4.7 **Trauma to the lower lip in a patient with traumatic brain injury to the central nervous system**

Bruxism

Bruxism is defined as non-functional clenching, grinding or rubbing of teeth during the day or night. Bruxism may be persistent throughout life, but is sometimes intermittent, and then often associated with emotional or psychological factors. Some authors have suggested that bruxism reflects a multifactorial interaction of anatomical, physiological and psychological variables. Determinant factors may be: genetic (rarely) – as in Rett syndrome (bruxism accompanied by constant wringing of hands), local – such as occlusal factors, or psychogenic – particularly caused by central dopaminergic mechanisms. Bruxism is thus common in learning disability, various psychiatric disorders, and drug use (antidepressants, amphetamines, ecstasy and others) (Fig. 4.8).

Bruxism usually manifests with night grinding of teeth, which is often noisy, or daytime bruxism, in which clenching is often prominent. Patients typically develop masseteric hypertrophy and tooth attrition incompatible with their age. The wear is of variable degree and has been ranked in increasing severity: ■ minimal attrition ■ wear parallel to the occlusal/incisal surface ■ loss of tooth cusp relief but without dentine exposure ■ loss of occlusal anatomy and exposure of dentine. Bruxists may also develop pain in the temporomandibular joint or masticatory muscles.

The goals of treatment are to reduce clenching behaviour, reduce pain, and prevent further tooth damage. There have been numerous approaches to try to help people unlearn their clenching behaviours, although these may be of limited success in individuals with learning disabilities. Nevertheless, methods to reduce daytime clenching tend to be more successful, since night-time clenching cannot be consciously stopped. Furthermore, in some people,

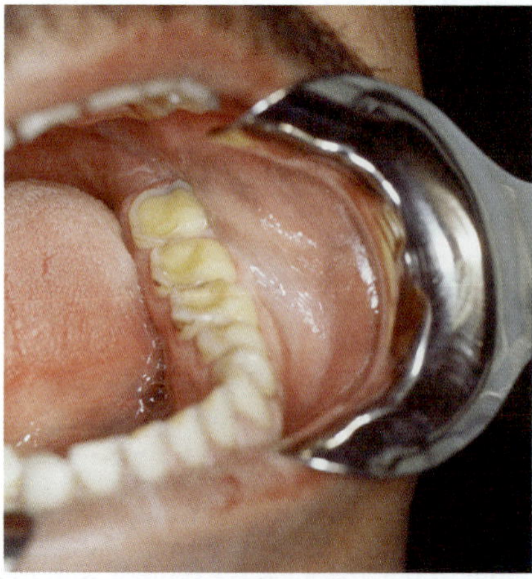

Figure 4.8 **Bruxism in a patient abusing amphetamines**

just relaxing and modifying daytime behaviour is enough to reduce night-time bruxism. An anxiolytic or tricyclic antidepressant may be of additional benefit.

Self-care steps include: ■ reducing daily stress ■ learning relaxation techniques ■ getting adequate sleep ■ relaxing facial and jaw muscles ■ massaging the muscles of the neck, shoulders and face ■ stretching exercises to help to restore a normal balance to the action of the muscles and joint on each side of the head ■ applying ice or wet heat to muscles ■ avoiding eating hard foods like nuts ■ drinking plenty of water.

There is no proven reliably effective intervention but the following can be used:

- Occlusal devices such as: ● hard guards covering the whole occlusal surfaces (Michigan splint or Tanner device) ● localised occlusal interference splints (LOIS).
- Occlusal adjustment; a controversial type of treatment as it is irreversible.
- Behavioural therapy and biofeedback. The most commonly applied techniques include: ● facing techniques ● training in imagination ● training in relaxation ● habit reversal ● aversive conditioning ● electromyographic biofeedback.
- Medication, such as: ● gabapentin ● propranolol ● bromocriptine ● botulinum toxoid.

As a next phase after splint therapy, orthodontic adjustment of the bite may be beneficial for some people.

Further reading ● Brown E S, Hong S C 1999 Antidepressant-induced bruxism successfully treated with gabapentin. J Am Dent Assoc 130:1467–1469 ● Da Silva L, Martínez A, Rilo B et al 2000 In: Alio Sanz J J (ed) Rapport XV Congress of International Association of Disability and Oral Health. Aula Médica, Madrid, p330–348 ● Demir A, Uysal T, Guray E, Basciftci F A 2004 The relationship between bruxism and occlusal factors among seven- to 19-year-old Turkish children. Angle Orthod 74:672–676 ● Malki G A, Zawawi K H, Melis M, Hughes C V 2004 Prevalence of bruxism in children receiving treatment for attention deficit hyperactivity disorder: a pilot study. J Clin Pediatr Dent 29:63–67 ● Nash M C, Ferrell R B, Lombardo M A, Williams R B 2004 Treatment of bruxism in Huntington's disease with botulinum toxin. J Neuropsychiatry Clin Neurosci 16:381–382 ● Scully C, Diz Dios P 2000 Oral dyskinesias and palsies. In: Alio Sanz J J (ed) Rapport XV Congress of International Association of Disability and Oral Health. Aula Médica, Madrid, p306–329.

Halitosis

Halitosis (oral malodour or breath odour), is a fairly common complaint, noted mainly in adults. Up to 30% of adults over 60 years old without disability have oral malodour but, although it is common in some people with disability – especially where oral hygiene is impaired and there is inflammatory periodontal disease – there is no published evidence.

Halitosis that is not due to eating various foods such as garlic, onion or spices, or to habits such as smoking or drinking alcohol, is most often a consequence of oral bacterial activity, typically from anaerobes arising from poor oral hygiene (Fig. 4.9), gingivitis, periodontitis, other oral sepsis or debris under appliances. Anaerobes produce the chemicals that cause malodour in many instances, which include volatile sulphur compounds (VSCs: methyl mercaptan, hydrogen sulphide, dimethyl sulphide), polyamines (putrescine and cadaverine) and short-chain fatty acids (butyric, valeric and propionic). Prevention of infective processes, improvement of oral hygiene, and sometimes the use of antimicrobial therapy can usually manage this type of halitosis.

In the absence of oral infection and nasal sepsis or foreign bodies, systemic causes which may be responsible for oral malodour include starvation, drugs and, rarely, systemic disease. Diabetic ketosis, respiratory problems, gastrointestinal disease, hepatic failure or renal failure may be responsible.

Management includes patient education, treating the cause, regular meals and good oral hygiene, possibly with antiseptics and tongue brushing/scraping. In recalcitrant cases, a specialist empirically may use a one-week course of metronidazole 200 mg tds in an effort to eliminate unidentified anaerobic infections.

Further reading

- Hartley M G, McKenzie C, Greenman J, El-Maaytah M A, Scully C, Porter S R 2000 Tongue microbiota and malodour; effects of metronidazole mouthrinse on tongue microbiota and breath odour levels. Microb Ecol Health Dis 11:226–233
- Loesche W J 1999 The effects of antimicrobial mouthrinses on oral malodor and their status relative to US Food and Drug Administration regulations. Quintessence Int 30:311–318
- Quirynen M, Zhao H, van Steenberghe D 2002 Review of the treatment strategies for oral malodour. Clin Oral Invest 6:1–10
- Scully C, Porter S R, Greenman J 1994 What to do about halitosis (Editorial). Br Med J 308:217–218
- Scully C, Rosenberg M 2003 Dental Update 30:205–210
- van Steenberghe D,

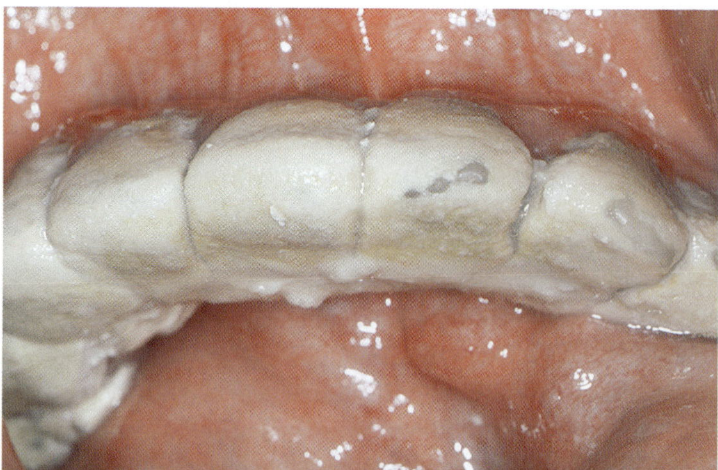

Figure 4.9 **Poor oral hygiene in an individual with learning disability, leading to a profound halitosis**

Rosenberg M (eds) 1996 Bad breath: a multi-disciplinary approach. Leuven University Press, Leuven • Yaegaki K, Coil J M 2000 Examination, classification, and treatment of halitosis; clinical perspectives. J Can Dent Assoc 66:257–261.

Retching

Stimulation of the glossopharyngeal nerve, by touching the posterior part of the tongue or palate (such as in dental impression taking) causes the protective reflex of retching. However, the cause of undue liability to retching is unclear and may have a psychogenic basis. There are several techniques available, used with varying results, to avoid retching such as salt on the tip of the tongue when taking impressions, or lifting the feet when having impressions taken. Desensitisation, hypnotherapy and acupuncture have been tried. Conscious sedation may also help some patients who retch.

Further reading • Bassi G S, Humphris G M, Longman L P 2004 The etiology and management of gagging: a review of the literature. J Prosthet Dent 91:459–467 • Fiske J, Dickinson C 2001 The role of acupuncture in controlling the gagging reflex using a review of ten cases. Br Dent J 190:611–613 • Noble S 2002 The management of blood phobia and a hypersensitive gag reflex by hypnotherapy: a case report. Dent Update 29:70–74 • Reid J A, King P L, Kilpatrick N M 2000 Desensitization of the gag reflex in an adult with cerebral palsy: a case report. Spec Care Dentist 20:56–60 • Wright S M 1979 An examination of factors associated with retching in dental patients. J Dent 7:194–207 • Wright S M 1980 An examination of the personality of dental patients who complain of retching with dentures. Br Dent J 148:211–213.

Index

B

C

D

E

F

G

H

M

N

O

P

Q

R

S

T

U

X

Z